To Jocelyn, Leslie, Melissa, and Rachel

"Drs. Klein and Wender have written a fine book about an important topic that has been badly neglected: biological psychiatry. In recent years it has become clear that there are some emotionally troubled patients who cannot be helped by psychological forms of treatment but who may show dramatic improvement when they are given appropriate medication. *Mind, Mood, and Medicine* describes such patients and their treatment in clear and practical language."

—Helen S. Kaplan, M.D., Ph.D.
Clinical Professor of Psychiatry
Cornell University College of Medicine

PAUL H. WENDER, M.D., is Professor of Psychiatry at the University of Utah and co-author of *The Hyperactive Child and the Learning Disabled Child*. He is also a past president of the Psychiatric Research Society.

DONALD F. KLEIN, M.D., is Professor of Psychiatry at Columbia University, Director of Psychiatric Research at the New York State Psychiatric Institute, and president of the American College of Neuropsychopharmacology. He is also a past president of the Psychiatric Research Society.

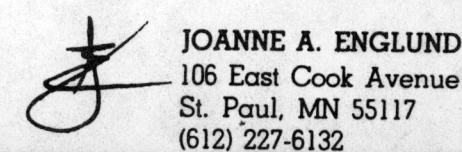

10-22-90

JOANNE A. ENGLUND
106 East Cook Avenue
St. Paul, MN 55117
(612) 227-6132

Mind, Mood, and Medicine

A Guide to the New Biopsychiatry

Paul H. Wender, M.D., and Donald F. Klein, M.D.

A MERIDIAN BOOK
NEW AMERICAN LIBRARY
NEW YORK AND SCARBOROUGH, ONTARIO

NAL BOOKS ARE AVAILABLE AT QUANTITY DISCOUNTS WHEN USED
TO PROMOTE PRODUCTS OR SERVICES. FOR INFORMATION PLEASE
WRITE TO PREMIUM MARKETING DIVISION, NEW AMERICAN
LIBRARY, 1633 BROADWAY, NEW YORK, NEW YORK 10019.

Copyright © 1981 by Paul H. Wender, M.D., and
Donald F. Klein, M.D.

All rights reserved. For information address Farrar, Straus &
Giroux, Inc., 19 Union Square West, New York, New York 10003.

This is authorized reprint of a hardcover edition published by
Farrar, Straus & Giroux, Inc. A hardcover edition was published
simultaneously in Canada by McGraw-Hill Ryerson Ltd., Toronto.

Designed by Irving Perkins Associates

 MERIDIAN TRADEMARK REG. U.S. PAT. OFF. AND FOREIGN COUNTRIES
REGISTERED TRADEMARK—MARCA REGISTRADA
HECHO EN WESTFORD, MASS., U.S.A.

SIGNET, SIGNET CLASSIC, MENTOR, ONYX, PLUME, MERIDIAN AND
NAL BOOKS are published *in the United States* by
NAL PENGUIN INC., 1633 Broadway, New York 10019,
in Canada by The New American Library of Canada Limited,
81 Mack Avenue, Scarborough, Ontario M1L 1M8

First Meridian Printing, October, 1982

    5 6 7 8 9 10 11 12

PRINTED IN THE UNITED STATES OF AMERICA

Gloria Parloff translated our words into organized English and was an invaluable intellectual resource. Kathleen Woznicki, Frances Ross, Janet Kearney, and Jean Greenwood were our indefatigable secretaries, who have proven that severe stress is insufficient to cause illness.

Both authors contributed equally. The order of their names is an artifact of the linear nature of our language.

We have avoided the clumsy locution "he or she" when sexual differences are not relevant, and instead have used the pronouns at random. The case histories are real case histories, except that identifying details have been changed.

P.H.W. and D.F.K.

Contents

1. **The Revolution in Psychiatric Treatment** 3
2. **Kraepelin, Freud, and Their Disciples: A Brief History of Twentieth-Century Psychiatry** 19
3. **Syndromes of Mental Disorder** 39

    MOOD DISORDERS 39
    Vital Depression, 43
    Manic States, 54
    Nonvital Depression: Neurotic Depression and Depressive Character, 58
    Masked Depression, 63
    Restitutional Devices, 66

    PERSONALITY DISORDERS 67
    Personality Disorder and Deviance, 70
    Shame, Guilt, and Rejection, 72
    Antisocial Personality Disorder, 75
    The Hyperactive Adult, 76
    Emotionally Unstable Character Disorder, 80
    Alcoholism and Drug Abuse, 82
    Hysteroid Dysphoria, 84
    Narcissistic Personality Disorder, 89
    Histrionic Personality Disorder, 89
    Conversion Reactions and Malingering, 91
    Avoidant Personality Disorder, 92
    Dependent Personality Disorder, 93
    Panic Disorder, Generalized Anxiety State, Panic Phobia (Agoraphobia), 94

Generalized Anxiety Disorder, 98
Simple Phobia, 98
Compulsive Personality Disorder, 99
Obsessive-Compulsive Disorder, 101
Explosive Personality Disorder, 102
Paranoid Personality Disorder, 103
Schizoid Personality Disorder, 103

SCHIZOPHRENIC DISORDERS   **104**
Acute Schizophrenia, 119
Chronic Schizophrenia, 121
Borderlands of Schizophrenia, 126
Antipsychotic Medication, 134

4. **An Intellectual Turning Point: The Drug Discoveries**   **141**
Malaria and Paresis, 143
Insulin Coma, 143
Convulsive Therapy, 144
Stimulants, 146
Major Tranquilizers (Antipsychotic Medications), 146
Minor Tranquilizers, 149
The Search for Better Antipsychotics, 149
Antidepressants, 150
Lithium, 152
Risks versus Benefits of Drug Treatment, 153
Drug Effects That Mimic Mental Illness, 157

5. **Nature, Nurture, and Psychiatric Disorders**   **163**
Family Studies of Schizophrenia, 166
Twins; Adoption Studies, 170
Phenocopies of Schizophrenia, 176
Disorders of Mood, 178
The Unnamed Quartet, 186
Genetics and Mental Illness: Evolutionary and Ethical Questions, 191

6. **The New Biology of the Mind and Its Psychological Implications**   **197**
Biopsychology in Disorders of Mood, 199
Biopsychology in Personality Disorders, 210
Biopsychology in the Schizophrenic Illnesses, 219

7. **The Threefold Nature of Unhappiness: Some Examples and Some Difficulties** — 229

8. **The Psychotherapies** — 259
   Intrapersonal Therapies, 284
   Interpersonal Therapies; the "Talking Cures," 289
   Multiperson Therapies, 294
   Behavior Therapies, 306
   Abreactive and Cathartic Therapies, 310
   State-Altering Therapies, 318

9. **What Path for the Sufferer?** — 329

APPENDIX: **The Use of Medication in the Treatment of Psychiatric Illness** — 343
   Tricyclics and MAO Inhibitors, 344
   Lithium, 346
   Major Tranquilizers, 349
   Minor Tranquilizers, 351

REFERENCES — 353

INDEX — 363

Mind, Mood, and Medicine

CHAPTER 1

The Revolution in Psychiatric Treatment

One day some years ago, a twenty-three-year-old woman we'll call Mary J. was suddenly struck by terror while walking down a street in New York City. She had a swimming sensation in her head as if she might suddenly fall or faint, her heart was racing, and she couldn't catch her breath. The horrifying conviction grew that she was having a heart attack or a stroke. She slumped to the sidewalk and appealed to passersby to help her get to a doctor. Although several pedestrians ignored her, assuming that she was drunk, a Good Samaritan came to her aid and attempted to flag down a taxi. The first few cabdrivers sped past impassively, not wanting to get involved with the nuisance of a sick or intoxicated passenger, but finally one stopped and took her to a hospital.

By the time Mary reached the emergency room, the overwhelming feeling of panic had subsided somewhat, but she was left in a state of stunned bewilderment as to what had hit her. At the hospital she was treated with indifference by the underpaid and overworked emergency-room staff. Since she was not unconscious, in pain, or obviously bleeding, and since she could talk in a reasonably connected fashion, she was shunted aside to wait until one of the interns on duty had finished stitching and stapling accident and assault victims. The emergency-room nurses responded mainly with irritation to Mary's timid complaints about continuing faintness and palpitations.

When she was eventually examined, the hospital staff found nothing to explain the attack. Heart, lungs, and blood pressure were all normal.

An electrocardiogram was negative. The usual blood chemistries revealed nothing. At that point she was told that it was probably just her nerves, which implied that she was a hypochondriac, or that her symptoms were too slight to complain about, or that she should stop bothering them and go see a psychiatrist.

Mary began to weep in confusion. "But what will happen to me?" she asked. "What is happening? Why do I feel this way? Something must be terribly wrong." She received no useful answers but was given some Valium. Within a half hour she did feel considerably relieved, but nervously called a friend to pick her up and take her home. With the help of the Valium, she eventually fell asleep.

The next day she felt perfectly well and was told by her friends that she probably had a twenty-four-hour virus or that maybe she was working too hard or that maybe she needed a vacation or a new boyfriend.

After a week of feeling quite normal, Mary panicked again while riding the subway. Not only did she have the same alarming feelings of fear, racing heart, choking, dizziness, and tremors, but she was stuck on an express train for five minutes and could not get out. Her fellow passengers edged away from her nervously when she began to whimper helplessly.

Finally, one helped her off and got her to a doctor. When the preliminary tests again showed nothing, the doctor began a more thorough examination, aware that her symptoms might be caused by hypoglycemia (abnormally low blood sugar), pheochromocytoma (a rare tumor of the adrenals), or hyperventilation syndrome (a tendency to breathe too fast and deeply). But all the tests were negative, and more Valium was prescribed.

Within the succeeding weeks the panics started to occur more often, in a crescendo, until every day was punctuated by terror. Now, with repeated panics, Mary developed chronic apprehensive anxiety. All day, every day, her stomach was in knots. She felt sweaty, slightly breathless, and constantly preoccupied both with the possibility of having another panic and with worry about her condition. She was afraid that the doctors were keeping something from her and that she would surely die in the middle of the next episode, or, since she had been told repeatedly that it was all in her mind, that she was going insane. She resisted the suggestions that she see a psychiatrist, dreading the possible confirmation of her worst fears.

Nevertheless, she could not fully suppress her suspicions of mental illness, for her attacks were now often accompanied by a strange unreal sensation as if she were living in a dream. Things around her seemed distant, small, thin, flat, as if the entire world were made of cardboard. From time to time she had the transient conviction that she could observe herself from a distance but was not voluntarily controlling her own behavior, as if she were a robot. Mary had of course heard about schizophrenia and knew that this meant being split from reality. She tried to describe the dream-like states to her friends and doctors, and one doctor, suspecting that she might have a rare form of epilepsy, sent her for an electroencephalogram to check the brain wave pattern. The EEG, however, was normal. Another doctor prescribed a stronger tranquilizer, Thorazine, but it made her feel sick and woozy and even more anxious. Several neurologists reviewed her carefully but agreed with the previous medical consensus that nothing seemed organically wrong with her.

At the same time that she was frantically seeking a medical diagnosis, Mary was beginning to change her style of living in response to the panics. She had already learned that help was not easy to come by from strangers, and that in certain circumstances, such as in subways or driving over bridges or through tunnels, she was effectively blocked from easy access to help. Without consciously planning it, she spent more and more of her nonworking time at home and traveled alone less and less. She gave up taking subways and buses and, despite the expense, used taxicabs more often. When she went to the theater, she required an aisle seat, and when she went to church, she sat in back so that if she had to run for help she need not embarrass herself and her companions.

Further, she began to believe that in some situations she was particularly prone to get panics, such as traveling alone, and that she was relatively immune to them if she stayed in her apartment. Confusingly, sometimes she could travel alone without panicking and sometimes she would have a panic even while sitting quietly at home; nevertheless, increasingly she restricted her activities to the area immediately surrounding home base.

She decided to give up her city apartment when her roommate told her that her clinging demands for reassurance had made her impossible to live with. In the hope of more sympathetic, safe surroundings, Mary returned to live with her parents in a suburb. At first this move seemed helpful: her panics decreased in frequency. However, her job required her to travel into Manhattan, and this, too, eventually became impossible because of the constant threat of panic during the long journey. She gave up her well-paying job as a department-store buyer, which had held out the exciting prospect of rapid advancement, and resigned herself to working as a salesgirl in a local store. This was a dead-end position, but Mary's repeated panics and sense of impending doom continued to prevent her from traveling a long distance to work. With the job change, she became extremely depressed, realizing that her plans for a rewarding career had been severely damaged.

After a while, even walking to her neighborhood job began to require great effort. The constricted life now did not seem to help and the panics returned full-force. Except for a few fear-ridden hours at her tedious job, Mary spent almost all her time at home. Too upset to concentrate, she gave up reading and spent mind-numbing hours before the television set.

She made increasing demands upon her family, crying and complaining bitterly. The family oscillated wildly between concern for her misery and resentment over the multiple restrictions that she was placing upon them. There was a scene every time they wanted to go out and leave her, and separate vacations were now out of the question. However, they lagged in urging psychiatric care because of the possible stigma on the family. Although they understood why some of their friends had sometimes consulted psychiatrists, they had the nagging feeling that if their daughter just pulled herself together she could overcome her difficulties. After all, it was something like her refusal to go to school at age seven, and she had outgrown that. And Mrs. J. vaguely remembered that she herself as a young girl had sometimes felt nervous about going downtown alone, but *she* had gotten over it.

After several doctors in turn told her that she didn't have a serious mental illness—she wasn't psychotic—but still ought to see a psychiatrist, Mary reluctantly came to the conclusion that she was probably neurotic. Having learned about Freud in college, Mary began to believe that her neurosis must be related to unpleasant, unconscious sexual and aggressive impulses, and that her panics must be her attempts to keep them repressed. The fact that she had always thought her own sexual interests and her few social animosities quite normal probably indicated how much she was repressing. Since support and tranquilizers had not helped, intensive long-term psychotherapy seemed her only alternative.

Once Mary decided that she had to see an analyst or become a permanent cripple, her parents readily agreed to pay for her treatment. From their exposure to psychology at college, from what they had seen in the movies and on television, from the experiences of their friends, they knew that though therapy was expensive and sometimes took a long time, at least it was effective. They would do the best for their daughter, and the best was obviously psychoanalysis.

Mary's analyst was a reserved, pleasant man whose confidence reassured Mary that she had done the right thing by going into analysis and that together they would get to the bottom of her difficulties. Mary's father, an accountant, could afford only two sessions a week, and the family's health insurance did not cover psychoanalysis. Although the doctor had recommended a minimum of three sessions, he agreed to give it a try on this attenuated basis.

Mary was told to lie down on the couch, to speak without reservations of everything on her mind, to free-associate—that is, to let her mind wander wherever it wanted to, and to try to remember her dreams so that she and the analyst could try to interpret them. When she asked for advice or guidance, her doctor gently reminded her that she was attempting to make a parent of him and that in order for her insights to have the requisite emotional impact she must work with him to discover them by herself. When she reported that she still took Valium, her doctor hinted that she was still hoping for magic and that the only real cure lay within. Further, by chemically deadening her anxiety she was interfering with therapy, since progress depended upon the expression of the unconscious wishes she feared. Clearly, she was resisting looking into her unconscious. Understanding the importance of facing her anxiety, Mary agreed to give up all chemical crutches. At times, when the anxiety was extreme, she guiltily took some Valium or a few drinks. When she confessed to her analyst, she accepted his interpretation of the lapses as evidence of her continuing resistance to the therapeutic process.

Mary freely associated about her job, her parents, and her former boyfriend. Much of what she said elicited only silence from the analyst, but she realized from his responses that she should say more about her sexual feelings and anxieties. As Mary opened up to the analyst, the following story unfolded.

About six months before her illness had started, she had moved to the city to begin her working career. After some initial homesickness, she had adjusted rapidly and happily to the freedom, excitement, and variety of the city. She went out regularly with a man she had known in college, but neither of them was considering marriage. However, being a wife and mother was clearly one of her major goals.

After some procrastination, Mary had started to sleep with the young man in her new apartment. She had anticipated being guilty and anxious and had been relieved and surprised that her sexual life had quickly become a warm, rewarding, and tender part of her life. Her attachment to her lover grew, although she recognized that he was erratic, impulsive, and somewhat self-centered. She was upset and wept when he told her that a job offer would require him to move to a distant city.

After his departure, Mary was surprised at how soon she was able to regain control over her emotions. She started to date again but had not yet found anyone to whom she was strongly attracted. Six weeks after she said goodbye to her friend, the panic attacks had started.

The period of Mary's life preceding the onset of her illness was explored in great depth during the analysis so that both the analyst and Mary could understand its hidden meanings. Was Mary's sexual adjustment really smooth and guilt-free? Hadn't she had difficulties arranging for her roommate to be away when she and her lover wished to be alone? Didn't she now doubt her ability to control herself sexually since she had gone to bed with him after only a few weeks of internal debate? Didn't the fact that she had not yet gone to bed with a new man indicate a fear of being sexually vulnerable, of losing control over her emotions, of turning into a promiscuous woman, a whore? Wasn't she anxious about an eruption of lust, of being in the streets where men might look upon her as a streetwalker, of being a loose woman, a degraded person? Didn't her panic attacks protect her from having to live as an independent single woman and make it possible for her to live as an over-aged child, dependent on her family? Didn't her demands that she never be left alone show that she feared separation and adulthood?

At still a deeper level, didn't her wish for a man represent her wish for her father's penis? Since this was forbidden to her by the incest taboo, didn't living as a dependent and invalid child in the family serve as a desexualized substitute for the repressed wish? Didn't her panic attack, the sudden rush of feeling that left her shaken and trembling, resemble orgasmic pleasure replaced by pain? Desperate to find some understandable meaning to her unbearable plight, Mary seized upon these interpretations and elaborated them into even more rococo structures. After two years, as progress continued to be slow, she heeded the analyst's suggestion to intensify the analysis by increasing the sessions to three times a week.

The school-phobia episode from her childhood was also reviewed. At age seven, after a happy summer spent with her parents, she suddenly became upset and refused to go to school. She said that she didn't like her new teacher, that some of her old friends had moved away, and that she didn't like her new schoolmates either. Each week day she woke up with a bellyache and cried piteously about having to go to school, although on weekends she seemed fine.

At school she began to worry about her mother's health. Maybe an accident would happen to her. Maybe her mother had been hit by a car and was dying somewhere. These thoughts plagued her until one day she burst out crying and rushed to the teacher, pleading to be allowed to return home. Her mother was called and came to school concerned about her daughter. For several weeks, Mrs. J. took Mary to school although the child begged to remain home. For a few days the mother actually stayed in the classroom, but eventually her household duties prevented her from continuing this, and after a brief worsening of Mary's fears, the whole thing blew over.

The episode provided more grist for the analytic mill. The analyst explained to Mary that fears are often associated with hidden wishes. If you fear that your mother may die, you may unconsciously wish for her death. Further, people unconsciously believe that such primitive wishes are magically effective, so that Mary was also unconsciously afraid that her wishes would actually result in her mother's death. She insisted on being with her mother, both at age seven and now, to reassure herself that her omnipotent wishes weren't harming her mother. Obviously, she both loved and hated her mother—again at unconscious levels.

Why should Mary hate her mother, who was a kindly, overprotective woman? It must be unconscious rivalry over the father, whom Mary now possessed once again as an invalid child. Similarly, Mary's panics and fear of panic actually represented her wish to lose control, to be sexually voracious and promiscuous, thus concealing her real wish to have just one man, her father. After three years, the analyst indicated that four times a week would be absolutely essential to counteract Mary's extremely strong resistances.

During the four years of analysis, Mary's illness waxed and waned. Sometimes months went by without a panic attack and Mary would make slow strides toward increasing her range of travel and thinking of moving back to the city. Eventually, she summoned up the courage to drive the family car, although not across bridges or through tunnels, which effectively restricted her from going into Manhattan. The unconscious sexual significance of bridges and tunnels was immediately obvious to the analyst, and after a while to Mary. Her fears concerning theaters plainly related to the fact that the theater is basically an exhibitionistic display of sexual activity; her similar fears about church were related to her primitive guilt about her sexual feelings.

Mary gratefully attributed her improvement to the accuracy of the analytic interpretations and her growing understanding of her unconscious wishes and defensive maneuvers. But, in the midst of her renewed confidence, she relapsed. A new volley of panic attacks forced her to give up even local travel. This was not surprising, though, for surely her relapse represented a regressive flight from the powerful analytic insights that had been revealing her primitive impulses. It was not the analytic method that was at fault; the patient was simply too resistant, perhaps due to a basic ego flaw.

Nonetheless, Mary's parents were becoming restive with her lack of durable progress. The fees were absorbing all of Mary's meager earnings and also depleting Mr. and Mrs. J.'s financial resources, but the parents' objections were interpreted as a clear example of familial resistance. Just as Mary wished to remain a sexless child because she could not have her father, so her father, with the unwitting compliance of his wife, was unconsciously conspiring to keep her a helpless invalid.

Then the father learned about another form of treatment from a social-worker friend. The social worker knew that psychoanalysis was the best form of treatment for neurotics, but recently a new treatment called behavior therapy had become very popular. Among patients with phobias it seemed quite effective, and Mary's panics did seem to be phobias. Mary's father investigated the method and thought it admirably simple and straightforward. The patient's phobia was understood to be due to some form of simple conditioning. Somehow the patient had become afraid of an object or situation and then had learned to avoid that situation. Both the avoidance and the initial fear were the products of learning and therefore could be unlearned. The simplest system—desensitization—was to pair the anxiety with a neutralizing incompatible response, such as relaxation. When the patient learned how to relax in the face of anxiety-provoking stimuli, then the fears would disappear.

Mary brought up the possibility of supplementary behavior therapy with her analyst, but predictably he saw the suggestion as yet another form of resistance. Mary's obvious wish to avoid looking further at her unconscious indicated that they were getting close to the end of therapy. Her surface feeling that she was no better was of no consequence, the analyst said, and it would be a shame if all their hard-won analytic gains were thrown away at the last moment.

Understandably, Mary felt torn. She was reluctant to leave analysis, with its complex and dramatic interpretations and insights, for the prosaic, apparently simpleminded behavior therapy. Further, she had become attached to her analyst and entertained possessive, erotic daydreams about him, which he related to her basic erotic wishes toward her father. Her father, however, increasingly skeptical about psychoanalysis, said that he would support her analysis for only another three months; he had not had a vacation or a new suit in three years and was fed up with the whole thing. Mr. J. remained adamant and at the end of the three months Mary was forced to make the switch. When she met her brisk new therapist, who immediately dismissed all the psychoanalytic complexities, her own accumulating doubts about analysis came to the fore and she felt some sense of relief. The behavior therapist said that Mary's trouble was that she had learned fear habits and that it was their job to get rid of them.

Mary was first taught to relax through simple verbal routines in which she was told to focus on each part of her body, feeling it become warm and heavy so that waves of relaxation streamed from her hands over her body and down to her feet. After this easy and pleasant exercise, Mary and her therapist constructed a ladder of fearful situations, starting with what least frightened her and building to a situation that would petrify her. First, Mary envisioned the relatively nonthreatening scene of herself walking to her job three blocks from home. Repeated pairings of this image with the relaxation technique she had learned enabled Mary to think of walking to work without the slightest anxiety; in addition, to her pleasure and growing excitement, she found that the real trip to the job became progressively easier. The next step was to imagine, along with relaxation, extended walks in the neighborhood with her mother; this in turn was followed by hesitant real walks, first with her mother, then only partway with her mother, and then daringly around the corner and out of sight of her mother.

During six months of weekly sessions, Mary became progressively more independent and outgoing. For the first time in years, she allowed herself to be driven into the city to see a movie. Her newfound confidence allowed her to ask for more responsibility at work. She began to contemplate moving into her own apartment in her parents' neighborhood. Perhaps someday she could return to Manhattan. She was delighted with her progress and became less anxious and demoralized.

She began to understand that the periods of improvement during her analysis had been only superficial responses of no real significance but that her improvement in behavior therapy was a permanent deconditioning of a maladaptive learned response. She could look forward happily to eventual complete cure.

Unexpectedly and disastrously, a shower of panic attacks returned. For the first time in months, Mary experienced overwhelming pangs of horror, fear, and the conviction that she was going to go crazy or die. Her confidence shattered, she retreated to an almost housebound existence, finding it difficult even to manage the few blocks to work.

The behavior therapist explained that she had undoubtedly pushed herself too fast and had placed herself in anxiety-provoking circumstances before the relaxation techniques had sufficiently deconditioned her. Strangely, however, Mary had not been suffering increased anxiety prior to her panic attacks and, if anything, had seemed almost anxiety-free, and positively cheerful.

In the face of Mary's resistance to renewing desensitization treatment, the therapist suggested a new and reportedly effective branch of behavior therapy called flooding, an ingenious application of the old principle that the way to teach someone afraid to swim was to throw him into the water. The therapist described how one poor unfortunate who was afraid of spiders conquered his fears by having a barrel of spiders dumped upon him. After a brief screaming fit, his fear of spiders disappeared.

The therapist admitted that flooding was somewhat difficult to reconcile with the relaxation, desensitization, and unlearning theory and that it might even seem to be the sort of traumatic experience that would make a person's fears worse. But he spoke of considerable success with the technique. Willing to try anything at this point, Mary agreed to be driven far from her home and left there to make her way back alone. As she was being driven away from home, she became tense and apprehensive, and finally had to be pushed out of the car. She returned home several hours later in a state of complete hysteria, and that was the end of that therapeutic effort and that therapist.

Mary and her parents were thrown into despair, feeling that the illness was intractable. Since two of the most widely respected forms of psychotherapy had failed, as well as tranquilizing medications, they believed that her prognosis was grim and that she could look forward only to a life of chronic, anxiety-ridden, neurotic invalidism.

One year later Mary was living alone in New York City, working well at her old job, developing an affectionate-sexual relationship with a young man, and looking forward to possible marriage. She was essentially symptom-free and had neither panic attacks nor the apprehension that she would become panicked.

Mary owed her improvement primarily to the discovery that antidepressant medication—a pharmacological agent different from tranquilizers—was effective with the kind of panic attacks to which she was subject. Weekly psychotherapy had at first helped her to adjust to her changing life situation as she had responded to the medication, but now was necessary only at infrequent occasions of particular stress. Although psychoanalysis and behavior therapy had not helped with her basic problem, once her panic was controlled by the medication she did find psychotherapy and relaxation techniques helpful with related problems.

Mary's case is not atypical. It is characteristic of a new and well-defined treatment for panic disorder that will be discussed in more detail later, in the chapter on kinds of mental illnesses. The point of presenting this case history is to focus attention, as forcefully as we can, on the startling fact that many patients with a variety of histories and symptom patterns, formerly treated ineffectively with psychotherapy alone, can now be treated effectively with medication and adjunctive psychotherapy. A virtual revolution is occurring in psychiatry. The public is largely unaware that different sorts of emotional illnesses are now responsive to specific medications, and unfortunately too many doctors are similarly unaware.

We now know that there is much more to biology and physiology in the explanation of emotional disorder than has been previously recognized. The tremendous increase in pharmacological preparations capable of helping people with emotional disorders has forced us to rethink what the bases might be for those disorders. At the same time, new basic information on the inheritance of emotional disorder and the genetics of psychiatric illness has become available through a new methodology, the adoption study. We can now make informed inferences about heredity and begin to answer the ancient question of whether behavioral illness is due to nature or to nurture. Finally, remarkable new developments in brain chemistry are enabling us to speculate on what some of the causal mechanisms of mental illness might be.

The causes, nature, and treatment of mental illness are a source of concern and confusion to everyone. Mental illness, which brings not only suffering but also disrupted lives to both the patient and the patient's family, is distressingly common. Unfortunately, disagreement about how to approach it is equally common: sects abound, each claiming that it has discovered the basic truth and the perfect cure, and that all others worship false gods.

Newspapers, magazines, and television convey a veritable babble of psychiatric and psychological tongues. Some claim that the illnesses are interpersonal in origin, the consequence of early traumatic psychological experience. Others aver that psychiatric difficulties are biologically caused—that they are true illnesses with well-defined, recurring characteristics, like mumps or coronary heart disease. Still others say that the words "illness" and "disease" are misnomers when used by psychiatrists, that there are no mental illnesses, only human beings who are adapting appropriately or foolishly to difficult life circumstances. Some even assert that the whole enterprise is useless—that individuals are unique and that classification of this kind is useless, demeaning, and possibly destructive.

Accompanying the debate about the causes and nature of mental illness is still greater chaos regarding its therapy. Thirty years ago there were only a few therapies, but today there are dozens; so many that no clinician can even know all their names, let alone their distinguishing features. In most communities no laws prevent anyone from defining himself or herself as a therapist, using novel procedures on people willing to be defined as patients, and thus inventing a new therapy. Not only do therapies abound but every day new ones seem to proliferate.

Since the outcomes of the various treatments are by no means equal, the choices made are of concrete importance. The selection of a therapist and therapy not only may affect how long a patient suffers but in extreme cases may affect how long he lives. Most people have been personally touched by suicides, and all have wondered if the sufferer could have been helped.

In some circles, psychiatry, unlike physics, is regarded as an area in which the casual student can generate as many useful thoughts as the expert. Literary critics, philosophers, popular psychologists, and hordes of analysands consider themselves qualified to expound upon matters of mental health. This self-confidence is no substitute for convincing evidence. The prevailing belief in the overall effectiveness of many of the popular panaceas is unfounded. Some forms of psychiatric illness should no more be treated by some supposedly well-established therapies than should cancers be treated by faith healers.

Given this "blooming, buzzing confusion," given the divisive schools of psychiatric thought, how is one to decide?

We claim no revelation of the absolute truth, but we do propose to present information that derives from repeatable experimentation and systematic observation rather than from speculation and conjecture. This information has been inadequately disseminated.

Complex as are the issues and problems that psychiatry faces, the painstaking, sometimes excruciatingly slow techniques of experimental science are making gains. The amount known, as compared to the amount we wish we knew, is still small. As with other areas of human concern, much nonsense, unfounded faith, and wishful thinking are likely to fill the wide interstices between islands of fact. To aggravate the difficulties due to ignorance, additional confusion is generated by a currently rampant anti-intellectualism. Unfortunately, meticulous attention to hard facts is less appealing to the media and the public than heart-tugging sentiment and instantaneous miracles.

In psychiatry, as in religion, it pays to know the faith of one's mentor. No one would ask ontological questions of a theologian without knowing if he or she is a Moslem, Hindu, Jew, or Christian, or a nominal or practicing believer. Similarly, the reader should know our biases.

Our biases are mixed: biological and psychological-cultural. We believe that a surprisingly large amount of aberrant human behavior can be explained without reference to the obscure, complex, and arcane. A large sector of the public, along with many psychiatric practitioners, believe that most mental illness is the product of early psychological trauma or conflict, compounded by intricate, subterranean churnings. We do not.

We shall elaborate our views in the course of the book, but the following tenets play an important part in our thinking. First, that the major mental *illnesses,* such as schizophrenia and severe disorders of mood, are primarily biological in origin. Even the less severe variants of these major illnesses—which are surprisingly common—have substantial biological components. We shall present data in support of the contention that there are both major and minor genuine psychiatric illnesses that are at least partially the product of inborn biological differences.

Second, that many human problems with which psychotherapists deal are not illnesses but are the result of what a wise psychiatrist (Ernest Southard) fifty years ago referred to as the "Kingdom of Evils" —ignorance, legal entanglements, vices, poverty, and self-constructed traps and blind alleys.

Some human misery, often erroneously called neurosis, is the predictable and easily understood product of an individual's family and other subcultural experience. That is, the values, attitudes, and expectations that he has been taught as a child and has dutifully learned conflict with his adult biological drives or with the current aspirations and values of society. Each society and each family (a society within a society) transmits to its children its values, attitudes, goals, and styles of behavior. A child may be taught to inhibit aggression or to act upon it, to humble himself or to be self-aggrandizing. Such variations in personality formation are *not* illnesses in any reasonable usage of that term. But they may nonetheless cause people considerable pain in adulthood and may require specialized reeducative care.

In a few patients, various modes of self-esteem protection by unconscious defense mechanisms seem to play an important role. To refer to these patients as neurotic is common practice. However, it should be realized that the term "neurotic" really has very little content, and people with very widely differing problems are often lumped together under this catchall. All psychotherapeutic schools direct their largest theoretical guns at these "neurotics," but more often than not the patients they treat suffer from illnesses that very likely have little to do with such unconscious conflicts. A few therapists eventually realize—as does Allen Wheelis in *A Quest for Identity*—that they have been taught a treatment for a rare, sometimes seemingly nonexistent, disorder.

In this book, we shall focus primarily on the role of biological factors in major mental illness and personality deviations, because the evidence substantiating the role of these factors in mental illness is not widely known. This evidence—which comes from studies of responses to medication, of inheritance patterns, and of brain chemistry—is of practical importance, because it often dictates the direction that should be followed in the treatment and research related to mental illness. It is also of theoretical interest, because it includes the first pieces in the solution of the greatest of scientific puzzles, the functioning of the brain.

The role of biological factors in both normal and abnormal psychological functioning has been comparatively neglected, not only because of genuine scientific disagreement and pendulum-like swings from one intellectual pole to another, but also because of the hopelessness that has been associated with the idea that behavior may have biological roots. This position is as difficult to accept now as was Freud's assertion, at the beginning of this century, that feelings, values, and intellectual outpourings were the result of unconscious forces beyond the control of conscious will. We think that an assertion of the importance of biological factors in thinking and feelings is as important as an assertion of the importance of unconscious factors.*

Psychoanalysis asserted that although behavior was under the control of the unconscious, one could acquire knowledge of it and thus—albeit somewhat laboriously—acquire control over oneself. The psychoanalytic position was basically hopeful—something could be done. The biological assertion is far more frightening, implying that cogitate as one will, analyze as one will, let it all hang out, desensitize it, look at it in the here-and-now, subject it to various operants, and still one may be unable to manage it.

---

*Freud usually argued that the discomfort produced by his discussion of the unconscious was further evidence supporting his assertion. This is clearly a "catch-22," no-fail method of proof. In contrast, we believe that the evidence for the role of biological factors in mental illness is no stronger if the reader rejects it. Such fairness undoubtedly represents scientific progress.

This is a far too gloomy outlook, however, for recent scientific advances have shown that certain medications may markedly help even organically caused conditions. Further, recognition of the persuasiveness of the biological evidence can lead to a more realistic structuring of life in accordance with any limitations that may be indicated.

We shall refer frequently to the varieties of ordinary human misery, so often seen by the psychiatrists, psychologists, social workers, and pastoral counselors. People with bad marriages or life-destroying jobs sometimes go to a therapist because they are convinced that they cannot change their circumstances; they hope that if they can change themselves life will be better. Deep psychotherapy, under these conditions, often focuses on long-term internal change, pursuing infantile trauma and repression.

Sometimes the patient is right. He needs help to overcome feelings of passivity and social inhibition that prevent assertive action. Bad marriages can be ended, constricting jobs can be changed. Psychotherapy for the self-defeating, inhibited person may have a great deal of value.

Sometimes the patient is wrong. His situation is miserable and nothing can be done about it by therapy or even by individual action. No one wants to hear that a situation is hopeless and few therapists will admit defeat, so the therapy continues, preserving the glimmer of hope. At times, the patient resembles an annuity.

Reality problems should be recognized for what they are. Value conflicts, financial problems, marital and family conflicts, and professional or job difficulties may require such remedies as domestic realignment, economic assistance, vocational rehabilitation, or social or political action. The contribution of psychotherapies to such problems is limited to helping the patient understand his position, helping him to acknowledge warded-off or disowned feelings, and dispelling unwarranted inhibitions that prevent constructive action. After that, the individual must deal with the problems himself and the solutions may at best be partial.

We hope to assist the reader in distinguishing such problems from biological illnesses and maladaptive learned patterns of behavior. We shall also indicate which psychotherapies as well as medications seem most promising in dealing with the various components of human misery.

In order to grasp the significance of these new kinds of data on mental illness, it is necessary to have some familiarity with several basic subjects: the history of psychiatric diagnosis and thought; the broad categories of psychiatric disorder—in particular, the disorders of mood, the personality disorders, and the schizophrenias; the variety of actions of the psychiatric drugs; recent progress in psychiatric genetics and in brain chemistry; the interweaving of psychological and physiological causation in mental illness; the implications of the physiology of mental disorder for the question of different kinds of unhappiness in man; and finally, the implications of all of these issues for a revised understanding of the functions of psychotherapy. This book will be devoted to the exploration of these concerns.

CHAPTER 2

Kraepelin, Freud, and Their Disciples: A Brief History of Twentieth-Century Psychiatry

"Mental illness" is a term broad enough to encompass external behaviors and subjective states ranging from the grossly aberrant experience of the psychotic to the mild idiosyncrasies and subjective discomfort of the neurotic and, beyond that, even mere dissatisfaction with the circumstances of one's life. Toward the end of the nineteenth century, two simplistic major explanatory schemes had developed to account for this gamut of psychological disorders. They may be termed the "exclusively organic" and the "exclusively psychogenic." Both had long histories and were the work of many contributors. The two schools of thought are the modern derivatives of two obvious facts ascertained in antiquity.

First, physical changes (trauma to the brain, physical illness, the ingestion of alcohol or psychedelic mushrooms) can produce profound changes in feelings, experience, and behavior. Therefore, mental states can be influenced by physical causes. Second, striking changes in feelings and behavior are produced by experiences that do not seem directly to affect the brain or body. Anxiety, depression, and fear are predictably generated by readily definable situations.

20 MIND, MOOD, AND MEDICINE

In simplified terms, the two exclusive approaches can be seen as evolving, on the one hand, from the work of Emil Kraepelin and, on the other, from that of Sigmund Freud. Both were physicians, German-speaking, and, incidentally, both were born in 1856.

Together, the two men have provided the basis for what we designate as a third major scheme—the biopsychiatric approach. This new way of regarding psychiatric disorders is partially based on three different perspectives: viewing psychological disorders as syndromes of illnesses—an elaboration and expansion of Kraepelin's ideas; viewing some aspects of the disorders as psychological complications, that is, as manifestations of psychological attempts by the patient to deal with his or her biologically based illness; viewing some psychological disorders as a reaction to or attempt to compensate for inborn psychological differences that are not in themselves illnesses. The role of life experiences and their interactions with particular vulnerabilities is also considered.

The concepts of "illness" and "disease" seem to be reasonably clear-cut and straightforward. But sophisticated medical thinkers are aware that these concepts are blurred around the edges. Although it is our intention to begin with the clear-cut central notions, first in relationship to physical and then to mental illness, inevitably we will be unable to avoid the gray areas.

The following definition perhaps best expresses the idea of illness: an *involuntary* affliction that produces distress or impaired functioning. Thus, "illness" refers to uncomfortable sensations, such as pain, itching, or malaise; impaired functioning, such as blindness or paralysis; or alterations that produce both discomfort and impaired functioning, such as fever.

Historically, some forms of malfunction did not require schemes of classification or profound sources of explanation—for example, broken bones. The causes of most illnesses, however, were obscure, and early attempts to classify them concentrated on single, discrete symptoms or signs. Symptoms are unpleasant *subjective* experiences; signs are *observable* abnormalities. Diagnostic terminology referred to conditions, such as fever, rash, and dropsy, defined by a single symptom.

Thomas Sydenham (1624–89) is given the credit for two major clinical innovations that enabled medicine to progress beyond the monosymptomatic approach. He began to categorize illnesses (1) on the basis of syndromes—recognizable *patterns* or clusters of symptoms and signs which ran together; (2) on the basis of their course, or evolving clinical history. For example, in the absence of any knowledge of the causation of arthritis (originally considered a monosymptomatic disorder), Sydenham was able to separate it into two distinct entities: gout, in which certain joints become inflamed but in time completely lose the inflammation; and rheumatoid arthritis, in which other patterns of joints are affected and in which basically the course is chronic, with increasing deterioration.

Even *before* the discovery of the causes of pathology, the syndrome approach often successfully isolated what later proved to be distinct diseases with distinct causes. Identification of syndromes also allowed specific treatments and predictions about the course of illness (prognosis).

In diabetes, for example, at one time physicians knew of two syndromes in which the patient urinated excessively. In both syndromes the patient was very thirsty and drank frequently. In one, the patient also lost weight despite a hearty appetite and ample food intake. For reasons that are obscure, some brave man tasted the urine of these two types of patients. One had sweet urine, a sign of diabetes mellitus—the common form of diabetes. In the other, now known to be a hormone deficiency of the pituitary gland, the urine was tasteless or insipid, a sign of diabetes insipidus.

Diabetes mellitus was found to be associated with high blood sugar, which eventually turned out to be the result of insufficient activity of the hormone insulin from the pancreas—that is, clinical observation of a syndrome had identified a distinct disease entity. Diabetes also illustrates the different kinds of signs that can occur in one syndrome. Some diabetics survive long after the onset of the disease, usually through the use of insulin. If the disease is inadequately treated or if it goes on for a very long time, the patient may develop complications: diseases of the nerves, poor circulation and ulcers on the feet, heart and kidney disease, and blindness. One diabetic may become blind and have nerve disease, another may have heart and kidney problems, and a third may not develop any of the signs at all.

With respect to prediction, diabetes provides the example of the power of the biochemical aspects of a syndrome. High sugar levels in the blood and urine indicate clinical diabetes. High blood sugar without sugar in the urine indicates a prediabetic patient, who can be carefully watched and instructed, in the interests of prevention.

Thus, such syndromes proved useful in identifying diseases and helping to search for their causes. All the signs and symptoms did not necessarily occur every time in a given syndrome. Identification of causes has in turn made possible diagnosis of syndromes even before clinical signs and symptoms appear.

Until the twentieth century, psychiatrists and alienists dealt only with the institutionalized mentally aberrant. These included the retarded, the organically psychotic (that is, those who were mad or insane on clearly physical bases, such as the victims of strokes or alcoholism), and the functional psychotics (that is, those who were "crazy" but in whom no underlying anatomical basis could be found). Thus, psychiatrists dealt with the grossly deviant, whose subjective experience was qualitatively different from that of the vast mass of mankind, and whose different experiences and behavior—even with the relatively primitive techniques of a hundred years ago—could sometimes be correlated with underlying abnormalities of the brain.

Many nineteenth- and early-twentieth-century psychiatrists assumed that all major mental disease was the product of brain disease. Indeed, a number of psychiatric disorders had been correlated with specific causes and with tissue injury to specific parts of the brain. Alzheimer's disease, in which the victim becomes psychotic and manifests premature senility, was associated with characteristic microscopic changes in the brain. One of the most common forms of psychosis of that period, general paresis—a disease that we now know is produced by syphilis of the brain—provided a clear model in which psychiatric symptoms, many indistinguishable from those seen in inexplicable mental disease, were correlated with demonstrable tissue changes in the brain; later pathologists were able to demonstrate the presence of the syphilis germ in the brains of paretics. Institutionalized patients in many parts of the world, such as the American South, suffered from a psychosis associated with pellagra, which had been described in the early eighteenth century; in 1915, pellagra was found to be caused by a nutritional deficiency.

The stance of Emil Kraepelin can be understood not only on the basis of such psychiatric observations but also in connection with the major evolutionary shifts that had taken place in the use of the scientific method in medicine. Microscopic anatomy, bacteriology, pathology, and physiology had all taken giant strides, and the psychiatrists of the day therefore harbored the justifiable expectation that if mental illness could be more clearly distinguished and described, a basic medical scientist would be able to identify structural and biochemical abnormalities underlying the manifest disease picture.

Of course, the basic scientist would be doomed to failure if several different diseases were lumped together. Since one illness might have one cause and another a different origin, it would obviously be impossible to find *the* underlying cause of the problem. The importance of the separation—splitting—has been clearly shown in the case of retardation. With modern biochemical and microscopic techniques, it has been possible to show that the group of the intellectually deficient is composed of a very large number of subgroups, each with clear and distinct causes, of which the best known are phenylketonuria (PKU) and mongolism. In Kraepelin's time, most of these were lumped together because the available analytic techniques were inadequate.

Physicians of the eighteenth and early nineteenth centuries had already identified three major groups of mental illness: madness (dementia praecox, or schizophrenia), disorders of mood (manic-depressive psychoses), and psychoses produced by demonstrable physical causes or injury to the brain. Based on the labor of his predecessors, Kraepelin made two advances. One, he introduced the syndromal approach of Sydenham, studying psychological illnesses on the basis of clusters of symptoms and final outcomes. Two, he collected life histories that included data on members of the patient's family, hoping that information on heredity—which he thought played a role in causation—would help to sort out groups of diseases.

With these additional observations, Kraepelin was able to systematize previous work. He identified a number of psychiatric illnesses that are caused by alterations in the chemistry or anatomy of the brain and body (such as illnesses caused by toxins, disorders of the thyroid gland, and head injuries). He also identified three clusters of illnesses that fit together on the basis of common symptoms and common prognoses but for which no identifiable physical abnormalities could be found. Two were the long-recognized dementia praecox (or schizophrenia) and manic-depressive psychosis; their symptom clusters were very distinct, and both illnesses developed in individuals who had theretofore been healthy. The third consisted of the psychopathies (disorders of personality).

In dementia praecox (dementing disease of the young), the patients became increasingly mad and disorganized and did not recover completely. In manic-depressive psychosis, those affected became either depressed or euphoric (or alternated between these two states), generally did not show disorganization of thinking, and eventually recovered fully. In the psychopathies, the patients were not mad but showed congenital deviations in personality structure.

Having identified these syndromes, Kraepelin and his followers applied the available elementary scientific tools to the search for anatomical or biological correlates of the psychiatric illnesses they had identified. When none could be found for dementia praecox, manic-depressive psychoses, or the psychopathies, the three clusters were labeled functional, or without *identifiable* physical causes, which once had been the status of all medical illnesses. (The word "functional" applies to our lack of knowledge and not to the status of the real world—it means "We do not know," not that there is no answer.)

Having been unable to find biological causes for these mental illnesses, the early psychiatric scientists turned to the methods of experimental psychology to study their patients. They investigated reaction time—one of the major psychological discoveries of the nineteenth century. They counted the numbers of family members who were ill. They tabulated the percentage of patients who recovered. Aside from their assumptions regarding causation, they theorized little or not at all.

Was their strategy of studying syndromes useful? Yes and no. At the time, identification of someone as having a particular syndrome provided some useful—if unalterable—knowledge about the course her disease would take, but little else.

Although Kraepelin is commonly identified with the organic point of view, he recognized that psychological experiences could trigger illnesses and affect their manifestations. For example, he described a woman who developed manic-depressive psychosis first following the death of her husband, next following the death of her dog, and finally after the death of a pet dove. Further, he did not assume that every symptom of mental illness was biologically caused by a single factor—that mental illness was like, say, measles, in which spots, fever, cough, inability to tolerate light, are all due to infection with a measles virus. Kraepelinians realized that a man could not have persecutory delusions of being followed by Freemasons unless he knew of the existence of Freemasons. (Nineteenth-century psychotics were plagued by Freemasons; twentieth-century American psychotics are plagued by Communists.)

Kraepelin also made the interesting observation that culture seemed to affect symptoms. Although auditory hallucinations were said to be a hallmark of dementia praecox, Kraepelin found that they were not inevitably present. For example, they did not appear in Javanese patients with dementia praecox. Clearly, culture—and thus learning—affected not only the content of symptoms but whether or not the symptoms occurred. Similarly, our own approach—the biopsychiatric—includes the idea that diseases are modified by learning; disease pictures with the same biological bases may show different psychological manifestations.

In opposition to Kraepelin were those who regarded mental illness as basically psychological in origin. The story of the development of the psychogenic approach is more complex, deriving from many more sources than the organic and with a far more intricate theoretical substructure. The nineteenth century was a period of intellectual ferment, and at the same time that the scientific approach to medical illness was expanding, a number of philosophers and psychologists—among them Gustav Fechner and Johann Bachofen—were becoming interested in the role of psychological factors in the genesis of mental disorders. Much of their writing was so vague and nonspecific as to convey little information, but it touched upon many topics that later were elaborated by Freud and his followers.

These ideas derived from ancient observations that both physical and psychological interventions can alter emotional states that have either physical or psychological causes. Opium and alcohol mitigate the pain of both fractures and grief. Similarly, human kindness or procedures such as hypnosis, meditation, and prayer can relieve not only the anxiety and depression caused by being fired but also that produced by menopause. In many instances, the subjective symptoms engendered by physiological and psychological causes are virtually indistinguishable—e.g., the anxiety engendered by final examinations and by epileptic brain storm—a fact that leads to completely comprehensible misunderstandings. If biologically based depression is indistinguishable from that produced by loss, frustration, or failure, it is not surprising that investigators may mistakenly explain all human depression on either one extreme basis or the other. A further source of confusion is the possibility that psychological stresses occur but go undetected, never fully reach consciousness, or are forgotten. All these considerations played a role in the emerging conceptions of psychiatry at the turn of the century.

At the time, a number of physicians, some of them neurologists, had become interested in the phenomenon of hysteria. Initially they worked in hospitals, but later they did most of their work with outpatients, shifting the focus from that customary with alienists. Jean Charcot, a famous French neurologist, began to investigate "grand hysterics" in a well-known hospital, the Salpêtrière. In hysteria, severely afflicted patients manifest symptoms and signs that seem to be psychologically produced but that mimic brain and nerve dysfunction and damage. Charcot's patients, who were clearly not insane, had epileptic seizures, paralyses, loss of sensation, and a host of other abnormalities for which no discernible physical bases could be found. Charcot found that Franz Mesmer's strange psychological procedure, hypnosis, could induce similar symptoms in asymptomatic hysterical patients and, as well, cure such symptoms in some patients. Thus, an apparently physical illness had psychological causes and responded to psychological methods.

Charcot's experiments with hypnosis legitimized this quasi-respectable procedure and encouraged others to try it. A number of physicians found that under hypnosis patients could remember important but forgotten episodes and that some psychological symptoms could be hypnotized away. These therapeutic uses of hypnosis were gradually expanded by attempts at psychotherapy without hypnosis, approaches employing such techniques as rest, persuasion, suggestion, and the establishment of a "beneficial relationship" between the physician and the patient.

As hypnotists and psychotherapists moved away from the realm of the hospital alienist, they began to treat the less ill: phobics with intense fears of certain objects or situations; obsessives preoccupied with unpleasant thoughts that they could not exclude (such as constant mental blasphemy of God); compulsives handicapped by their repetition of meaningless acts; and finally, the anxious or mildly depressed. For the most part, these patients were not disoriented, hallucinated, or deluded. In general, they were able to function adequately and had a relatively realistic appraisal of their surroundings.

The psychological treatment of nonhospital patients, whose problems were not severe, eventually set the stage for treatment of people whose difficulties did not seem related to illness at all—major problems in living, problems arising out of the patient's character, and problems arising out of confused value systems. These patients seemed to have no cluster of symptoms running a predictable course, and a medical approach, with its concern about underlying diseases, seemed grossly inapplicable. The resultant confusion about the appropriate domains of psychiatry, philosophy, and religion, a major issue to which we shall return, was a later development, but we can see its beginnings here.

The late nineteenth century was also a time of psychological investigation without a therapeutic focus. During this era, Krafft-Ebing wrote his classic work on sexual aberrations and Havelock Ellis published his volume on sexuality in the anthropological context.

It was in this atmosphere of growing scientific rigor, increased interest in psychological functioning, and greater openness about the study of sex that Freud became interested in mental disorders. He had studied with Charcot in Paris, and upon his return to Vienna began to collaborate with an internist, Josef Breuer, who had been employing hypnotic techniques in the treatment of a hysterical patient. From this beginning, Freud branched out to study nonhospitalized neurotics with a variety of difficulties.

Charcot had observed that the hysterics' symptoms corresponded to the patients' own ideas of how the nervous system functioned. A hysteric who believed that one nerve received sensations from a glove-shaped portion of the hand would develop a glove-shaped loss of feeling; actual nerve damage never produces such a pattern of loss of sensation. Thus, the patient's *ideas* influenced his or her symptomatology.

This hypothesis seemed to be reinforced by Freud's work with hysterics and obsessives. Depending on accounts by his patients, at first he believed that hysteria was caused by seduction in childhood, and that obsessive and compulsive symptoms were caused by seducing others while one was still a child. When Freud realized that hysterics' and obsessives' confessions of seduction were not true—they had told him of their fantasies or had confused fantasies with reality—he saved the theoretical day with a startling piece of psychological legerdemain: it was not the experience but the fantasied experience that caused the neurosis. Not what had happened to the patient but what the patient imagined had happened. (Why he imagined such things still had to be explained.)

The Standard Edition of Freud's works occupies twenty-four volumes, and countless books have been written by others summarizing and explaining Freud's theories. To summarize them briefly is impossible, but we will attempt here to indicate the essential elements of his thought, which became the core of the psychogenic position.

First, Freud believed in the dynamic unconscious. Many eighteenth- and nineteenth-century philosophers had believed in a vaguely specified unconscious, realizing that many of the workings of the mind, including but not limited to portions that regulated the physiology of the body, were beyond conscious awareness. Freud's postulated unconscious includes motives, wishes, memories, and fantasies—often of a sexual or aggressive nature—which the individual cannot willingly—consciously—accept. Freud at first tried to discover the nature of the mind's unconscious contents by hypnosis, but he soon found, as had many psychotherapists before him, that a substantial fraction of patients were not hypnotizable. In an attempt to circumvent this barrier, he devised two techniques: free association and dream interpretation. In the former, he requested that the patient report every thought—no matter how trivial or unacceptable it seemed to be—to the analyst. This uncensored and full account of the contents of consciousness would, Freud felt, eventually allow the pressing, dynamic, unconscious contents to achieve expression. Similarly, he believed that interpretation of dreams could lead to an awareness of the patient's unconscious.

Later Freud hypothesized that resistances blocked easy access to the unconscious, and that these barriers had to be removed in order to reach the unconscious.

Initially, Freud believed that psychological symptoms were produced by blocked drives, primarily of a sexual or aggressive nature (analogous to the discomfort produced by an overfull bladder). An early formulation attributed anxiety neurosis to sexual intercourse that was unnecessarily prolonged or stopped short of orgasm. The dammed-up sexual energy was ostensibly transmuted into anxiety.

Though never abandoning this simple theory, Freud came to attribute most symptoms to a compromise between repressed drives (drives that were kept out of consciousness because of their unacceptability to another portion of the mind) and the forces exerting the repression. In all cases, the symptoms not only represent a defect (a failure to express the drive) but also are an elaborate compromise that blocks the drive from attaining its fantasy object—that is, whatever the person unconsciously desires—while at the same time allowing it some symbolic gratification—that is, some substitute satisfaction. Let us present an example. A nineteenth-century female hysteric might develop the following symptoms: epileptic-like, convulsive movements of the pelvis, together with an anesthesia of the lower portion of her body. The Freudian explanation would be that she harbored intense sexual desire for her father. An awareness of this desire, much less its expression, would be intolerable. As a result, she unconsciously discharged some of her sexual energies in the pelvic movements and at the same time, by the hysterical anesthesia, effectively prohibited herself from experiencing sexual gratification. In addition, these signs and symptoms rendered her an invalid, which meant that she would receive additional attention and love from her father.

In another example, an obsessive-compulsive neurotic might unconsciously want to do away with his burdensome wife and children. This wish might be manifested, every time he left his home, by the need to return to make sure that the gas stove had been turned off and the door locked. He would return immediately to check, turning the gas on again and then making sure he had turned it off, and likewise unlock and lock the door. Ostensibly, these compulsive acts gratified his wish to obliterate the family (he was going through the motions of administering lethal gas and leaving the family vulnerable to thieves) and at the same time kept the wish from consciousness by symbolizing extra care. Freud termed the mental processes that executed such compromises "defense mechanisms."

Specifying the number of Freud's innovative ideas is akin to specifying the exact number of causes of the French Revolution, but we do want to emphasize three more of his contributions to dynamic psychology. First, he made explanatory use of everyday, common-sense phenomena of psychological life—such as envy and jealousy. Obviously, since the inciting causes of anger, satisfaction, self-appreciation, and the like can be discerned by anyone very early in life, thinking in terms of empirical cause and effect in human emotion was hardly innovative. What was innovative was their use by a physician to explain psychopathology. It is of interest that Freud sometimes felt he had to defend himself for writing his case histories in a form more like a novel than like a scientific report.

Second, in explaining more complex, unconscious patterns of family relationships, he pointed out that such patterns occur in mythology and had been explicitly represented at least as early as the time of the Greek dramatists. Foremost among these was the Oedipus complex, the rivalrous wishes of the son in competition with the father for the love of the mother. This was considered an inevitable stage in male development, and the failure to resolve the conflict was invoked to explain a multitude of symptoms.

The third striking innovative feature was an emphasis on sexuality, particularly childhood sexuality. Freud called attention to the fact that young children were not the pure creatures idealized by the Victorian imagination but were rather intensely interested in urination, defecation, penises and vaginas. In addition, Freud asserted that the manner in which children had dealt with their infantile sexuality helped to determine their later personality problems.

It is easy to see the dramatic appeal of Freud's ideas. With the concept of the unconscious, he was able, he thought, to make the meaningless and the accidental explicable. Our trivial actions had become mysterious and awe-inspiring and the mundane interesting. With the technique of free association he thought he could bring concealed wishes and fears into the bright light of consciousness and dispel mephitic influences. His use of mythology to name and exemplify what he saw as universal laws of psychological functioning was remarkably persuasive, and his emphasis on the importance of childhood and adult sexuality inevitably attracted attention and excited the adulation of the avant-garde. In combining these ideas, Freud diverged widely from traditional, organically focused, medical psychiatric thought. A wide gulf had been opened between the biological and psychological approaches to the causes of mental illness.

Freud's undoubted major contribution was his in-depth concrete inquiry into the lives of individuals. With his methods, he encouraged people to speak their innermost thoughts and reveal aspects of themselves and their relationships that they would otherwise never have done. On the basis of this technique, he compiled a mass of observations concerning the interplay of psychological forces in the lives of healthy and sick persons. Some of his observations and inferences have been substantiated and some have not, but with them he constructed a massive theoretical superstructure—an inverted pyramid of theory erected upon an apex of fact. His biographical and literary approach was invaluable for creating hypotheses, but despite his own devotion to science, his methods were inadequate for testing these ideas. Freud's faithful observations were true to the science of his time but do not meet the requirements of today's researchers for the evaluation of psychological hypotheses and therapeutic outcome. His theoretical structure is beloved by many of his followers, but Freud himself was aware that the facts he had observed and not the theories he had promulgated were the most important. Referring to his speculations concerning the structure of the human mind, he wrote: "For these ideas are not the foundation of science, upon which everything rests: that foundation is observation alone. They are not the bottom but the top of the whole structure, and they can be replaced and discarded without damaging it" (1914, Vol. 14, p. 77).

While the Master expressed reservations, showing a healthy regard for fact and a contempt for premature theory, many of his followers have gone from conjecture to dogma. Before discussing Freud's intellectual descendants, however, it is important to emphasize that while they moved further and further away from concerns about the relationship of biology and the mind, Freud never did. Beginning his professional life as an investigator in laboratory neurology, Freud had been fascinated by recent advances in scientific methodology and based his theoretical models on neurophysiology. He believed that psychological illnesses ranged from those in which biological factors were predominant and experience mattered little to those in which biology played a small role and experience a determining one. He understood that his explanation of hysteria was incomplete—that although ideas might underlie hysterical symptoms, there was a biological predisposition for what he referred to as the "mysterious leap from the mind to the body." Not everyone developed hysterical symptoms and signs, given similar experience. Likewise, when Freud propounded his theories of innate sexual and aggressive drives, he conceded that basic, quantitative biological differences among people might be important in the origin of symptoms. In his last important paper, "Analysis Terminable and Interminable" (1937), Freud stated his belief in the significance of biological contributions to deviant behavior. He regretfully confined himself to the psychological approach because that was the only way he knew of to explore mental abnormalities. He used psychological techniques because he thought they were the best available—not because they necessarily struck at the root of the problem.

To give a detailed account of the delta into which the mainstream of psychoanalytic thinking flowed and broke up would be beyond the capacity of the authors, the tolerance of the reader, and the main point of our argument. The following is greatly abbreviated.

The institutionalization of psychoanalysis might perhaps be dated to 1902, when a small group of people gathered at Freud's home for weekly discussions on problems of psychoanalysis. Dissenters appeared almost immediately, beginning with Alfred Adler. Like a religion, psychoanalysis has continued to break into a number of closely related but warring sects, each believing itself the defender of the true faith.

The splits continued as psychoanalysis moved to the United States. Adlerian views have crept into much of current psychodynamic thinking, although most of those who employ his ideas do not realize their source. Adler downplayed the importance of the unconscious and the conscience (or superego), placing great emphasis on the role of obvious experiential factors in the formation of personality, particularly experiences in the family. Much behavior, he claimed, was generated not by repressed sexual drives but by feelings of inferiority and by the individual's need to maintain and increase his self-esteem. Adler also viewed behavior as pulled by future plans, as opposed to being pushed by past forces. Still another of his ideas was the manipulative aspect of symptoms. By being psychologically crippled, one could control the actions of one's loved ones—a theme later picked up and expounded in detail by the transactional analyst Eric Berne, author of *Games People Play*.

The other major dissenter from Freud's original group was Carl Jung, who broke away in 1914. Jung, who had been working with sexually satisfied middle-aged patients, turned away from considering sex and aggression as determinants of human behavior. His work represents an attempt to preserve a religious view of man and contains elements of self-transcendence and quasi-mystical notions such as archetypes (universal symbols) and the racial or collective unconscious (unconscious ideas inherited by everyone).

Freud's ideas crossed the Atlantic in the early days of the psychoanalytic movement, and he was invited to give a series of lectures at Clark University in Massachusetts in 1909. American psychiatrists were impressed by Freud's work, translated it, and went to study with him. This communication continued and increased in the ensuing years and was intensified during the 1930s, when the Nazi threat caused a massive exodus of European analysts to the United States. In the United States, psychoanalysis diverged strikingly from the original Freudian position by an increasing deemphasis of biological factors and a concomitant emphasis on psychology and culture. Unlike Freud, many of the American psychogeneticists not only explained neurosis completely on the basis of experience but also proposed that more serious mental illnesses, the psychoses, could also be completely explained on the basis of an individual's own experiences.

Like traditional Christian theologians, Freud believed that the natural, yet to be acculturated infant was not a Rousseauian noble savage. He or she was a selfish, unprincipled scoundrel who slowly and painfully had to be trained into being civilized. When Freud's ideas were transported across the Atlantic, the infant changed into what John Locke had called a *tabula rasa,* or blank slate, for experience to write upon. This viewpoint matched that of American behaviorism, earlier propounded by John Watson, who claimed that children were almost infinitely malleable. Further, the specious belief that emotionally and intellectually all men are created equal has a democratic ring to it, appealing to prevailing attitudes in the theoretically classless United States. Emotional and intellectual equality is, however, not a prerequisite for the democratic political man; if anything, equality of opportunity—in the broadest sense—is even more important for unequal man.

After World War II, the number of schools of psychogenesis and of practitioners of psychotherapy began to grow exponentially. Freud had argued that nonphysicians should be taught psychoanalysis, and in Europe many prominent psychoanalysts were not M.D.s (Erich Fromm and Erik Erikson are in this tradition). It was one of Freud's great disappointments that the American psychoanalytic movement remained firmly in the hands of M.D.s, who for many years refused to allow non-M.D.s into psychoanalytic institutes. Nevertheless, as Freudian practices and ideas spread and moved into the academic world as a part of personality theory, a modified version of psychoanalysis called psychoanalytic psychotherapy began to develop. Some psychoanalysts left the ranks of orthodoxy, and the evolution of a nonmedical therapeutic approach, based on the relationship between the therapist and the patient, also appealed to psychologists and social workers. They recognized it as closely allied to aspects of their disciplines and began to incorporate its ideas into their clinical work.

Simultaneously, Kurt Lewin and his colleagues, who were at first primarily interested in ways of decreasing prejudice, were studying group processes. This stream later blended with emerging group therapy, led to the foundation of the National Training Laboratories, and evolved into numerous other forms of group exploration of behavior and feelings. At approximately the same time, the psychologist Carl Rogers began to use a nondirective approach to counsel clients, profoundly influencing American clinical psychology in the 1950s. Rogers concentrated on empathy rather than interpretation, and much of his work was with college students who were not severely disturbed but were attempting to resolve the question of who they were and where they were going. His development of a simple form of counseling for relatively healthy people also had strong impact on the encounter-group movement.

In the ensuing years the scene became one of generalized chaos, with the introduction of over a hundred therapies in a period of twenty years: transactional analysis, gestalt therapy, primal scream, bioenergetics, psychosynthesis, marathons, nude groups, and scores of others. Among the diverse therapies are even some that might be called antipsychiatric.

One can better understand the origin of some of the numerous and varied currents of antipsychiatry by recalling what had happened with the theoretical and practical application of the psychogenic point of view. First, psychotherapy was increasingly used for nonsymptomatic conditions in which people complained about *ineffective behavior and understandable feelings of unhappiness:* conditions that are not diseases. Second, the emphasis on the psychological origin of disturbed behavior implied that mental illness was radically different from other illnesses. These themes—and allied themes, such as moral responsibility—have been seized by two well-known antipsychiatric psychiatrists, Thomas Szasz and R. D. Laing. Both are able to maintain their contentious positions by careful neglect of facts. Szasz has held that mental illness is a myth, asserting that the words "illness" and "disease" are pejorative terms applied by the mainstream of society to those who are nonacceptably deviant. As we elaborate our thesis in this book, we will document the errors in Szasz's position. Primarily he overlooks the biological and genetic contributants that place many kinds of mental illness in the realm of true disease. By failing to distinguish between the more and the less severe conditions seen by psychiatrists, Szasz has practiced some fine sophistry. If mental illness is a myth, it is a myth with a genetic component.

The position espoused by Laing is that psychiatric conditions are the explicable responses of normal souls to painful and destructive family circumstances. Again, this is a half-truth that strikingly resembles the ideology common among adolescents (young and old) that all their troubles are due to their parents. *Some* psychological difficulties are undoubtedly the product of faulty, deviant, or unpleasant experiences while growing up. Like Szasz, however, Laing makes the illogical transition from "Some A are B" to "All A are B."

A third antipsychiatric response reacts against the position taken by some early Freudians that since everything results from individual intrapsychic experience, social deprivation is unimportant. Delinquency, for example, was related to a distorted family life, and realistic deprivations and social influences were ignored. This stand obscured *realistic unhappiness* by camouflaging it as psychological disorder. The same argument has been used by analysts against revolutionaries, whose attempts to overturn the establishment have been described as symbolic enactments of their oedipal conflicts with their fathers. This explanation also requires one to believe that the followers of revolutionaries are also acting out *their* oedipal conflicts and that ruling classes somehow contend with Oedipus differently. Unsurprisingly, left-wing theorists have assailed Freudian thinking as still another obscurantist attempt by the ruling classes to belittle the legitimate claims of the oppressed. Related protests have come from a variety of groups—women, blacks, Chicanos, homosexuals—who believe that their psychological distresses are not illnesses but normal responses to their debased, persecuted station in life. Out of such criticisms has emerged the point of view that adequate social reform—good housing and schools, full employment, enforcement of civil-rights legislation—would mean the disappearance of much mental illness. Of course, much unhappiness *is* a result of prejudice, discrimination, and lack of opportunity. But these oppressions do not immunize the deprived from the kinds of mental illnesses that afflict the nondeprived.

Finally, some current antipsychiatric views are simply anti-intellectual—deriving from the belief that science and technology and even rational thought itself interfere with the direct experience of truth and beauty. This position is imbued with the belief that technology has brought us a vast range of troubles and that spirituality may offer escape from an overemphasized rationalism that has shut out half of man's nature. This is a recurrent position, a return to nature familiar at least since the Taoist philosophers of ancient China. Its value is not subject to discussion here, but factually it errs. The laws governing biochemical reactions and the evidence for the inheritability of certain psychiatric disorders, and the value of medication for some illnesses, are not altered by such views.

Kraepelin and Freud stated their beliefs clearly enough. Were they more than beliefs? Is there any evidence to substantiate their theories? Kraepelin was atheoretical. He noticed that people with certain groups of symptoms tended to have similar histories, to recover or become progressively more ill. That much was true. The rest was faith. He had no evidence that these illnesses were the product of abnormal biological functioning. The critical tests have come more than half a century later. As we shall see, in at least three important instances his hypotheses were correct.

What about Freud? Was he right? That depends on which aspects of his theory are being considered. Freud did four things. First, he collected intimate, introspective data over time. By seeing a few patients intensively rather than many patients superficially, and by adopting a permissive rather than a critical position with regard to his patients' confessions, he acquired information about subjective states that biologically oriented psychiatry failed to obtain. Indeed, he reported many odd things: that many hysterics claimed to have been incestuously violated, that many paranoid people were concerned with homosexuality, that some psychologically disturbed people reported crude aggressive impulses and startling incestuous ones, that many young children were surprisingly interested in and stimulated by sexual matters. Numerous fragmentary attempts to document these observations have been inconclusive and at times contradictory (see Fisher and Greenberg, 1977).

Second, Freud developed in free association a technique for exploring personality which has clearly produced unexpected data. Employing it, psychoanalysts have observed that people do report things they would not reveal in casual conversation and do discover recurrent preoccupations of which they were unaware. This anecdotal material casts new light on personality, but its relation to the origins of psychopathology is unclear.

Third, and this is what concerns us here, Freud claimed to have discovered the causes of some psychiatric illnesses by means of psychoanalysis. Have these theories, these hypotheses, ever been verified? No.

It is often assumed that the validity of these theories is demonstrated by Freud's fourth innovation, psychoanalytic treatment, but the relationship between the therapy and the theory is tenuous, and after eighty years the scientific evidence for the specific effectiveness of psychoanalysis is minimal and contradictory (see Fisher and Greenberg).

Critics of the exclusively organic approach have assumed incorrectly that the organic model of the mind is no more complicated than a clock, which tells the correct time, runs fast, runs slow, runs erratically, or stops. Such criticism is greatly oversimplified and sets up a straw man. Even Kraepelin did not employ the exclusively organic approach in pure form. For example, he realized that both the presence of hallucinations and their content were influenced by psychological factors.

Just as Kraepelin did not employ an exclusively organic approach, Freud did not employ an exclusively psychogenic one. His theory included the possibility of constitutional differences among people. Yet many of his followers have continued to assert that mental pathology derives overwhelmingly from life experience and that inborn differences among individuals are largely irrelevant.

We are suggesting a synthesis of these viewpoints that consists of the following major beliefs. Many illnesses have a hereditary predisposition. Further, a wide spectrum of deviant behavior, generally not considered to be illness, has important biological contributions.

Important psychosocial issues, such as separation anxiety, choice of mate, rejection sensitivity, and so forth, must be viewed in the framework of the specific biologically evolved nature of man, who is a social primate and often a rational one.

We do not deny—in fact, we affirm strongly—that social and psychological processes are vital in understanding the complex behavior of the mentally ill. Psychosocial theory helps us to distinguish among primary symptoms of disease and the adaptive and maladaptive reactions to suffering from a disease. Further, psychosocial theory helps us distinguish disease from other unhappiness.

One must be skeptical of all forms of therapy, biological or psychological, until they have demonstrated their worth. The biopsychiatric approach sees no necessary antagonism between these two forms of therapy. In many instances they seem compatible and complementary. This, too, is open to study.

In summary, the biopsychiatric approach takes into account what is known about heredity, brain dysfunction, and our species characteristics. It does so without neglecting what we know concerning human learning and the role of experience.

Although we are hesitant about using mechanistic metaphors, the computer might be an appropriate model for our approach. Unlike the clock, a computer can perform complex activities in a variety of ways.

Advanced computers can actually develop new approaches to problems with experience. Thus, they manifest both learning and goal-seeking. Similarly, and again in distinction from the clock, there are several ways a computer can malfunction. Its parts can malfunction; its wiring can be faulty; or it can be fed the wrong instructions. Its systems can mesh under some circumstances and clash under others. A clock can malfunction by going slow or fast or stopping, but it takes something with the complexity of a computer or a brain to give you a really good wrong answer.

One of our statistician friends marveled at a computer printout by saying, "You know, it would have taken ten thousand mathematicians thirty years to make this mistake."

Drawing on nineteenth-century science, Freud saw behavior as pushed by factors in the past. The computer model can expand that picture to include concern for desired outcomes, preferred futures, especially when one considers that the programming instructions are coming from the individual as well as from the environment; in a sense, the cybernetic computer model introduces legitimate teleology.

In order to understand how this new complex view of the mind was developed and how the new drug therapies actually work to correct malfunction, it is necessary to consider the psychiatric illnesses in some detail. This we shall now do.

CHAPTER 3

Syndromes of Mental Disorder

The welter of conditions that have been described as mental disorders can be classified in many different ways, none of them completely satisfactory. We have chosen to present the most common disorders in three major categories: disorders of mood, personality disorders, and the schizophrenias. This classification system will have its share of overlapping, but that is a reflection of the nature of the field and of the numerous still unanswered questions concerning the disorders themselves.

MOOD DISORDERS

Disorders of mood include a loose collection of depressed emotional states—such as sadness, demoralization, disappointment, and grief—and a few states of exaggerated euphoria. In describing them, we will from time to time make use of a concept from biological research, the *phenocopy*, which we find particularly useful in the study of mental illness. Phenocopies are phenomena that are superficially alike but result from different causes. Depression, for example, may arise from a biological malfunction, from actual losses, deprivations, or rejections, or from personal limitations. The difficulty in sorting out such causal factors is a source of enormous confusion in the diagnosis and treatment of disorders of mood.

The confusion is further compounded by the fact that depression, like anxiety, is an emotion of everyday life. The feeling of being blue, down in the dumps, gloomy, or unhappy is a normal reaction to many of the inevitable afflictions of human existence. One of the goals of the psychiatrist is to try to distinguish such reactions from depressive patterns that can be considered mental illnesses—that is, true disorders of mood (often called affective disorders).

Before we describe the illnesses themselves, it will be useful to say what we mean by mood. A distinction between moods and feelings is analogous to the distinction between climate and weather. Moods are relatively enduring; feelings are comparatively short-lived. The importance of mood is that it regulates our disposition to action. In this we shall see that it may very well have evolutionary utility. In normal people under normal conditions, mood varies between moderately subdued (down) and moderately euphoric (up). Mood reflects our evaluation of the enduring features of our life—ourselves and the overall structure of our life circumstances. People in happy, optimistic moods are likely to engage in outgoing, exploratory, pleasure-seeking, and risk-taking behavior. People in subdued, pessimistic moods are likely to be unresponsive, cautious, and self-protective. Feelings may be regarded as a sort of fine tuning in healthy people, reinforcing or counteracting the current mood. Mood tends to be stable. A person may become quite depressed or elated upon hearing news of a particular loss or gain, but if his overall evaluation of himself is not affected, those feelings are generally short-lived.

The relationship between mood and self-evaluation is complex. Each affects the other. If we view ourselves as capable of routinely producing important rewards and engendering rewarding circumstances, then our attitude is self-approving and the accompanying mood is pleasant. Such an optimistic mood produces expansive activities. Since normal, mature self-evaluation reflects our actual capacities, these activities have a good chance for positive outcomes. Capable people in favorable surroundings can benefit themselves by increasing their involvement with their environment. Sometimes less capable people can also increase their chances of success through cheerful moods.

The opposite state of affairs holds for the person with a subdued or retiring mood. Such a person is often called depressed or pessimistic, and frequently has difficulty responding happily to good tidings. Further, he may view not only his current but his future surroundings as unrewarding. We *observe* that such people often have low self-esteem and see themselves as incapable. Sometimes these self-evaluations are inaccurate and thus augment the chances of failure. If, however, the evaluations are accurate, it is sometimes reasonable for such people to cut down on their attempts to extract rewards from the environment—for example, it may make sense to adjust employment goals downward in terms of realistic capacity. Doing less diminishes the exposure to both unmanageable risk and the possibility of making bad situations worse. Conservative, withdrawn, self-protective behavior may in fact minimize possible losses.

Mood can therefore play an important role in regulating behavior. The expansive activities of the self-assured, optimistic person probably maximize his chances of rewards, at the cost of increased but usually mild risks. The more limited person who acts defensively does not maximize his possible gains, but by minimizing his potential losses he may be making the best of a bad bargain. Mood thus provides an automatic, overall strategy—optimism or pessimism—that often fits the realities of the world. But people who are exceedingly and enduringly pessimistic or optimistic and whose moods and self-evaluation are very much at variance with reality destroy the adaptational (and evolutionary) value of mood. Many of them are suffering from forms of biological emotional illness: vital depression and mania.

Two other qualities—energy levels and the pursuit and experience of pleasure—tend to change with mood. Some people are singularly energetic, active, spontaneous or lively, and emotionally responsive, capable of joyfully undertaking a task and persevering toward the goal in the face of opposition. At the opposite pole are those who are listless and apathetic, lack spontaneous initiative, have difficulty in undertaking a pursuit that promises to be rewarding, or if started, cannot continue in the face of opposition.

Energetic feelings are usually pleasant and frequently associated with well-being, mastery, and high self-esteem. (In the extreme, one can feel unpleasantly driven.) Listless feelings are unpleasant, especially when circumstances demand action that cannot be undertaken. They frequently accompany low mood and low self-evaluation. In general, therefore, mood, outlook, energy, and the ability to pursue and experience pleasure move in the same direction.

In the variety of mental disorders that go by the name of depression, however, there seem to be some subdivisions in the usual relationships between pleasure and mood. The pursuit of anticipated pleasure and the experiencing of pleasure—the joys of the chase and those of the feast—are distinct. One may be affected while the other is not. These differences seem to be helpful in distinguishing among the various kinds of depression, and also seem related to the correct selection of antidepressant medication.

Many people, even those in a depressed state, respond pleasurably to a new positive experience—a vacation, a new lover, a better job. Those who appear to be unable to anticipate or pursue pleasure nevertheless recognize a good thing when it comes along. The degree of such responsiveness is variable, and what may be sufficient to raise the spirits of one may be insufficient for another. Nonetheless, for such people, within the range of the usual depressed feelings, mood is not entirely autonomous but responds to environmental changes. In others, however, depressed mood is not responsive to environmental change, and this is often an important indicator of a possible biological component in the disorder.

As a symptom, depression is also seen in numerous psychiatric conditions other than disorders of mood, including psychoses, phobias, and anxiety states, some chronic physical illnesses (endocrine abnormalities, liver trouble, multiple sclerosis), and menopause. It is analogous to fever, which may occur in infectious disease, cancer, or serious physical injury.

Thus, it is important to reemphasize that, as with anxiety, the use of one word, "depression," is misleading. There are at least three major states to which the word is applied. The first we would call demoralization, a pervasive state in which one is overwhelmed by feelings of ineffectiveness and helplessness. It can result from any of life's defeats and is accompanied by an expectation of future failure of one's efforts. Demoralization can accompany either of the other two states labeled depression (since depression itself produces a feeling of incapability), but it can also occur independently. Because demoralization is a generalized state that goes beyond specific symptoms and can derive from a variety of illnesses, maladaptive situations, and life circumstances, we will delay detailed consideration of it until a later chapter; when we consider the three major sources of unhappiness.

The second state is depression with a small *d*—that is, nonvital depression—often called neurotic depression. It may be produced by defeat, disappointment, or loss of a loved one. The major feeling is not having what one wants and thinking that one is unlikely to get it. This type of depression is referred to as sadness or being blue, and *may* be accompanied by demoralization if the patient feels that his own efforts are not equal to his problems. Another version of nonvital depression is depressive character, which is typified by a continuing mildly depressed mood.

In both demoralization and nonvital depression, the person *retains the ability to experience pleasure.* If life events go well (a raise, a new car), he may feel better or even happy. But the ability to experience hopeful interest and to pursue future gratifications may be somewhat impaired. Both of these forms of depression differ from the third form, vital or physiological depression, in which even the *ability to experience the pleasure of a usually satisfying consummation is lost.* To this depressive, food has come to taste like cardboard and sex becomes a mechanical, pleasureless routine, even if the person was previously a gourmet and a rake.

Vital Depression

We will begin our detailed description of disorders of mood with the most important form of depression—the depressive disorder that is probably physiological in cause and to some degree genetic in origin. Psychiatrists disagree on the appropriate name for this illness, but we are using the recognized term "vital depression" because of the apparent physiological basis. Physiological depression is one of the most common and most unrecognized of psychiatric illnesses. Since depression is an emotion that occurs normally as a reaction to some life events, depressive illness is frequently explained incorrectly on psychological grounds. This is most important. There are approximately 30,000 suicides per year in the United States, and it is likely that a large fraction, perhaps a majority, are committed by physiologically depressed persons. This is especially tragic because depression is among the most treatable of severe psychiatric illnesses, and the risk of suicide in severe depression may be between 5 and 15 percent. Unlike the schizophrenias and many of the psychologically determined disorders, it frequently can be controlled and reversed by the use of medications available to every family physician. Prompter and more accurate recognition of the disorder, by both the lay person and the practicing physician, could reduce and alleviate a substantial amount of human misery.

In the nineteenth century, European psychiatrists, who were beginning to systematize ancient observations on mental disorders, focused some attention on persons who sometimes developed a profound depression of mood, frequently accompanied by changes in bodily functioning. The terminology of the time was confused, but such illnesses were frequently referred to as melancholia. It was noted that melancholic or depressive illnesses might develop either in reaction to unfortunate life experience or, seemingly, spontaneously. Toward the end of the nineteenth century, Kraepelin observed that some depressives had other periods in which they exhibited qualitatively opposite behavior, referred to as mania. During these episodes, the affected person became euphoric (or high), overactive, impulsive, irritable, sexually hyperactive, excited, and excessively energetic, required less sleep, spoke incessantly, and might develop delusions and hallucinations. Kraepelin labeled such persons manic-depressive and their illness manic-depressive psychosis.

Kraepelin assumed—we now think erroneously—that everyone who manifested serious, recurrent, depressive episodes was manic-depressive; even though not all depressives experienced periods of mania, their long-term outcomes were similar—spontaneous improvement and good functioning between episodes. This, he felt, distinguished the illness from schizophrenia, which progressed to chronicity.

Current information suggests that there are at least two major forms of affective disorders: the unipolar affective disorders, in which patients suffer recurrent episodes of depression but never mania; and bipolar affective disorders, or manic-depressive illnesses, which show periods of both depression and mania. The distinction is an important one in that the two groups differ with respect to genetics and responsiveness to treatment.

The unipolar form seems by far the more common. It often occurs for no apparent reason and thus is called endogenous (inner-caused). Such depressions are regularly accompanied by so-called vital changes. The patient will say that she went to bed one night feeling fine and awakened the next day feeling miserable. In nonvital, reactive (to a life event) depressions, the patient is likely to feel "rotten" but does not usually show major alterations in physiological functioning. In the endogenous depressions, several kinds of vital changes frequently occur. There is often a specific alteration of sleep pattern. The patient falls asleep with relative ease but awakens in the early morning and spends several restless hours before arising. Further, he may start the day feeling terrible but improve slowly and show some elevation of mood as the day progresses. At times, for unclear reasons that may not be associated with the customary loss of appetite and decreased food intake, the patient has a noticeable weight loss. Loss in sexual interest, impotence or frigidity, constipation, dry mouth, coldness of the extremities, and dryness of the skin sometimes accompany vital depression. Investigators of physiological malfunctioning in vital depression have also found evidence of hypothalamic dysfunction. For instance, the sleep cycle during depression is typically disrupted. The rapid eye movement (REM) period that accompanies dreaming occurs much earlier during the night than it does in healthy people.

Recently, it has been demonstrated that many patients whose episodes of depressive illness seem to have been precipitated by a life event (e.g., a death in the family) nonetheless develop vital changes. Such patients are called endogenous-like. Some investigators refer to all precipitated depressions as reactive, but this obscures the physiological component.

The down mood itself in endogenous depressions, particularly the milder ones, is different from ordinary sadness. The affected patient may honestly say that he is not sad, even wishing that he were able to cry, but complains of loss of interest in life, a loss of zestfulness and the ability to experience consummatory pleasure, and a decrease in optimism, self-confidence, and self-esteem. As the illness becomes more severe and hopelessness grows, the patient may become preoccupied with ideas of suicide. Rather than the typical feelings of aching loss that accompany grief, the mood may be colorless and has been described as one of painful anesthesia—painful because the patient remembers that life used to be pleasurable, and anesthesia because of the general numbness. (Such patients may actually have an increased threshold for painful external stimuli.) Other frequent symptoms are helplessness, boredom, a decreased capacity to love, total indecisiveness, and guilt.

Interestingly, the presence or absence of guilt seems to be dependent on the surrounding culture rather than the illness. In contemporary Western Judeo-Christian society, physiologically depressed persons may berate themselves endlessly. They tirelessly lament their past sins, their worthlessness, and their responsibility for the real and imagined problems of themselves, their families, and—if they are also psychotic—of the world and universe. However, historical and cross-cultural data do not indicate that guilt is an inevitable accompaniment of depression. Melancholia has been known for millennia, but until the sixteenth century there seem to be few cases on record of exaggerated guilt feelings; in Asia and Africa guilt still is rare in depressives, except among the Westernized (see Murphy, 1978). Many psychiatrists have regarded guilt as the *cause* of depression, but the variable data cast doubt on this formulation. In physiological depression, guilt may be an *effect* of depression occurring in a culturally molded personality. We shall expand on this point later.

In the early stages of depression the affected person may increasingly cling to loved ones; the constant company and attention of a spouse, lover, or parents seems to ameliorate the psychological pain. Since at times only a few of the symptoms—such as ennui and excessive dependency—are present, and since they can vary in severity, mild illnesses are difficult to distinguish from the ordinary problems of living or reactions to specific situations. A further complication is that anyone can at any time find a reason for being depressed if he looks hard enough. It's been observed that "depression is that state of mind in which any intelligent human being finds himself when he stops kidding himself." Conversely, one might wonder how much fashionable existential anomie, often justified by elaborate philosophical reasoning, is simply the product of underlying and unrecognized physiological changes.

Vital depressive reactions tend to be self-limited—that is, they tend to disappear in time; however, the possibility of suicide must always be kept in mind. Since the introduction of effective methods for the treatment of depressives, studies of their untreated course are no longer done, but data collected earlier indicate that the duration was often from several months to a year or two. Although finite, the periods tend to be recurrent, and anyone who has suffered one such episode is much more at risk for vital depression than is a member of the population at large.

The preceding descriptions of depression are skeletal. To make them more vivid, and to illustrate some of the variations that can occur, we will present several patients' histories. An older psychiatrist once remarked to one of the authors: "When you learn to listen, all depressions sound alike." The remark was an astute observation of a property that is typical of medical diseases—an unchanging repetition of specific core complaints. Their patterning and intensity may differ, the discomfort may be colored by the patient's stoicism or ability to report subjective experiences, but to the trained ear the common note sounds throughout.

William M.

A successful lawyer in his late forties, William M. had been in individual psychotherapy, most recently for two years, with a skilled psychologist, because of lifelong feelings of intermittent depression. Despite considerable professional success, he had always regarded himself as a failure. Unlike his brothers, uncles, and father, he had little interest in athletics, was somewhat shy and socially uneasy, and his father held him in low regard. Academic success, a reasonably happy marriage, well-adjusted and successful children, and a career of moderate accomplishments and continuing upward mobility had done nothing to eliminate his low self-esteem. Because of these chronic feelings of inadequacy and intermittent depressive periods, he had decided to reenter psychotherapy, during which the origins of his attitudes toward himself were uncovered and explored. The discrepancy between his opinion of himself and that of others was highlighted, and his chronic distortion in perception was repeatedly called to his attention. Although he developed considerable insight, neither the feelings of inadequacy nor the intermittent depressions were relieved. In the second year of this course of psychotherapy, his feelings of depression intensified and he discussed with increasing anxiety his increasingly frequent thoughts of driving his car off the road at high speed. At this point he was referred for psychiatric evaluation.

On the basis of the patient's reported self-image, the psychiatrist anticipated meeting an awkward, socially inept, defeated man; instead, he was surprised to find William M. good-looking, urbane, witty, intelligent, and psychologically sensitive. Over the previous half year or so, he had become anxious and fearful about the most ordinary things. He found himself awakening at three or four in the morning, able to go back to sleep for only ten or fifteen minutes at a time, tossing and turning until the alarm rang, preoccupied with wishing that he was dead. At work he was increasingly afraid to accept assignments. With his professional associates, his wife, and his children, he had become critical and irascible. Although he had previously been fairly sensual, his sex drive had diminished markedly. He had lost interest in all aspects of living that had formerly provided him with considerable pleasure. He considered himself a fraud, a useless member of the human race, and a burden to those around him.

No other members of his family gave any history of having had mood disorders, although his father had been a heavy drinker. William M. found it extremely difficult to believe that his outlook might stem from a biochemical abnormality, but being compliant and eager for help (a feature that often vanishes as depression grows deeper), he assented to a trial of antidepressant medication.

A few days after he began to take the drug, his sleep patterns returned to normal, and as the dosage was increased during the next two weeks, his appetite and interest in sex returned. The dose was further increased over a period of three or four weeks, and by this time all his recent complaints had disappeared. He no longer thought of suicide, he enjoyed his family, profession, and sexual activities, and his self-esteem had returned to its pre-illness level.

Since successfully treated depressions often relapse if the medication is discontinued too soon, the medication was continued, and a remarkable effect was noted. The patient's low self-esteem, which had been present since his earliest childhood, began to disappear. He began to reevaluate his aptitudes and assets in a thoroughly realistic manner. The insights gained in psychotherapy, which heretofore had had no emotional impact, were now accompanied by a different attitude toward himself. It was as if William M. had been subtly depressed throughout his life and as if his low self-esteem had been a superficial manifestation of the depression. The medication had relieved not only his recent illness but a depressive state of mind that had existed for nearly fifty years.

After nine months, the dosage of medication was gradually lowered and discontinued. The severe depressive complaints did not return, but gradually the patient's low self-esteem began to reappear. At this point, he accepted the idea, difficult though it was to do so, that his lifelong attitudes as well as his phase of serious depressive illness might both be the result of a biological illness. He realized that he had been unrealistically unhappy throughout his life and that the medication had induced an entirely different philosophical outlook.

The patient now presented a difficult therapeutic problem. Information concerning the long-term effects and possible risks of the kind of antidepressant medication William M. was taking is still inadequate. The patient was fully aware of the benefits but not in a position to make an informed decision as to the relative values and risks of continuing the medication. After being apprised of the lack of data on long-term effects, William M. decided that he preferred to take the medicine under close medical supervision, understanding that it might possibly diminish his life expectancy or increase his risk of developing medical illness. Since the medication was normalizing a central derangement, it was also possible that his health might be improved. Accordingly, he had a medical examination and periodic medical follow-ups while continuing to receive antidepressant medicine. Intermittent attempts to discontinue the medicine during the next three years resulted each time in his regressing to his premedication state. Contact with the patient was discontinued when he left the country on business.

Although depression is supposed to be a self-limited disease, occurring intermittently and disappearing by itself, psychiatrists are becoming impressed with evidence for continuing depressive effects that respond to medication. William M. seems to be in that category. For such patients, antidepressant medication might be considered in the same category as insulin in the treatment of diabetes—continuous replacement of a lifelong deficiency.

As indicated in the case history, we do not know the hazards of long-term treatment with antidepressant medicine. In persons with partial conduction defect, a rare form of heart disease, it may increase the risk of death. We have no systematic information about the very prolonged use of the medication with patients without that heart defect, although many clinical anecdotes attest to its safety. As in physical medicine, we can only inform the patient of available knowledge and of probable prognosis with and without the treatment.

The following case illustrates a milder depression, precipitated by life events.

Margaret T.

In her mid-thirties and unmarried, Margaret T. was a personnel manager in a high technology industry. For many years she had functioned with dedication, efficiency, and compulsiveness, and had risen to an important executive position. About a year before the initiation of therapy, her boss, whom she had adulated, had been replaced. She described his successor as erratic, disruptive, hyperenergetic, and incompetent. Since the beginning of his tenure, she had become increasingly unhappy about the management of the office (which constituted most of her life) and had suffered from recurrent anxiety attacks. As her concerns at work had increased, she had developed insomnia, despair about her future, and occasional thoughts of suicide.

Her past life revealed her to be a strong person—in her own words, "something of a Rock of Gibraltar"—who had overcome many difficulties in moving upward in the world. Her mother had died when she was an infant and her father when she was an adolescent. She was forced to move from relative to relative, and had had to endure considerable economic deprivation. Nevertheless, throughout childhood she was conscientious, uncomplaining, hardworking, and reasonably happy. Following high school, she managed to complete her education through scholarships and part-time work. Her major satisfactions came from occupational achievement, but she also had several close friends. In her twenties, she had had a number of casual relationships, almost purposefully conducted, with men with whom she could not become permanently involved. She did not complain of any previous psychological difficulties but she had had intermittent physical complaints over the years—bouts of diarrhea and constipation of unknown origin, and inexplicable aches and pains in her arms and legs, vaguely designated as rheumatic.

She also seemed to be strong-willed. When she thought that she was drinking "too much" (several drinks at cocktail parties), she gave up alcohol entirely. When she decided that her heavy smoking was bad, she stopped abruptly and permanently. When she thought that she had become too fat, she went on a stringent diet and promptly lost twenty pounds. After a little while, thinking that she was becoming something of a social butterfly, she decided to work harder and to involve herself only in meaningful relationships.

This degree of self-control seemed to have the effect of restricting her pleasure in life. The most unusual feature of her current life was her intense but platonic relationship with Phil, a bachelor of her own age to whom she had been close for nine years. They saw each other several times a week, dined at each other's homes, did after-hours work together (much like college students doing homework), and were very fond of and dependent on each other though they had progressed sexually no further than "necking." The patient attributed this to her friend's lack of assertiveness and to her puritanical reaction to her previous casual ways. Her physician had treated her anxiety and gastrointestinal difficulties with minor tranquilizers, which had helped a little but still left her suffering considerable distress.

Aspects of the patient's story suggested two obvious—and different—sources of difficulty. First, although her depression had developed in apparent reaction to life difficulties, it had many aspects of vital depression—insomnia, weight loss, diminished efficiency, an unrealistic decrease in self-esteem, and suicidal thoughts. Equally obvious were the possible situational factors in the depression—the absurd relationship with her inamorato, and the long-standing tension over her new boss.

Conjecturing that Margaret's friend Phil was excessively timid, had some serious sexual problems, or somehow had maneuvered himself into an unsatisfactory but unchangeable position, the therapist arranged to see him in couple therapy. Phil was an efficient, compulsive, somewhat timid man, who had unconsciously conspired with Margaret to construct a vicious circle in which the expression of sexual interest by either was feared as a possible cause of rejection by the other. He had had somewhat less sexual experience than average, had been rejected for sexual advances in the past, and was determined not to risk destruction of this otherwise gratifying relationship by the introduction of such a possibly disruptive activity. Both Margaret and Phil admitted, somewhat shamefacedly, that they had—much to the therapist's relief—attempted to pet, but the experience had not been satisfactory. Phil's knowledge of female anatomy and sexual physiology was minimal, but he welcomed the opportunity to correct his lamentable educational deficit and seemed eager to learn through doing. He seemed to react with an immediate release of tension to a discussion of concrete sexual problems with an interested, nonjudgmental, and reasonably expert listener. This impression was verified when the couple informed the psychiatrist that they had experimented with their newfound knowledge with most satisfactory results.

At the same time, the possibility of endogenous depression was not ignored. Margaret's multiple somatic complaints over the years were consistent with masked depression, the condition in which nondepressive symptoms might derive from biological abnormalities similar to those that cause clear-cut depression. Together with the couple therapy, she was begun on a temporary course of antidepressant medication, and within three weeks lost her depressive symptoms: her sleep patterns returned to normal, she began to gain weight, she resumed taking responsibility at her office, and she married Phil.

The struggles with the boss continued. Probably quite realistically, she decided they were insoluble and arranged to transfer to another department, where she was warmly accepted. The marriage seemed to work out well: the couple continued to do their homework together, enjoyed traveling together, and had a normal sex life.

One year after discontinuing medication, Margaret suffered another depressive episode. She appeared for treatment promptly, and the problem responded satisfactorily, receding in a few months. In succeeding years, similar depressions recurred, and she began to regard them as the physical illnesses they were. In cases of this kind, many psychiatrists now treat recurrent depressions with maintenance drug therapy.

The last case that we will present in this section illustrates the difficulty of detecting biological depression, the range of disorders that may have biological components, and the possibility that such depression may begin very early in life in a different form.

Donna L.

Donna was a twenty-one-year-old college student referred by a colleague because of her breakdown in Africa. She had taken a leave of absence from college to spend two years in the Peace Corps and during that time had become profoundly homesick and incapable of managing either her work or her personal life. Depressed and panicky, she had traveled a few thousand miles to visit her brother, who did his best to calm Donna down and shortly thereafter sent her home.

When Donna was first seen by the psychiatrist, she was almost mute, lamenting her life failure, and preoccupied as to whether her college would accept her back as a student. She radiated an attitude of anger with a theme of "I want to be helped but I'll be damned if I'll let you help me." She virtually refused to allow the psychiatrist to see her parents, since "they may have made me what I am but now I've got the problems."

The parents were gentle, confused people who had always indulged their daughter and been browbeaten by her. Donna had always been insatiable and impossible to please, and they had done their best to placate her. To casual inspection it seemed that she had been spoiled, but the bewildered parents guiltily and mistakenly blamed themselves for her unhappiness.

Donna had learned to inhibit partially the critical manner she adopted with her parents, and she had functioned passably with peers and had done well academically. Physically, she had the potential of being attractive but dressed and groomed herself in an uncomplimentary way.

Donna's continuing difficulties had led her parents to seek psychotherapeutic assistance for her in high school, but the year of therapy had yielded no appreciable benefit. She recognized that her inability to experience pleasure was different from the emotional capacity of others, and had explained it by telling herself that she had been chronically short-changed at home. This explanation had been of no help to her.

During Donna's breakdown in Africa, she had manifested all the typical symptoms of endogenous-like depression: appetite and weight loss, insomnia with early-morning arising, and loss of energy. An inquiry about the possibility of such symptoms in her earlier life disclosed that she had suffered numerous but shorter, less intense episodes. She was begun on a trial of antidepressants, and her major depressive complaints quickly resolved. She was still left with secondary personality problems that had been long in the making and that were not expected to respond to drugs. The therapist hoped to have her develop an appreciation of the physiological factors contributing to her attitudes and values, and then planned to place her in group therapy, where she might learn something about the image she projected to others. With continued antidepressant medication, she might begin to experience a normal amount of pleasure and extricate herself from the living patterns into which her physiology and her reactions to it had jointly taken her. Such psychotherapy was precluded, however, by her return to college, where she continued medication.

Donna did well academically in her senior year, and has since entered the life of a postgraduate nomad. She has not entered psychotherapy. It remains to be seen whether medication will continue to afford her stability and whether such chemically induced stability of mood and access to pleasurable rewards will permit her to benefit characterologically from more or less normal experience.

Prolonged depression—and certainly depression with endogenous-like characteristics—is thought to occur rarely in childhood. Donna's case, in which depression seems to have been present intermittently from early on, is part of a growing body of data suggesting that depression, like schizophrenia, may be a lifelong illness and that the manifestations are different at different ages. Recent experimentation by one of the authors (Klein) indicates that children with school phobia, who have marked separation anxiety and become extremely fearful on leaving their mothers (behavior reminiscent of the dependent clinging of adult depressives), respond with decreased separation anxiety when they receive antidepressant medication. Antidepressant medication is rarely used in the treatment of children in this country, but in England it has been prescribed for a variety of childhood psychiatric problems, including phobias, anxieties, and transient depression. No one has followed the history of such children long enough to come to firm conclusions, but it is conceivable that many grow up to suffer depressive illness in later life. The obvious inference is that depressive physiological abnormalities may exist in childhood.

Cases like Donna's also illustrate the necessity of further study to ascertain the frequency of less serious but biologically determined depressions. The lifetime risk for serious affective illness has in the past been estimated at about 1 to 3 percent. However, a recent community survey in New Haven found that in this population sample major depression was the most common psychiatric disorder, with a current prevalence in about 4 percent of the population ("major depression" approximates our term "vital depression"). The investigators also estimated a lifetime prevalence (the appearance of major depression sometime during the course of a lifetime) in about 20 percent of the population (Weissman and Myers, 1978).

In view of our present inability to separate such depressions from those that occur for psychological reasons, the practicing psychiatrist is placed in a difficult position. Some mild depressions may be biological in origin, while some that are seemingly more severe may not. Since the physician cannot be certain which depressions are biological and which are psychological, he is likely to err in his treatment. One strategy would be to offer all patients with symptoms suggestive of biological depression a trial of antidepressants. For the less clear-cut case, a time-limited trial of psychotherapy and a trial of antidepressants seem of equivalent value. Unfortunately, the failure of a mildly depressed patient to respond to antidepressant medication does not prove that the depression is psychological in origin, but may relate to choice of drug, dosage, or individual metabolic peculiarity. Resolution of these problems at the practical as well as at the theoretical level awaits further research.

Manic States

Mania or manic states may occur as discrete episodes or may alternate with periods of vital depression. When mania is mild, the patient is often merry, enthusiastic, and full of ideas and infectious good humor. In the next stage, his physical and intellectual activity increases, he apparently can experience more enjoyment, and frequently he displays excessive optimism concerning future achievement. Because the first stages of mania involve attractive attributes, recognition of illness is often delayed. Later, more negative and exaggerated traits begin to appear—increased motor restlessness, excessive talking, euphoria, irritability, a ready tendency to anger, insensitivity, and bossiness. As mania becomes more severe, the afflicted person may become frenetically active, grandiose, angry, suspicious, disorganized, and pressured in thought and behavior; finally, in full-blown cases, hallucinations and delusions may occur.

The extreme symptomatology does not occur in all manic patients. Milder instances are more common. When sustained, they constitute probably the only psychiatric illness in which the patient feels better than the rest of mankind. Who would dislike feeling energetic, euphoric, sexy, creative, and optimistic, and requiring little sleep? But the sum of human happiness is generally not increased by mania. The manic's family suffers, since in addition to being infectiously good-humored, the manic is likely to be thick-skinned, egocentric, irritable when crossed, and rude. His inability to anticipate bad consequences (the polar opposite of the depressive, who views the future as dismal and doomed) undoubtedly contributes to unrestrained and self-centered demands. As a rule, the manic's increased pleasure is overbalanced by the consequences imposed on those around him.

The following case history provides a glimpse of acute mania.

Bob W.

Bob, a graduate student in his early twenties, was brought to see the university psychiatrist by his roommates because of inappropriate ebullience and activity, and a breakdown of practical judgment. Previously, Bob had interrupted his graduate career briefly, to intern with a large corporation in a foreign country. He had enjoyed the experience immensely, functioned effectively, and returned to school eager to resume his studies. Socially conscious, he had upon his return become active in an organization concerned with pacifism and the promulgation of the universal language Esperanto as a means of breaking down the barriers among peoples. Even within the United

States, language, he felt, was an issue, for the white majority could not really communicate with blacks or Hispanics. Rather than trying to teach each the language of the other, he reasoned all would be more amenable to learning a language none of them spoke.

With the help of the organization, he began a program for interested medical students and law students. Pursuing these activities, his roommates recounted, he had become very excited and eager to enlarge them. In his efforts to obtain funds, he had first appealed to community leaders, but gradually, his roommates realized retrospectively, had begun acting grandiosely. They finally recognized the magnitude of the problem when they returned home one evening and found the small study packed with office equipment, together with a recently hired typist. Soon letters were going to congressmen, senators, and the governor. Although the recipients recognized the sensible elements of Bob's plans, they also perceived an unrealistic tenor to the requests. Nevertheless, Bob's enthusiasm continued to expand. He became convinced that suitable crash courses, not only in Esperanto but in all foreign languages, together with most academic subjects and several skills, such as playing the violin, could be taught painlessly and rapidly, in a few days at most. He rarely stopped for meals and soon lost fifteen to twenty pounds. To relax, he would go dancing at discotheques in the early morning hours. His roommates became exasperated when he awakened them late at night to suggest a jaunt downtown.

In grammar and high school, Bob had been a compulsive, hardworking, outstanding student. He had been stable, moderately outgoing, and well liked. So far as could be determined, none of his relatives had suffered from disorders of mood. His manic episode occurred before lithium treatment became common, as it is now, for mania and bipolar illnesses, and he was placed on antipsychotic medication. Within about a week, his excessive energy disappeared. He began to eat and sleep normally and to lose interest in his unrealistic plans for benefiting mankind, even though he retained some faith in the basic ideas.

As Bob's judgment returned, he became embarrassed about his illogical plans and returned to his previous somewhat dull life at graduate school. Following his graduation, he was lost to follow-up, and his subsequent history is unknown. Like all manics, he was in danger of suffering recurrent episodes. At present a young person with such a history would be considered for prophylactic lithium for an indefinite period, with appropriate cautions about possible long-term consequences.

The confusion and difficulty in diagnosing mild, atypical, and semi-masked forms of mania is illustrated by the case of David.

David B.

David was a physicist in his late twenties who consulted a psychiatrist because of his sexual voyeurism. Ever since preadolescence, he had suffered from an intermittent need to spy on women. In childhood this had been easy, but as he grew older he became increasingly anxious and fearful about his behavior. It had become so blatant that he worried about being arrested and the possibility that his career and life would be ruined.

Although he was moderately active heterosexually, he complained of periodic impotence. Skillful at sports and the captain of his college baseball team, he found, nevertheless, that he could not perform with requisite aggressiveness as an athlete. Having taken up squash and golf, he realized that he played at his best when he was losing, and that once he began to win, his performance would deteriorate.

David's childhood and family background seemed relatively normal but was overshadowed by an extremely vigorous, hypermasculine, dominating father. David had also played more than a typical share of games of "show" with a younger female cousin and her friends, and had on principles of equity, allowed them to inspect his genitals as well. It is difficult to know whether these early activities were the cause of his later fixation on looking and being looked at or whether they were the first sign of an excessive interest in a normal childhood activity.

As with William M., feelings of inadequacy characterized David's life. These may have resulted from his relationships with his overbearing and successful father, but we shall see that later data also opened other possibilities. After describing his voyeurism, David acknowledged after several sessions of psychotherapy that his major passion was not that but rather the desire to exhibit himself. Exhibitionism is often considered by psychiatrists to be a sign of a feeling of sexual inadequacy. Presumably, the sudden revelation of one's genitalia to a shocked female provides a reassurance of masculine adequacy. David's inability to be consistently assertive heterosexually—as well as on the squash court or golf course—was likewise compatible with the thesis that he had a sense of inferior masculinity.

Operating on this belief, the therapist tried several modalities that together seemed to ameliorate many of David's symptoms. An exploration of his past allowed him to recognize his exaggerated estimation of his self-aggrandizing but insecure father and his underestimation of himself. His periods of exhibitionism occurred during periods of heterosexual drought, and the latter were caused by his anxiety about possible impotence. The use of mild tranquilizers and the cooperation of his current (though sporadic) sexual partner, who readily agreed to a Masters and Johnson technique of not pushing him sexually, rapidly eliminated his impotence. When his relationship with this woman ended, his renewed confidence in his prowess resulted in several conquests and the total disappearance of his impotence, his voyeurism (which had been a minor problem listed first because of embarrassment), and his exhibitionism.

At this point, however, it became apparent that his excessively apologetic attitudes were interfering with relations with others in his job and aggravating his feelings of inferiority. He was unable even to ask the laboratory telephone operator to place a long-distance call for him. When he role-played speaking to the operator, he displayed an almost profound degree of humility. Role-playing appropriate assertiveness toward telephone operators, bosses, roommates, and girlfriends gradually resulted in his acquisition of a moderate degree of social strength.

As these other symptoms also abated, another problem of which he had always been aware began to emerge in the therapy. Every few weeks or months he would enter periods of mild grandiosity at the laboratory, during which he would initiate money-making schemes based on devices which he thought he could but had not yet constructed. Although these plans were generally rational, his overenthusiasm and excitement antagonized others. The periodic, psychologically inexplicable nature of the episodes, together with the excitement that characterized them, suggested some form of mania, although euphoria was not present.

A reexamination of his father's history revealed that the father had had a lifelong record of an unusually high energy level. He slept only four or five hours a night, was continually initiating successful business ventures, and, unlike his son, had always been a successful Don Juan. It was possible to see the father as having been chronically hypomanic (low-level mania) and to see the son as having periodic, abortive, manic episodes. Accordingly, it was decided to give David a trial of lithium therapy. Treatment with lithium did eliminate the periods of excitement and consequent occupational difficulties, and may have further diminished some of the patient's feelings of inadequacy. It was difficult to be certain about the latter because psychological treatment and the passage of time had produced considerable benefit.

It is possible, as with William M., that David's feelings of inadequacy were the product not only of a difficult upbringing but also of an early and continuing manifestation of periodic depression. Further, if the voyeurism, exhibitionism, and impotence were related to feelings of inadequacy which had biological components, they too, in a sense, were physiologically derived.

This patient illustrates several useful points: (1) the complex way in which psychological experience can interact with and derive from biological predisposition; (2) the way in which psychological symptomatology may mask an underlying physiological abnormality; and (3) the way in which psychological and biological treatments can be used in a complementary manner.

At present there are no laboratory tests that permit us to make a psychiatric diagnosis. Therefore, there is no way of determining whether David's mild mood shifts were psychological or biological in origin. Until biochemical correlates of these presumably biologically caused mental illnesses are discovered, one can only infer the existence of an illness on the basis of typical signs and symptoms.

Neither of the case histories that we have presented as examples of manic states shows bipolar depression at its worst. The mood swings can carry the afflicted patient from extreme euphoria to near-suicide or to actual suicide. Fortunately, lithium is of considerable help with this serious illness.

Nonvital Depression: Neurotic Depression and Depressive Character

The concept of neurotic depression is relatively enduring and relatively confused. Initially, the term was employed to designate patients who were depressed but not psychotic—in this sense equating "neurotic" with "less severe." Later, "neurotic" was applied to depressions secondary to life experience—equating "neurotic" with "reactive." Others used the term "neurotic depression" to signify depressions, whether produced by actual life experience or not, that were not accompanied by changes in body physiology—equating "neurotic" with "nonvital." Still others held that "neurotic" signified unconscious intrapsychic conflicts that occasionally welled over into depression. Finally, some contrasted neurotic depressions with psychotic depressions in which the afflicted persons developed delusions and hallucinations. Plainly, this is a term worth discarding, as the American Psychiatric Association has considered.

Our use of the term "neurotic depressive" combines the reactive and nonvital definitions, referring to persons who become or stay depressed, usually in the context of distressing events or chronic maladaptation, but do not show the usual physiological alterations, do not respond to ordinary somatic therapies (tricyclic medication or the older somatic therapy, electroconvulsive treatment), and lastly, *do* seem reactive to current experiences. Their depressive mood of sadness and hopelessness may be quite intense, but unlike those suffering endogenous depression or the precipitated depression with endogenous-like symptoms, these people often feel better after receiving tender care or social stimulation. We believe that the nature of the mood changes is different in the neurotic depressed patient. In vital depression, the core experience is loss of the ability to enjoy consummatory pleasure. In neurotic depression, the feelings are more typically blueness, sadness, or unhappiness, and difficulty in anticipating pleasure, but consummatory pleasure itself is possible. The neurotic depressive may not feel like hunting, but he will enjoy the feast if someone else brings back the pheasant.

Although the physiological alterations characteristic of the vital depressive do not appear in the neurotic depressive, the patient sometimes undergoes a different kind of sleep disorder, encountering difficulty falling asleep rather than awakening early in the morning, or escaping into sleep and sleeping more than normal. Some, rather than eating less, seem to use food as a sedative and may eat compulsively. Patients characterized by episodes of apathy, overeating, and oversleeping, who nevertheless can respond positively to good events, have been referred to as atypical depressives because they differ so sharply from vital depressives. A subgroup of the atypical depressives, labeled hysteroid dysphoria, manifests strikingly unusual personality traits and is therefore discussed under "Personality Disorders."

It is important to realize that mild does not imply "neurotic." Mild biological depressions respond to medications, not to life experiences, but are sometimes miscalled neurotic. As we have indicated, it is often difficult to identify chronic, mild vital depressions. On the other hand, depressions that are *not* associated with physiological shifts—whether they are mild or severe—do not generally respond to antidepressant medications or to electroconvulsive treatment. They do respond somewhat to changes in life experiences and to psychotherapy. In planning treatment, it is the quality, not the severity, of the depression that is important.

In addition to those who are miserable in response to one or a series of distressing circumstances, some people are categorized as having depressive character; their whole lives seem to be characterized by a depressive state of mind. Although they have periods in which they feel better or worse, their average level of functioning seems to be one of continuing depression and anhedonia, a diminished ability to experience pleasure or emotion. Anhedonic persons report that almost nothing produces feelings of intense pleasure. Like the color-blind, they do not know directly what they are missing, but perceptive anhedonic patients have a strong conviction that they experience pleasure at a lower level than others do. They report that nothing—success, marriage, sex, children—provides the pleasure or kicks that they have been led to believe they should have.

We do not know how common neurotic depression and depressive character are. The frequency of these problems in the population has not been subjected to extensive study, and surveys have not adequately discriminated depressions in terms of their duration, extensiveness, and degree of life stress. Certainly, they are extremely common. Most such depressives probably wind up not in the office of a psychiatrist but in that of a general practitioner or clergyman or in the living room of a family friend.

The treatment and natural history of neurotic depression are additionally difficult to determine because several different psychiatric illnesses are often erroneously included in the category. First, there are the anhedonic, mild, borderline schizophrenics, whose illness tends to be lifelong. Current antipsychotic medications act against psychotic disruptions rather than against pervasive anhedonia, and antidepressants are generally of no value with this group. A second group are the hysteroid dysphorics, mentioned earlier. Their symptoms tend to appear when they are rejected and to remit and disappear when their intimate personal relations are flourishing. Their depressive symptoms respond to only one type of antidepressant, which we shall discuss later. A third group comprises adults who had been hyperactive as children. Many seem subject to a lifelong fluctuation of mood. Although their downs are often precipitated by easily observable psychological stresses, some negative moods occur spontaneously. They respond to neither form of major antidepressant but do respond to treatment with stimulant medication.

All three of these illnesses will be described in more detail later in the chapter. We strongly suspect that psychotherapy by itself is of little value for all these misidentified neurotic depressives, as well as for the mild vital depressive frequently misidentified as in this category. The other neurotic depressives do respond to psychotherapy, however, as indicated by the following two case histories.

Carole G.

Carole, a twenty-six-year-old married woman, was admitted to a hospital after five suicide attempts during the preceding year. At admission she was an obese but attractive woman, with obviously dyed black hair. She was moderately depressed, seemingly no longer suicidal, and able to express humor appropriately. She was easily accessible, and approached the interview situation in a confident, comfortable manner. She quickly developed rapport with her psychiatrist.

Carole's problems had begun—or, more correctly, intensified—at age twenty-three, when she gave birth to her second child, a daughter. The pregnancy had been difficult and the newborn baby was colicky and exhausting to handle. Carole felt tremendous resentment against her daughter, became extremely depressed and agitated, and felt trapped by her children and her older, passive, dependent, inadequate husband. Her insecurities and dissatisfactions were aggravated by her mother, who continually criticized how she cared for her children. The mother also berated her son-in-law, going so far as to instruct him in table manners and to coerce him into making decisions she favored. During the succeeding three years, Carole's problems and depression persisted despite repeated attempts at somatic therapies, including antidepressant medication and electroshock treatment. With her despair growing in the face of her seemingly unresolvable problems, she had spiraled downhill during the year preceding her admission to the hospital. Her quandary could easily be seen as related to her life experiences, a conclusion that was supported by her history.

Carole was one of three children of an affluent family. Both parents were psychologically removed from their children: the father stressed a philosophy of self-sufficiency and strength; the mother demanded independence, but ruled the children with an iron fist. Carole had been a "good" child who could develop closeness with neither her siblings nor her peers. One of her most salient memories was of a prolonged, severe beating by her father when he had discovered her playing doctor with a school friend at age eight. Throughout adolescence she felt distant and hostile toward her parents and shy with boys. In retrospect, she thought she had married largely to free herself from a cold nest. Although at first she said that she and her husband had had a good sexual relationship, later she acknowledged that she found sex "disgusting and dirty," that her sexual life was totally unsatisfactory, and that she had always been anorgasmic. Although she absolutely did not want to have children, the mechanics of contraception were left to her husband. As a result of what she considered his typical ineptness, she had become pregnant within six months of marriage.

After repeated attempts at pharmacotherapy had proved unsuccessful in the hospital, she was begun in intensive supportive and exploratory psychotherapy. In this therapy she was able to recognize a central conflict: her fear of giving up her dependent position and the attention of her family, but also her anger at being told what to do. She was concerned about the resentment she felt toward her children and feared she was an inadequate mother. She could not tolerate her underlying wishes to be cared for and nurtured—wishes that had never been fulfilled during her own childhood and adolescence.

As Carole continued in psychotherapy, she became increasingly defiant toward her entire family, allowing only occasional visits from her parents and husband. Eventually she was able to relinquish some of her dependence and act with greater autonomy. After discharge, she became more independent and self-sufficient, and assumed responsibility for organizing her own life. She separated from her husband, obtained a well-paying job, achieved professional advancements, and developed a more loving relationship with her children. Her social life became active, and though at first she often dated ineligible men (too old, married, or inappropriate in some other way), she finally began to select more suitable companions. Sexually, she became regularly orgasmic. As Carole assumed greater responsibility for her life and began to understand how to go after the satisfactions that she desired, her prolonged depression gradually disappeared.

Carole's history emphasizes the fact that some depressions are extremely severe, prolonged, and unresponsive to somatic treatments and yet show a noticeable and enduring response to psychological intervention.

Psychotherapy was also useful in the next case history, helping the patient to develop insight into the basic source of her dissatisfaction and into her self-deceit.

Rebecca S.

Rebecca was a professional woman in her late twenties who consulted a psychiatrist because of increasing marital problems. Over the past several years, she had become quite anxious, had lost much of her previous enthusiasm for living, and had undergone considerable friction with her overbearing spouse. Her psychological difficulties had not been accompanied by any physiological alterations.

Rebecca had been intellectually and psychologically precocious, independent, and effectual, but at an early age had married a man twelve years her senior. Within a few months of marrying, she discovered that she had made a major error. Her husband was opinionated, authoritarian, and intrusive, regulated her household activities minutely, and could tolerate no differences of opinion. Whenever they disagreed on a minor practical point or "intellectual issue," he would badger her for days until she feigned agreement.

Faced with clear-cut evidence of a catastrophic mistake in judgment, Rebecca nevertheless decided to "make the marriage work" and pursue her own career interests. For a while she was able consciously to suppress her dissatisfaction and to function fairly well. She would not admit to herself that her life was not as rewarding as it might be, and rationalized that "life is like that."

After ten years of marriage, for reasons that were not entirely apparent, her ability to suppress diminished. She accepted a job beneath her abilities, her self-esteem declined, she became somewhat disorganized, and she began to manifest diffuse dissatisfaction. It was at this time that she entered psychotherapy. With but a small number of individual psychotherapeutic sessions, she was able to acknowledge to herself the full extent of her dissatisfaction with her marriage. For some reason, she was finally able to abandon her self-induced ignorance of the depth of her deprivation and resentment, and shortly thereafter she divorced her husband. Several years later she married again, this time happily, and became fully productive.

This young woman illustrates a set of all too common circumstances. The depression was not the product of deep unconscious forces but of evident dissatisfactions. Rebecca had recognized her own intensified emotions but had not been able fully to acknowledge their obvious cause in her unhappy marriage. Psychological treatment catalyzed an already developing self-awareness, permitted an accurate and honest appraisal of the situation, and enabled her to take actions that freed her from her difficulties.

Masked Depression

In 1621, Robert Burton wrote in *The Anatomy of Melancholy:* "The tower of Babel never yielded such confusions of tongues as this chaos of melancholy doth variety of symptoms." Many twentieth-century psychiatrists would agree, since they believe that there is an ill-defined group of psychiatric disorders that do not look like but basically are manifestations or relatives of depression. This group of disorders is sometimes referred to as masked depression, which means that the cause of the disorders, whether psychological or physiological, is the same as that seen in more typical depression even though the manifest symptoms differ. Psychiatrists disagree as to what symptom constellations should be included, but the following have been suggested: (1) miscellaneous, physiologically inexplicable pains, particularly recurrent rheumatoid aches of the extremities, often occurring at night and often diagnosed as arthritic; (2) anorexia nervosa, a disorder that occurs predominantly in young women and is characterized by a pronounced loss of appetite or refusal to eat and a profound and sometimes life-threatening weight loss; (3) recurrent self-destructive behavior such as accidents or even polysurgery; (4) certain forms of recurrent states of panic and anxiety (discussed in the section on panic phobias); (5) certain forms of impulsive behavior, such as kleptomania, repeated wandering (some persons say that they are only happy when they are on the move), and some kinds of repetitive sexual behavior.

Other abnormal behaviors might be added, but this list is sufficient to convey the general concept. None of these symptoms superficially appears to be depressive, but since they occur in psychological circumstances that might produce depression (such as loss of a loved one) and sometimes respond to treatment with antidepressant medication or electroconvulsive therapy, they are considered depressive equivalents. Because research evidence indicates that antidepressant medication does not lift the mood of normal people who are not clinically depressed, psychiatrists infer that ill persons without depressive symptoms who nevertheless respond to antidepressant medication suffer from the same physiological abnormalities as do more typical depressives.

Obviously, in the absence of any independent way of ascertaining whether depression truly exists, such as a blood test or a measure of brain activity, labeling these disorders as masked depressions must remain speculative. At a practical level, it is important to be alert to the possibility that some behavioral malfunctions that do not appear to be typical depressions will respond to antidepressant medications. Since psychotherapy is nonspecific, its effectiveness with a disorder suspected of being a masked depression is of no diagnostic help. As our knowledge of the biology of depression increases and as we develop objective (nonpsychological) methods for diagnosing depression, we may discover that the spectrum of the depressive disorders is far larger than we had anticipated.

The case history that follows illustrates one of the protean forms of masked depression.

Clark W.

Clark was a thirty-one-year-old computer scientist who complained of a compulsive need to call and date women. A brilliant man, the youngest Ph.D. in his field in his university's history, he spent approximately four hours a day on the phone initiating and cementing relations with women. He seemed an obvious candidate for *Playboy*'s Man of the Year. However, the prize might have to be rescinded, since Clark himself regarded his sexuality as compulsive and was anxious about his behavior. His frenetic sexual life interfered with his many other interests—he was an accomplished jazz saxophonist, an enthusiastic initiate of the complex Japanese board game Go (his interest in chess waned after he became state champion), and a mountain climber.

Clark had sought psychotherapy for this difficulty several years in the past, attending sessions once a week for several months. He felt as if he had achieved some insight, but there was no change in his behavior. A trial of minor tranquilizers initially relieved his anxiety, but after several weeks he became tolerant to their effects.

Clark had been a shy, obese child and adolescent. He justifiably regarded himself as sexually unattractive and had not begun to date until he was twenty. He had had a plethora of early symptoms, including episodes of compulsive stealing in adolescence, stuttering, tics, and several bouts of separation anxiety in elementary school. On going to camp, visiting his grandmother, or spending time with a friend in the summer, he had suffered from severe homesickness. His parents and siblings had a complex, disturbed series of relationships that would have provided Eugene O'Neill with material for several plays. In passing, he mentioned that his father and an older brother had had several nervous breakdowns whose nature was unclear but which had responded to electroshock treatment and to drugs.

Clark's problems did not appear to be those of a typical depressive, but the childhood history of separation anxiety and the compulsive desire for companionship hinted at a depressive component. Clark was asked to obtain a psychiatric history from his father and brother, and found that both had indeed had recurrent, typical, endogenous depressive episodes.

A trial of antidepressant medication was therefore begun, and Clark experienced a remarkable response to the treatment. His compulsive womanizing, excessive dependency, and several other pathological characteristics all simultaneously disappeared. Further, one could be fairly certain that his response was not due to any placebo effects of either psychotherapy or medication, since he had already had both in some form in the past without substantial benefit. In addition, whenever antidepressant medication was diminished or stopped, his symptoms reappeared.

Clark clearly illustrates chronic neurotic problems secondary to an inferred underlying depression. Their chronic nature was of special interest since his father's and brother's depressions had been recurrent, with symptom-free intervals. The use of his family's history to substantiate the suspected diagnosis was indicated because depressives manifest much more depressive illness and suicide among their family members than do nondepressives. Increased rates of alcoholism and various forms of impulsiveness—sometimes symptoms of masked depression—are also found among the relatives of depressives. We shall return to the question of the various possible forms of depression in the chapter on nature and nurture.

Restitutional Devices

Depressed patients, like psychiatric and medical patients of all kinds, generally initiate compensatory techniques to offset the effects of their ailments. Just as the phobic patient avoids what he is afraid of and the hard-of-hearing person watches the lips of others, so the depressed patient often drinks or takes drugs or searches for diversions in order to attempt to diminish depression. Most prominent and most destructive is the use of alcohol. Alcohol is not a good antidepressant, but some depressives report a temporary alleviation of their distress when drinking. Some become fearful of abusing alcohol, because it alone affords some relief. In fact, this relief might account for the increased number of alcoholics among the relatives of depressed patients. Some might be chronically and minimally depressed persons whose treatment rather than disease has been diagnosed.

Abusable stimulant drugs, such as amphetamines, are also used at times by the depressed, although these are more likely to be used by the chronically demoralized. Although marijuana may intensify both good and bad feelings, recent studies have shown it to be ineffective in severe depression. This was not news to some of our own knowledgeable graduate students: "Everyone knows that grass is sometimes a bummer when you're down."

Among psychological maneuvers that may be used to reduce depressive feelings are compulsive social activities, such as running to parties and frenetic dating; excitement and thrill seeking, such as skiing, auto racing, and mountain climbing; compulsive sexual behavior (a judgment that must depend on the person's usual sexual behavior); and excessive work activity (work being known by all as a fairly good local anesthetic). The list could be enlarged extensively. Many such activities do not seem antidepressive, but they may be hiding the underlying disorder. The therapist may mistakenly concentrate on, say, the compulsive need to work or the sexual shenanigans, miss the basic depression, and proceed with an inappropriate treatment.

PERSONALITY DISORDERS

The term "neurosis," like the term "psychosis," is a poorly defined residue of the early development of psychiatry. In general, it simply means, "ill-defined, mild but not psychotic." The patient is having some kind of emotional or behavioral trouble but has not broken with reality by developing delusions or hallucinations and does not show gross disorganization of the personality. Yet the first edition of the *Diagnostic and Statistical Manual* of the American Psychiatric Association specified that the positive common denominator for the neuroses was "anxiety which may be [consciously] directly felt and expressed but which may be unconsciously and automatically controlled by the utilization of various psychological defense mechanisms (depression, conversion, displacement, etc.). . . . It is produced by a threat from within the personality (e.g., by supercharged repressed emotions, including such aggressive impulses as hostility and resentment), with or without stimulation from such external situations as loss of love, loss of prestige or threat of injury." This definition depends upon the acceptance of a specific theory of neurotic development with which many psychiatrists disagree, including the authors of this book. The idea that all anxiety is so produced seems incorrect and is reviewed in our section on panic and anxiety states. The extent of the disagreement can be seen in the fact that the third edition of the A.P.A.'s *Diagnostic and Statistical Manual,* recently published, no longer contains this description of the neuroses and tends to consider many illnesses formerly labeled in this way—such as hysteria—as more closely allied to the personality disorders. We concur with this conclusion and identify the syndromes discussed in this section as personality disorders. In some of these syndromes one sometimes sees unconscious defense mechanisms that some might call neurotic, but usually other causes for the behavior are more likely.

If it is difficult to define neurosis, it is even more difficult to define personality disorders. The basic characteristic of such a disorder tends to be a lifelong pattern of inappropriate action or behavior that is chronically maladaptive. The person is continually in trouble and at the same time is so inflexible that he cannot constructively modify his actions.

This definition of personality disorder seems quite obvious, yet turns out to be elusive. In talking about personality, we say that John is cheerful and Mary is pessimistic, or that Jane is honest but Jim is crooked, or that George is adaptable but Howard is rigid. Plainly, what we mean by these adjectives is that each person is predisposed to act in a predictable, enduring way. If Jane is honest, then given a wide variety of circumstances involving temptations to cheat, lie, or steal without fear of punishment, Jane would not succumb. Further, long-term stability is implied. If Jane is honest at the age of ten, she'll be honest at forty.

Surprisingly, these presumptions are incorrect. The belief that people's behavior can be predicted accurately from knowledge of their personality is simply wrong. The common belief to this effect stems from the fact that we usually deal with others during a short span of time and under relatively unchanging circumstances. If you want to predict how Erwin is going to behave tomorrow, your best bet is to examine how he behaved yesterday under the same circumstances, but not how he behaved five years ago under somewhat different circumstances.

An enormous, complex literature testifies to the difficulty of behavior prediction on the basis of personality. For example, during World War II, the Office of Strategic Services (OSS), which was then our espionage and sabotage organization, attempted to predict who would make an effective spy or saboteur. Psychologists and psychiatrists assumed that this predictive task lay well within their abilities, but psychiatric interviews, projective testing, and mock missions all were lamentably unsuccessful when measured against actual field performance.

Some of the unstructured projective tests used by the OSS—such as the Rorschach (inkblot) or the Thematic Apperception Test—enjoy the reputation of cutting through superficialities to get to the real roots of behavior. In the Rorschach test, ten symmetrical, abstract inkblots on cards are presented to the subject, who freely associates to the blots, stating various perceptions—say, dancers, bats, trees, faces, or parts of bodies. Afterwards, the psychologist interviews the subject, inquiring about the details of the blots that led to the perceptions. For instance, a patient may have identified a cat in one blot because a couple of thin lines looked like a cat's whiskers. Such a response could be interpreted to indicate that the patient might make arbitrary—even delusional—decisions about the world on the basis of minimal evidence.

In the Thematic Apperception Test, subjects are asked to tell stories about pictures of people in ambiguous situations. One such picture shows a young boy looking at a violin. If the subject tells a story involving the child's wish to become a great violinist, this is taken as evidence of concern about achievement; a story about the child's resentment of being forced to practice the violin could lead to the guess that the storyteller is resentful of discipline.

These tests, however, have failed to produce any more substantial predictive information than can be gained from a simple interview, which is not much. Their continued widespread use is a tribute to the power of self-serving wishful thinking by professionals and blind, uninformed hope by patients.

One of the difficulties with being critical about personality testing is that it is easy to convince people that you have a profound grasp of their nature by the use of mysterious procedures and sufficiently vague and laudatory results. If after an impressive preliminary battery of techniques you tell someone that he is basically warm and tender but has learned to conceal these emotions for fear of being hurt, he is unlikely to disagree.

This P. T. Barnum-like effect of personality tests has been illustrated by a clever experiment. Psychologists Arthur Bachrach and Evan Pattishall took a number of astrological columns, routinely pitched at the proper note of complimentary generality, and extracted the personality descriptions. A class of college students was given a personality test—one of the usual paper-and-pencil inventories (Do you salivate at the sight of mittens?). The students handed in the inventory, and the next day each was provided with an "individual" personality analysis. These, however, had been devised by randomly assigning the astrological statements, without regard to what the students had actually said about themselves, or for that matter, their Zodiac signs. When asked to comment on the accuracy of the personality analyses, the vast majority of the students were astonished by their depth, insight, and aptness.

In sum, the current technology for personality assessment does not allow strong, accurate predictions of behavior, despite the many attempts made to develop measures of deep underlying source traits that would predict behavior under varying circumstances and over time.

Tests that deal with the range of intellectual, perceptual, and psychomotor abilities have somewhat better predictive power, although motivated cooperation is necessary. Clearly, if a job requires a high level of intellectual capacity, a more limited person is unlikely to do well at it. Of course, a bright person might also not do well both on the test and on the job, because of motivation, attitude, or environmental peculiarities.

If it is so difficult to predict behavior in terms of personality variables, what success can we expect in attempting to describe personality disorders? We believe that another element enters into the identification of personality disorders that makes the situation different—the element of inflexibility. The difficulty in developing useful personality descriptions for normal people results primarily from their changeability and adaptability. People change developmentally and biologically with time. Further, they are able flexibly to change their tactics given new situations and new life demands. One of the outstanding things about the human species is its adaptability. All other animals live comparatively stereotyped existences.

For persons afflicted with personality disorders, however, adaptability has been reduced by the development of inflexible tactics. Disordered persons can be recognized as such because of the constant clashes between them and their environment, indicating that they have not been able to modify their behavior and goals to suit the requirements of varying circumstances.

For example, the suburban mother who tries to keep her kitchen floor highly polished while the children are running in and out of the snow has failed to adapt to the changing standards accompanying servantless and children-oriented households. The bridegroom who continues to consult his little black book after the honeymoon has similarly failed to change as the situation requires. Mechanical adherence to such behaviors in the face of varying circumstances and issues should be considered as possible evidence of maladaptive disorder.

The second example epitomizes Oscar Wilde's *bon mot,* "I can resist everything except temptation." Here the paradoxical inflexibility is the predictable refusal to deny any impulsive gratification, with consequent alienation of family, friends, employers, lovers, and the law. Such people will be described further under antisocial personalities and several of the other categories.

Thus, personality disorders are recognizable precisely because people who have them are not adaptable and regularly run into conflict. In the following descriptions of specific personality disorders, the inflexible nature of the patients will consistently emerge. As with mental disorders as a whole, the overlapping nature of many of the personality disorders often makes it difficult to categorize them precisely. Sometimes, as in depression, the response to a particular medication is the best clue to a patient's diagnosis.

Personality Disorder and Deviance

The inflexible, maladaptive patterns of behavior that we have defined as personality disorders are generally recognizable by adolescence or even earlier. Continuing throughout most of adult life, these pervasive character traits are exhibited in a wide range of important social and personal contexts.

Personality traits are more often a source of distress to the environment than directly to the person involved, which has led to a debate over the possibility that so-called personality disorders may simply reflect the pursuit of goals that are not acceptable to society. According to this view, the disturbing behavior does not represent a disorder as much as a deviance, a set of unpopular preferences or standards. Much ink has been spilled over this issue.

We take the stand that to consider someone ill requires the belief that something has gone wrong with his biologically evolved regulatory processes. This viewpoint also includes the possibility of pathological reactions to particular kinds of parenting because of faulty biological endowment. We recognize that these are inferences since it is not now possible to examine the hypothesized brain processes. Nonetheless, if someone's behavior is so inflexible as to continually land him in trouble, so that his own goals are not achieved—whatever these goals may be—it seems fair to hypothesize that there may be an underlying disorder that prevents relearning and redirection. We also believe that certain life styles in themselves are contra-survival, such as drug addiction and alcoholism, and that these self-destructive behaviors can also be understood as due to flaws in the evolved pleasure and incentive regulatory systems. We shall discuss these postulated mechanisms and their psychological concomitants in detail later.

However, we do want to differentiate clearly between people with personality disorders and those who simply have unusual interests or goals, especially when these interests or goals are supported by some subcultural groupings. It would not surprise us if somebody raised in a Mafia household or community becomes a Mafia soldier who kills on orders, since such behavior has been defined for him as being both right and admirable throughout his formative period. Such a person does not have a personality disorder; he doesn't kill blindly and he tries not to kill under conditions where he will be caught. He has rejected the legal codes of our society and therefore our society reasonably defines his behavior as criminal but not as mentally ill. Similarly, many people who espouse unconventional social, political, or religious ideas are not victims of personality disorder but innovators in areas of reasonable dispute.

Many patients with personality disorders are aware of the difficulties resulting from their traits but are unable to modify them, even with great effort. They may, therefore, appeal for help to psychiatry. In other cases, traits that lead to difficulties are not regarded by the patient as undesirable; such patients may indeed define themselves as being only deviant and may object strongly to the idea that they are ill. Patients of this kind who enter treatment usually do so as a result of family coercion or legal pressure and are seldom good candidates for psychotherapy. In contrast, there is appropriate medication for some personality disorders, and if the patient takes it, the medicine works whether he believes in it or not. The types of personality disorders that may benefit from medication will be indicated below.

Shame, Guilt, and Rejection

The anguish of shame and guilt is clearly related to man's being a social animal and occurs after an individual has broken a social regulation. Since such regulations vary widely from culture to culture, the transgressions that elicit shame and guilt also vary widely, but the capacity for such controlling feelings seems universal. However, some societies seem to emphasize guilt and others shame.

Shame is directly related to social exposure, ridicule, humiliation, embarrassment, and being caught. Many acts that people perform nonchalantly in private, such as picking their nose or primping before a mirror, would be embarrassing if observed. Shaming tactics are used somewhat by parents, but are the outstanding mechanism of peer pressure since peers are not usually in a position to use physical punishment. Scapegoating in children is largely shaming behavior ("Nyaah, nyaah, Billy can't climb the tree").

Shame is particularly linked to the development of excretory control. Publicly losing control over bowels or bladder is intensely shameful. Plainly, the training adult does not wish the child to develop the feeling that having a bowel movement is in itself wrong or bad, but rather that it must be done under socially defined, secluded conditions. Nonetheless, many adults have great difficulty in using public bathrooms, especially if there are no booth doors.

Shame is not autonomous but is responsive to changing social definitions. On induction into the army, recruits may feel shame about using an open latrine. This is rapidly dispelled in the barracks atmosphere, which demands such behavior. If society either changes its views of shameful acts or sets up specialized areas where these acts are no longer considered shameful, the feeling of shame is quickly relieved. This probably accounts for the recent pornography explosion, since inhibition of sexual curiosity was apparently primarily reinforced by public opprobrium. When the opprobrium began to diminish, shame was insufficient to overcome latent interest.

Guilt, on the other hand, is far more complex. Certain acts are defined as bad or wrong, and people who commit these acts are bad people, whether the acts are done in private or in public. The inculcation of such ideas in a developing child takes place by assault, blackmail, exhortation, modeling, or a combination of these methods. Adults are handled in the same way, with the addition of occasional rational discussion.

Physical punishment as a socializing method has a number of drawbacks, probably the most important one being that it teaches the developing child a great deal more than intended. The child learns not to get caught, the basis of antisocial deceptive practices. The child also develops fearful and helpless or angry and hateful feelings, and the wish to retaliate in kind. Further, punitive acts structure the child's view of the world into one polarized around dominance and submission. Remarkably, many people who have had a harsh upbringing defend these methods as the only correct way. Adoption of such childrearing techniques may be related to a person's own ambivalence as a child, when she not only rebelled against the authoritarian rule but also affirmed it in order to identify with the power and protection of the parent, and to look forward to achieving such power eventually. Yet, whether socialization by physical punishment results in the formation of a stable conscience remains an open question, since the overriding learning may be to learn how to deceive.

Blackmail, another major socializing practice, usually involves the threat of withdrawal of love, which arouses extremely powerful feelings of desolation and abandonment. Under such circumstances, the developing child is faced with two problems. It is relatively simple to inhibit the particular behavior that led to this dire threat, but the more crucial task is to become the *kind* of lovable person whom the parents will never abandon.

Thus, more than simple impulse inhibition, active self-editing plays a basic part in personality molding. The child's impulses become subject to preliminary internal review—a process often referred to as the workings of an internalized conscience. If the child commits an act that she herself judges as an offense, she punishes herself by no longer considering herself worthy of loving care, an anguished state of low self-esteem. On the other hand, doing the correct thing builds up the child's self-esteem.

Internalized conscience has the unusual property of being quite refractory to the social environment, since what is being striven for is not merely current social approval but the approval of the glorified image of the parents perceived by the young child. The little boy who feels guilty for masturbating is not simply ashamed (although he would be if caught) but feels that he is a bad person for doing a wicked thing. In such a situation, shame and guilt are inextricably mingled.

Guilt is an internalized state that leads to fear of punishment but does not depend on being caught. Further, guilt leads to regret and remorse, the feelings of sorrow and disappointment over one's sins. The tendency to punish oneself when guilty may be derived from actual disciplinary punishments experienced during childhood. Insofar as the person punishes herself, she makes less likely the far greater punishment in store from the parents—or from the Heavenly Father. But, most clearly, guilt is self-condemnation, painful in itself.

The specific punishment is probably also of great consequence. If the punishment anticipated is loss of love, then guilt may produce the pangs of imagined separation from the indispensable figures in one's life. Significantly, the Christian mystics referred to hell as the awareness that one has been severed from God's presence because of worthlessness. The insightful mystic clearly says that the flames and torture of physical punishment are only the externalities of guilt. The central issue is separation and loss because one's sins prevent a loving union with the source of one's being.

Shame and guilt processes of this kind play a role in some personality disorders. In others, questions arise concerning a possible deficiency in the manner in which initial attachments develop—a weakness in the bonding tendency itself. If so, would shame or guilt occur, or simply the avoidance of punishment through deception? And what if even the mechanism that allows anticipation of punishment didn't work too well? These points may apply in such disorders as antisocial personality and hyperactivity in adults.

Closely allied to shame and guilt but distinguishable from them is the sense of interpersonal rejection. The feeling of rejection comes about when one has positive expectations toward another and then is disappointed by a noncaring act. If the rejection seems a response to some transgression, then both guilt and shame may arise. However, rejection often occurs for no apparent reason or simply because one does not meet another's wishes or expectations.

If there is a tendency toward guilt or shame, interpersonal rejection will frequently lead to a flare-up of such emotions on the assumption that one has in some way offended the other and that if proper restitution is made, reaffiliation will occur. But some people are so extraordinarily sensitive to rejection that even if they do not believe they have done something offensive, they will be depressed at somehow not measuring up to standard. There are wide variations in the intensity of such feelings, and it is possible that they can have either psychological or biological origins. Sensitivity to rejection might be the outcome of early massive teasing and withdrawal of approval by capricious parents. On the other hand, the personality disorder hysteroid dysphoria, characterized by extreme pervasive rejection sensitivity, gives many indications of having a biological basis.

The issue of rejection sensitivity also relates to the idea of an ego ideal. As we said, a person who is prone to guilt is involved in self-editing—preventing herself from doing anything that will make her unlovable. At a slightly higher stage of development, she may become concerned about making herself positively lovable. In attempting to conceptualize the kind of person who would be censure-proof, she may seek guidance from parents, peers, religion, television experts, and so forth. This can lead to tension over the discrepancy between one's perception of how one actually is and how one would like to be. Too great a discrepancy is a source of chronic misery. As we mentioned, self-evaluation in early life is usually acquired from parental evaluation, and modified through peer evaluation. Only with growing maturity does our self-evaluation develop a greater component of realistic appraisal, derived from how we have met the tests of life. Revisions of self-images and ego ideals are the central issue in many psychotherapeutic practices, as will be discussed in the chapter on therapy.

Antisocial Personality Disorder

An inability to conform to social norms is apparent in some people in early adolescence or even during childhood; they seem deficient in shame and guilt. The problem is not related to lack of intelligence, for they obviously have the ability to learn what is expected of them. The enduring theme in their behavior is a failure to develop or sustain lasting, close, caring relationships with family, acquaintances, or sexual partners. What relationships they do form are exploitative and callous, with no allegiances or a sense of identification, reciprocal obligation, or sharing.

The normal person forms bonds to families, acquaintances, and sexual partners, so that there is a sense of participatory pleasure in others' joy and of participatory pain in others' distress. At the least, we tend to help our helpers. These capacities are frequently referred to as sympathy or empathy and seem common in higher social animals, as shown by observation of other primates.

The failure to care results in self-seeking and often reckless behavior, sometimes complicated by aggressiveness and even pleasure in another's pain. The type of difficulty that an antisocial person gets into depends on his developmental phase. Early demands for conformity and obedience to discipline are made in the period of bowel and bladder training, and it has been reported that many antisocial personalities have difficulty in achieving bladder control. This is not, however, a symptom of antisocial personality; enuresis (bed-wetting), which tends to run in families, is common in many kinds of people.

In childhood, the difficulties are usually at the level of accepting discipline from parents, relating to peers, and conforming to school restrictions. Gang stealing, fighting, truancy, and resisting authority are typical preadolescent signs.

In adolescence, unusually early aggressive or sexual behavior, excessive drinking, and the use of drugs are frequently added. In adulthood, these behaviors continue, but after age thirty the more flagrant aspects diminish for some.

Antisocial personality is much more common in males than in females and tends in males to have an earlier onset. An older term for someone with this disorder was "psychopath," deriving from a nineteenth-century term, "constitutional psychopathic inferior." More recently, American psychiatry has been using "sociopath," which reflects the unsubstantiated belief that social conditions contribute to this behavior. No doubt, social contagion plays some role, but what is important in identifying the disorder is the lack of affiliation, even within a gang setting.

Such people are the proverbial black sheep of their families and a source of distress to everyone who feels some responsibility for them —in particular, parents and spouses. They often end up in jail and probably constitute a large proportion of the repeaters (though the vast majority of criminals never get caught).

Psychotherapy for persons with this disorder has been very disappointing. There is some evidence, as we shall discuss later, that the disorders of the antisocial personality and the hyperactive adult may belong to the same family of diseases. Since hyperactivity does respond to medication, the possible relationships between the disorders suggest obvious implications for research.

The Hyperactive Adult

For a number of years, the authors of this book have been doing research on and writing about a very common psychiatric illness of childhood, hyperactivity. Although for the most part we are not going to discuss psychiatric illnesses of childhood in this book, we will say something about hyperactivity because we have both discovered that it may be related to a range of personality disorders in adult life.

Hyperactive children, who constitute 5 to 10 percent of school-age children of normal intelligence, manifest behavioral and cognitive-learning problems in varying permutations and combinations. In addition to hyperactivity, the children usually manifest inability to focus attention (resulting in the frequent complaints of a short attention span, inability to complete tasks at home or at school), instability of mood, lack of response to rewards and punishments, and a volatile temper (see Wender and Wender, 1978).

The cognitive-learning problems are mainly in the areas of reading, spelling, and arithmetic. A high percentage of the reading problems in middle-class schools are probably related to inadequate teaching procedures for dyslexic youngsters.

A remarkable feature of hyperactivity is that the children's behavioral problems respond to stimulant medication—the amphetamines (the most common brand is Dexedrine), methamphetamine, and methylphenidate (trade name, Ritalin). These medications are sometimes colloquially called "speed" or "ups." Over 80 percent of well-diagnosed hyperactive children show a dramatic response to such medication. They slow down, become better organized, begin to adhere to parental prescriptions and proscriptions, and become less volatile.

The widespread treatment of hyperactive children with stimulant medication has been a subject of considerable debate because in some adults the drugs are habit-forming and abusable. One point of view also maintains that exuberant children are being chemically straitjacketed to prevent their rebellion against an intolerable school system. The available evidence strongly suggests, however, that hyperactivity is a true disease, often genetic in origin, and often associated with neurological impairment and congenital stigmata, and that hyperactive children become neither high nor addicted to "speed." In the authors' extensive clinical experience with drug-abusing adolescents who had been hyperactive as children, not one had been medically treated with stimulants. It probably would have been better for them if they had.

For a long time, child psychiatrists thought that the problem went away as hyperactive children grew up, in part undoubtedly because the children disappeared from the child psychiatrists' or pediatricians' offices as they grew older. Recent studies have indicated that perhaps two-thirds of hyperactive children do have significantly fewer problems as they grow older but the others continue to have difficulties—that is, about a third of hyperactive children seem to be much more likely than normal children to wind up as delinquents or psychiatric patients. Adoption studies also show that the parents of hyperactive children have higher rates than normal of alcoholism and antisocial personality (sociopathy), suggesting that some hyperactive children may grow up to have such problems.

Approaching the problem from the other end, Wender and his colleagues (Wood et al., 1976) have investigated adults with problems resembling those of hyperactive children—restlessness, impulsivity, short attention span, hot temper, an inability to finish tasks, and refusal to abide by normal rules and regulations. Because of the similarity of the syndrome to hyperactivity, Wender and his co-workers gave the parents of these adults questionnaires, asking them to describe their offspring when they were children. A large number of the parents did describe the patients as having been hyperactive children. Wender has followed up sixty or seventy of them. Interestingly, the adults under investigation had previously had psychiatric diagnoses quite similar to the diagnoses of the parents of hyperactive children—alcoholism, drug abuse, and antisocial personality in the men, and depression and mood lability in the women (genetic patterns will be elaborated in the chapter on nature and nurture).

Ellen B.

Ellen was a thirty-three-year-old mother of four who complained of anxieties, irritability, emotional instability, inability to tolerate minor frustrations, and chronic marital problems. She wept continuously throughout her first interview, claiming that her life had brought her little happiness. She had first come to the clinic on the recommendation of a child psychiatrist, who while evaluating one of her sons for hyperactivity had noted similar difficulties in her.

The patient remembered problems going back to childhood. During grade school, she did well in arithmetic, but reading and spelling were problems. She remembered being so fidgety in the first and second grades that the teacher had to turn the pages of her books for her. In the third grade she was placed in a special school for children with learning difficulties, despite an IQ in adulthood of 115 (upper 15 percent of intelligence). Throughout grade school, she also had difficulties with her peers because of a quick temper.

There was improvement in high school, where she began to have friends. Reading continued to be difficult and she avoided it as much as possible. Although she participated in many social activities, she had the nagging feeling that she derived less pleasure from them than did others. She married when she was twenty-two, only to have problems with her husband from the start. These were compounded by the birth of four children in rapid succession. Both she and her husband had intermittent individual psychotherapy and couple therapy over a ten-year period, but there was little improvement in their relationship. Problems diminished somewhat when the husband learned to leave her alone when she became angry.

Ellen's parents had separated while she was an infant. Her father, whom she did not know, was quick-tempered. Her younger brother, although intelligent, was a poor student and a behavioral problem in school, and later had difficulties with the police. Thus, the family history suggested hyperactive-like problems in her close relatives.

Ellen received stimulant medication under controlled circumstances in which neither she nor her therapist knew whether she was receiving active medication or a placebo. While receiving the active agent she felt much calmer, no longer overreacted to minor problems, and was happier and better able to organize her household. Her husband was aware of a marked change almost immediately, especially in her ability to control her temper. In follow-up after several years, she had continued to receive medication and to maintain her level of improvement.

Ruth K.

Ruth, a twenty-year-old divorced woman, came for therapy because of her concern that she was abusing her child, which she related to excessive temper and poor ability to tolerate frustration. She also suffered from chronic anxiety and alcohol abuse.

She had been told that as an infant and grade-school child she had been extremely active, belligerent, and hot-tempered. When she entered junior high school, her family began to live with her grandparents, a change followed by an increase in family disputes and a further deterioration in her adjustment. She now started to cut classes and to run away from home. This was shortly followed by experimentation with and abuse of several drugs. During this time, she fell in love and wanted to marry, contrary to her parents' wishes. Frustration and discord led to two suicide attempts. When she became pregnant, her parents allowed her to marry during her junior year of high school. In a short time, arguments and fights led to separation from her husband. When the child was born, Ruth became worried about her temper and her inability to deal with the stress of being a mother. One manifestation was excessive punishment of the child, which became physical abuse.

Ruth described her father, an alcoholic, as having an explosive temper, and he met many of the criteria for the diagnosis of antisocial personality. Her mother was described as very nervous. One of her brothers was clearly hyperactive, and her son may also have been hyperactive.

Ruth began a trial of medication and showed a favorable response; she became less irritable and anxious, was able to control her temper, and could deal with her child less punitively. Shortly thereafter, she entered group therapy, began vocational training, and developed a stable relationship with another man. At one time she stopped taking her medication and quickly fell back into her old patterns. Resuming the drug therapy produced immediate remission of her symptoms. At a year's follow-up, a satisfactory therapeutic response had been maintained.

The Wender study of which these patients were a part used the double-blind technique (a method in which neither the psychiatrists nor the patients know whether a drug or a placebo is being administered) to give a stimulant medication to the adults with hyperactive problems. About two-thirds had a positive response to the medication, and about half of those (one-third of the total) manifested as dramatic a response to medication as did hyperactive children. The placebo patients showed slight improvements. The experiment is now being repeated in a more sophisticated fashion.

If these first results are borne out, the finding will be of great practical importance. The alcoholism, antisocial personality, and mood lability (and associated incapacitating somatic complaints) that characterize many of these adult hyperactives have been notoriously difficult to treat effectively by psychotherapeutic means. Their response to stimulant drugs could be an encouraging therapeutic advance. Amelioration of the patients' distressing problems would also be of help to their families, who suffer greatly from the disorganized and insecure life style that accompanies the illness.

Many of the patients were also diagnosed as having minor or chronic characterological or neurotic depressions, which usually do not respond to antidepressant medication. Surprisingly, the stimulant medication also decreased the depression, and the effect was different from the euphoria or elation sometimes associated with stimulants. People who abuse stimulants rapidly become tolerant to their effects and within a period of months may require doses hundreds of times greater than initially required to produce the same degree of euphoria. These patients, like hyperactive children, did not develop a tolerance to the stimulant medication and continued to benefit from the same small doses even a year later.

Emotionally Unstable Character Disorder

Klein and his colleagues (Frederic Quitkin and Arthur Rifkin; see Rifkin et al., 1972) have long been interested in a common but poorly recognized syndrome, found largely in adolescents, called emotionally unstable character disorder. The illness consists of short periods of tense, empty unhappiness, accompanied by inactivity, withdrawal, depression, irritability, and sulking, alternating suddenly with impulsiveness, giddiness, low frustration tolerance, rejection of rules, and shortsighted hedonism; the alternations can occur several times a day for no apparent reason. Such young people react with excitability and ineffectiveness when confronted with minor stress, their judgment may be undependable, and their relationship to other people may be fraught with fluctuating emotional attitudes.

The patients' affective lability is often not noticed immediately as core pathology because of their complicated self-presentations. These can range from a fragile, immature, dependent image that elicits protectiveness to a wise-guy manner that expresses independence and lack of need for care. The patients are perplexed about their life goals, stating that they do not know who they are, what they are, or what they want to be. They are also confused about issues of dependency, intimacy, and self-assertion, often reacting in a disorganized, flighty, and despairing fashion. There is a pervasive feeling of exclusion from normal life and peer groups, with the conviction that they are basically, irreparably bad. To use a current and unenlightening cliché, they suffer from identity diffusion.

They are rational, relevant, and coherent except for agitated or fearful periods during which speech and behavior become scattered and disorganized. Participation and activities fluctuate considerably, but the patients are often creative, skilled, and original. Their disorganization, in combination with frequent habitual use of intoxicants or psychedelic agents, often leads psychiatrists into misdiagnosing them as borderline schizophrenics.

Many of these patients have childhood histories of impulsiveness, hyperactivity, and low frustration tolerance, resembling in some respects the histories of children with hyperactive impulse disorders. Further, on neurological examination, many of them have a high incidence of signs usually associated with brain damage or at least immaturity.

The drug lithium has a valuable stabilizing effect on their tendency to sudden mood oscillations. The possible relationship of this group of disorders to childhood hyperkinesis is complicated by the fact that there is little evidence that lithium is good for the child with hyperactive impulse disorder. In addition, many of the adolescents with emotionally unstable character disorder have had unremarkable, nonhyperactive childhoods and develop their characteristic oscillations only at puberty.

Psychotherapy has not been particularly effective for patients with this disorder, and research into the effectiveness of other kinds of drug treatment is continuing. For some of the patients, maturation brings diminished symptoms. Others sometimes gravitate into highly structured situations—such as strict religious groups—in an attempt to stabilize their lives.

Alcoholism and Drug Abuse

Although alcoholism and drug abuse are so incapacitating that they are usually considered independent syndromes, they are frequently accompaniments of other mental disorders or of particular social and cultural conditions. Unfortunately, the rate of success with treatment is low. Libraries are filled with theories and suggestions that have failed to help individuals and societies to control the destructive aspects of this behavior. On the whole, we have little to add to this discouraging picture, but we do have a few new formulations that may hint at possible directions for research.

Drugs that lend themselves to self-administration primarily affect the individual's state of feeling, at least temporarily, in a positive direction and thus can be used to combat unpleasant feelings. The sedative drugs, including alcohol, have a long history of use in Western culture, especially during rituals and celebrations; alcohol is used in most cultures for its disinhibiting effect—an effect that is commonly attributed to release of repression but perhaps may be better understood as the relief of anticipatory anxiety (the expectation of pain—in this case, of social discomfort). In a later chapter we shall explore the possible mechanisms for this effect, but none of the theories adequately explains the destructive grip of alcohol.

Whereas the production of pleasure by alcohol and sedative agents often seems to be secondary to their value in relieving feelings of anxiety and guilt, drugs such as opium (heroin, morphine) and stimulants (cocaine, amphetamine) produce extremely powerful and new pleasurable feelings. The literature on these agents is too complex to include in this book, but their immediate effects can be related to the two kinds of pleasure discussed in the section on depression—pursuit and consummation. The stimulants artificially increase the sense of excitement associated with pursuit, and the opiates produce an artificial effect akin to consummatory drive satisfaction. These ideas, too, will be elaborated later.

The use of stimulants and opiates seems particularly likely if one is living a nonrewarding, ungratifying life, and in that sense is realistically unhappy and has little to look forward to. Since this is a familiar situation in inner-city ghettos, it is not surprising that drugs flourish there. In this respect, part of the problem of drug abuse is akin to the problem of crime—a reaction to the deprivations of slum life. Just as becoming a criminal may be considered an alternative form of upward social mobility when standard forms are unavailable, so becoming a drug addict is sometimes seen by the culturally deprived as a step upward. Beyond the pathological manipulation of mood, there is also the realistic fact that this is one of the few ways that slum dwellers can get into the big money (prostitution is another).

Marijuana is a more difficult subject to approach, both because it is socially more widespread and because the full scientific estimate of its long-term effects has not yet been completed. Since its effects are still under dispute and at one time were highly exaggerated, the question of whether its use and abuse should be treated is greeted with disdain by most users. Occasional use by healthy adults seems to have negligible impact, but accumulated studies point to the following medical evidence as reason for caution in its use: short-term effects—increased pulse rate, memory and problem-solving impairment, increased reaction time, and impaired coordination (the combined effects on driving are particularly important); long-term effects (with substantial daily use)—lung irritation, possible impairment of aspects of reproductive function, and psychological impairment (such as apathy in teenagers).

Currently, the major controversies about marijuana are as much legal as medical. The uncertainty concerning effects is given as a reason to keep marijuana on the list of agents whose use is subject to criminal penalties. This is considered an inconsistent attitude by some, since marijuana critics do not ask for the criminalization of alcohol and tobacco, whose deleterious effects have been established beyond any reasonable doubt. The prohibition of alcohol failed, critics will perhaps answer, but it is best to retain what degree of prohibition remains —that is, the prohibition of marijuana.

Recent data indicate that criminal penalties have failed to keep the use of marijuana from spreading to all levels of society. Instead, there has been an erratic, unjust application of criminal penalties to a small percentage of those breaking the law. A tacit decriminalization does seem to be in process, in that law-enforcement officials now tend not to harass the occasional social smoker but continue to pursue the big-time pusher. It might be less hypocritical if this decriminalization was made explicit by changes in the laws, and this has happened in a few communities (see Blachly, 1976). In the meantime, investigations should continue on the long-term effects of marijuana.

The marijuana question epitomizes the complex social problem of how paternalistic the government should be—that is, to what extent the government should forbid its citizens doing something that may be harmful, though they are willing to accept the risks. The problem, of course, is that accepting the risks makes sense only if sufficient information is available about what those risks are. A further complication is that risks that are seen as individual are in actuality social, affecting families, strangers (e.g., those involved in automobile accidents caused by drug abusers), and the public health and welfare budget.

The control issue continues to be a frustrating one in the case of heroin, where government-supported methadone maintenance programs simply substitute a legal addiction for an illegal one. Apparently, the methadone programs are leveling off, with less than half of the opiate addicts enrolled. We read this as indicating that these programs are of value primarily to the older addict, who would rather accept methadone than continue in the hassled world of the heroin addict. Young addicts, still in the honeymoon phase, see methadone as for losers.

However, those who propose drug-free programs of psychotherapy and sociotherapy do not show convincing evidence of effectiveness. Residential groups such as Synanon have had some success with the few addicts who are sufficiently motivated to adhere to the rigid program, but the success is achieved at the cost of the addict's becoming permanently embedded in the structure of the organization.

Both opiate addiction and alcoholism are national disasters, with alcoholism the far greater burden. Recent research into the cause and prevention of alcoholism has very heavily emphasized social and psychological factors, but the recent discovery through adoption and other genetic studies that there is a genetic component to alcoholism (a discovery consistent with previously observed ethnic variations in alcohol use) seems to us to call for rethinking by investigators of alcoholism. Increased biological studies are surely warranted.

It may be true that the ghettos and the monotony of lower-class life (and increasingly the monotony of middle- and upper-class life) provide fertile breeding grounds for substance abuse, but only certain segments of the exposed populations become either alcoholic or addicted. There may well be biological components in the behavior of those who progress from social user through the stages of abuser, dependent, and addicted.

Hysteroid Dysphoria

Hysteroid dysphoria, mentioned briefly under depression, is an illness, found largely in females, that is characterized by dramatic, applause-seeking behavior and extreme and sudden mood swings. Of special note are the seemingly specific medication-response patterns of many of the patients. The patients' general state, often characterized as hysterical, is an extremely brittle, shallow mood ranging from giddy elation to desperate unhappiness and a sense of leaden paralysis and inertia. The mood level is highly responsive to an external source of admiration and approval and crashes bitterly on rejection, especially a romantic one. These women may appear hopelessly bereft when a love affair terminates, then meet a new, attentive man and feel perfectly fine and even slightly elated within a few days. When elated, they minimize or deny the shortcomings of a situation or personal relationship, idealizing all objects of their affection. When at the opposite emotional pole, they express feelings of desperation out of all proportion to actual circumstances. Their life seems a continual roller-coaster ride.

Although these patients refer to the dark aspects of their moods as depression, the essential characteristics of the vital depressive mood are absent; the patients' mood and ability to experience pleasure are responsive to improved circumstances. They are prone to oversleep and overeat, especially sweets and chocolate, and are chronic dieters. Although they may express themselves in tones of despair, often within a few days they become activity-oriented and successfully strive to engage in new rewarding situations.

Their personality characteristics are distinctive and striking. They tend to be expansive, fickle, emotionally labile, irresponsible, love-intoxicated, shortsighted, egocentric, intrusive, narcissistic, exhibitionistic, flamboyant, vain, clothes-crazy, seductive, manipulative, exploitative, illogical, and an easy prey to flattery and compliments. Their general manner is histrionic. In their sexual relations, they are possessive, grasping, demanding, romantic, and foreplay-centered. When frustrated or disappointed, they become reproachful, tearful, abusive, and vindictive, threaten suicide, and often resort to alcohol.

Although they sometimes speak fervently of suicide, they rarely follow through. They speak frequently of loneliness but are not dominated by separation anxiety and related symptoms. If they are in the company of a dull and unadmiring man, they remove themselves as quickly as possible, whereas the patient dominated by separation anxiety accepts any type of companionship. Psychotic depressive states can occur in these patients but are most unusual.

The description we have given may seem misogynous, but merely reflects the exaggerated "femininity" seen in the disorder. Women with a normal range of emotional responses use a wide variety of seductive but discreet social tactics to establish the pairing that is understandably one of their primary goals. This is not much different from male adoption of currently favored hair and beard lengths and well-advertised shaving lotions. The hysteroid dysphoric patient, however, is a caricature of femininity because her disorder drives her to attempt to repair her unhappy mood by inflexibly exaggerating the seductive maneuvers employed by normal women in our society. It is the driven, maladaptive quality and repetitiousness of the behavior that indicate the underlying disorder. Although these patients are sometimes diagnosed as being borderline schizophrenics, it seems more accurate to describe them as affectively vulnerable.

Both major classes of antidepressants have been tried with these patients, but one (the tricyclics, to be described later) has negative effects, at times producing racing thoughts, somatic distress, and feelings of depersonalization. The other major group—those that inhibit a brain enzyme called monoamine oxidase (the MAO inhibitors, also to be described later)—are probably of value. They are rarely used by most therapists, however, since the dysphoric states are fleeting and antidepressants take several weeks to have an effect. But this ignores the prophylactic stabilizing effect of medication in the disorder.

Lois L.

When Lois L. began outpatient treatment, she was twenty-five years old, unmarried, a strikingly attractive and highly talented but usually unemployed entertainer. She came to treatment complaining of a long, varied, and anorgasmic series of sexual liaisons; dramatic shifts in mood from elation to crying jags that lasted several hours; and a pervasive feeling of depression.

Lois's father had died when Lois was nine, but she remembered him vividly as a handsome, capable, completely admirable businessman with a great sense of humor. Her mother, in contrast, she described as cold, indifferent, narcissistic, infantile, and subject to unpredictable rages. She punished her two daughters in a bizarre fashion, hurling knives at them over minor difficulties and beating them if they returned home late from a date. Only Mr. L. had been able to insure some degree of normalcy in the home.

From a very young age Lois was bright, pleasant, and histrionic, with outstanding singing and dancing talent. She was very early upset by her mother's lability but admittedly adopted some of her flamboyant techniques for controlling people.

Lois and her sister, three years older, were always beautifully dressed and well-mannered. Her parents were also concerned about her tendency to gain weight and constantly pressured her to diet.

She reported little of early sexual development except that her father once caught her masturbating and laughed. Mortified, Lois did not masturbate again until adulthood.

At the time of Mr. L.'s death after a year of illness, Mrs. L. was in complete collapse, and Lois lived with relatives for a while. Lois showed no marked grief after his death but often screamed in her sleep. She also became quite dependent on her sister.

At school, Lois was a good student and popular. By fourteen she was very well developed, big-bosomed, and her intensive involvement with boys began. By age sixteen she had become a successful showgirl, with excellent reviews—a role she enjoyed hugely. But she could not hold a job and became romantically entangled with a succession of agents, directors, and performers. Her mood fluctuated with the relationships and contributed to her professional unreliability.

At twenty-two, Lois started psychoanalysis because of her anorgasmic relationships, recurrent suicidal thoughts, fatigue, weight gain with no appetite, anxiety, and panic at being alone. Shortly thereafter she became pregnant, had an abortion, and switched from psychoanalysis to a year of supportive and directive treatment with a psychologist. She made social progress but still felt miserable, and a boyfriend urged her to try mescaline group psychotherapy, which emphasized fantasy and the release of hostility. After eight months of that, she wound up nonfunctioning and suicidal, despite some powerful cathartic experiences and a few welcome periods of euphoria and calm sensuality. A trip to Europe with a new boyfriend revived her. After her return she began outpatient treatment.

During ten months of psychotherapy her life continued as usual, with the same succession of intense but fleeting sexual relationships, spasmodic employment, recurrent mental and physical complaints, and increased use of marijuana. At that point a tricyclic antidepressant medication was begun in the hope of modifying her depression. It was ineffective, and a major tranquilizer was substituted. For the next seven months a combination of drugs (including diet pills) and twice-weekly therapy barely held her together. At the death of a wealthy older lover she became very upset, temporarily stopped all medication except diet pills, and became panicky and terrified. A variety of different major tranquilizers were tried over a period of two months, but she remained fearful, depressed, and socially withdrawn. Combinations of tranquilizing drugs and changed dosages were not helpful, and she began to feel worse than ever—overwhelmed, hysterical, and suicidal. When continued drug changes did not work, she was given a short course of electroconvulsive therapy, with only temporary benefit. A new affair and the return of an old boyfriend temporarily perked her up, but rejection by a third boyfriend reduced her to a suicidal state again.

At this point, a trial of an MAO inhibitor was decided on, and other medications were stopped. The first week, several of her complaints diminished, but she still felt lost. The second week, with the dosage increased, her sleepiness decreased and, surprisingly, she worked several nightclub engagements. By the third and fourth weeks she was working regularly, had reemerged socially, and was feeling well enough to reduce therapy to one visit every two weeks. During the next seven months the medication seemed to help her mood, her reliability, and her sexual response, although her personal relationships still continued to be transient. A five-day trial discontinuation of the medication produced sensations of shifting identity, and the medication was resumed.

Three years after entering treatment, at age twenty-eight, Lois discontinued treatment, found a steady show job in another city, and formed a long-term relationship with a musician. For a while she used the medication irregularly, and eventually only when under stress. During the next six years she went from heavy marijuana use to yoga and Eastern philosophy, to meditation and vegetarianism, and from singing to modeling. By age thirty-four she had become expert at Indian music. She could now control her moods much more, but it is unclear what the source of her improvement was—successes in life, maturation, a steady love, vegetarianism, yoga, friends, and/or experience. She believed the medication had been useful when she was under stress and that psychotherapy had given her some insight into her dependency as the source of her erratic and driven life.

In general, when treated with MAO inhibitors, the hysteroid dysphoric patient often manifests increased stability of two kinds. There is less tendency to overevaluate approval and admiration, and the patients do not become as dysphoric and upset when they experience rejection or loss. Eventually, some of them no longer find it necessary to fling themselves into fruitless, self-destructive, unrewarding romantic involvements. With a decrease in the need for psychological anesthesia, there is also a lessened use of alcohol.

Drug termination often leads to a recurrence of emotional lability. A rational goal is to maintain medication until the patient's life is organized well enough to ensure adequate external sources of self-esteem. At this point, weaning from medication may be attempted. Because the drugs do not cure, however, there often is a resumption of the old roller-coaster pattern. Many patients need maintenance medication to suppress their underlying biological problems.

Narcissistic Personality Disorder*

Persons with narcissistic personality disorders seem to have particular difficulty with the regulation of self-esteem. It is often difficult to decide whether mild forms of this disorder should be considered illnesses. Some people behave in a relatively inflexible, self-seeking way but on the whole attain what they want from life and are not themselves in any pain. They are often a source of distress to those who share their lives, but not to such a degree that they are recognized as ill.

In the narcissistic personality disorder, which sometimes seems close to the antisocial personality disorder, people have an inflated sense of self-worth, so that they take it for granted that others will cater to them. They may not be indifferent to the welfare of others, but their concern for others is limited.

Their behavior varies between mild callousness and outright exploitation. The inflated sense of self-worth also enables them to justify failures by facile rationalizations, blaming others, and even outright lying. The more self-admiring among this mixed group also seem akin to hypomanic people in that they generally appear youthful, vigorous, and cheerful. They may also spend hours primping, which is often a prelude to exhibitionistic behavior.

Many narcissistic people do not themselves seek psychiatric help but are sometimes persuaded by family members to make at least an appearance in a psychiatrist's office. Treatment under such circumstances is useless.

When the devices for propping up self-esteem fail, or when unrealistic expectations do not materialize, the person with a narcissistic personality disorder may seek treatment. The results of psychotherapy are ambiguous.

Histrionic Personality Disorder

The histrionic personality disorder resembles both the narcissistic and the hysteroid dysphoric personality disorders, and it is often difficult to tell them apart. The narcissistic personality seems to have an unreasoning self-admiration, however, while those afflicted with histrionic personality seem to have an unreasoning lack of self-esteem and

---

*The term "narcissistic personality disorder" is used here in a descriptive sense, as in the 1980 edition of the American Psychiatric Association's *Diagnostic and Statistical Manual*. In approaching these difficult patients, some therapists find the psychoanalytic formulations of Heinz Kohut or of Otto Kernberg useful. Systematic evidence for either Kohut's or Kernberg's theoretical position is minimal.

a distaste for themselves. They do not have the rejection sensitivity or medication response of the hysteroid dysphoric.

Histrionic personalities are constantly striving to be far more than they are. They are not consciously aware of the problem, but may be lost in daydreams of incredible success and admiration. There is continual attention-seeking and active maneuvering to get stage-center. Their lives are punctuated by interpersonal conflicts and attachments of staggering poignancy. What seems most characteristic, however, is that their intensely emotional self-presentations are often perceived by others as lacking genuineness, as if they were playing a role or self-dramatizing. Since their moods are abrupt, short-lived, and reversible, they are often referred to as shallow, manipulative, and phony.

The attention-seeking of the histrionic personality may take the form of seductiveness, yet there is often a lack of sexual responsiveness to ordinary heterosexual activity. They are often viewed as teasers, and seem more interested in romance and petting than in intercourse—that is, they like the chase but not the feast.

Such people sometimes have a surprisingly small store of practical information and show a lack of interest in the prosaic facts of life. They may not know who is running for President, or when the last war was, since such information does not relate to their preoccupations.

In dealing with other people, they are often perceptive enough to be highly manipulative, and are capable of coaxing others into actions and commitments that are not in their best interests. But with regard to themselves, they are obtuse, unself-critical, unreflective, and blame-avoidant. They are also highly suggestible and as a result often adopt passing fashions, or become overconcerned with their physical health.

A major characteristic is their inability to be satisfied with a stable relationship. They are intolerant of inactivity, crave novelty, and unremittingly search for excitement. For this reason, life with them is stormy and ungratifying at best. When a histrionic personality has driven supportive others away through unreasonable demands, then suicidal gestures, tantrum behavior, hysterics, and extreme threats are common. In keeping with the other aspects of their personality, they may malinger, feigning physical illness or different kinds of mental illness in an attempt to achieve control over a losing situation.

In group therapy or in a hospital situation, they can be placated by being given leadership functions, but these techniques do not transfer to the nontherapy situation. The prognosis for change is poor.

Conversion Reactions and Malingering

Some of the mysterious, seemingly physical illnesses that people with personality disorders occasionally develop, involving paralysis, anesthesia, blindness, deafness, and convulsions, are technically known as conversion reactions. Conversion reactions—which were common in Freud's hysterical patients—are usually explained on a psychoanalytic basis as the symbolic expression of an unconscious conflict. It is difficult, however, to distinguish this behavior from that of the motivated malingerer who uses physical illness to justify parasitism.

Psychiatrists debate this issue endlessly. The controversy is similar to that over whether there is anything specific about the hypnotic state or whether all hypnotic phenomena can be understood as intensely motivated role-playing. In hypnosis, the latter conjecture is supported by the fact that hypnotic subjects who are told that they are three years old actually act, in measurable ways, as if they were six—the youngest age most people consciously remember (for more details, see the section on hypnosis in Chapter 8). The major difficulty in distinguishing between conversion reactions and malingering is that victims of conversion reactions seem to believe fervently in their own incapacity.

An illuminating clinical anecdote concerns a patient in a state hospital who was seemingly blind but had no observable organic defects and never bumped into anything. In an investigation of this apparently hysterical blindness, the patient was placed alone in an experimental room and told that his task was to press a button at specific time intervals, trying to estimate when the right time to press was. An auditory signal would indicate when the button had been pressed at the right time, and he would get a reward whenever he did so. The introduction of a visual cue as to the right time—increased light, which supposedly the patient could not see—frightened the patient and his score deteriorated at first. When his score then improved, but not beyond that without the visual cue, the investigators observed him through a peephole. He was holding his head down on the table, with his arm covering his eyes, and pressing the button without the aid of the light cue.

The psychiatrists interpreted this as an unconscious defensive adaptation to maintain his hysterical blindness. Eventually, as the experimenters increased the visual cues, the patient suddenly demonstrated that his sight had returned, and he was discharged from the hospital. The initial group of psychiatrists believed that their experiment had somehow shown the patient that he could really see, and that therefore his hysterical defense mechanisms had become superfluous (Brady and Lind, 1961).

Another group of psychiatrists chanced upon the same patient a few years later in a different ward in the same hospital, again "blind" and denying that he had ever had any improvement in his vision. This time a somewhat more sophisticated maneuver was used. The patient was brought to a room and told to tap one of three levers; again, he would be rewarded for striking the right lever. Over each lever was a light, which went on when that was the correct lever. The patient regularly tended to strike one of the two levers that was *not* lit and therefore rarely got a reward. At this point a confederate, a ward aide, was brought into the act. While escorting the patient to and from the experimental room, he groused about how much he disliked the doctors, the job, the hospital, and authority in general. After some weeks, he secretively pointed out to the patient that if he were really blind, he would be hitting the right lever by accident one third of the time. Not hitting the right lever that often showed that he really wasn't blind. The patient promptly shifted to hitting the right lever one third of the time, which seemed to indicate that he was impersonating blindness (Grosz and Zimmerman, 1965).

Avoidant Personality Disorder

One group that may easily be confused with those diagnosed as suffering from schizoid personality disorder (which will be discussed later) but that has a vastly superior prognosis consists of people who have what we call avoidant personality disorders—a fancy phrase for extreme shyness. Their essential attributes are shyness and social inhibition, secondary to a propensity for becoming easily embarrassed and ashamed. Their fear of humiliation puts a crimp into attempts to form friendships unless they are given unusual guarantees that they will be uncritically accepted. Children often mock each other and can be unmerciful to the vulnerable, as these people surely are, which early aggravates their tendency to withdraw from opportunities for close relationships.

The avoidant personalities, in contrast to the schizoid personalities, strongly desire affection and acceptance, and once they loosen up, are often socially skilled and charming. However, they may be so overanxious to please that they may seem insincere and incur rebuffs; this increases the likelihood that they will have few friendships, and they often suffer from feelings of loneliness and isolation.

Not surprisingly, they are highly self-critical and self-deprecatory, but they also harbor much covert resentment. At times they may overcompensate for their vulnerability and actively repel attempts to engage them. Their self-protective motto seems to be: "You can't fire me. I quit."

This shy pattern is quite common in children and young adolescents and seems a remarkably benign one. Follow-up studies indicate that the great majority of such children and adolescents develop into normal adults. Probably such people make up a considerable proportion of the successful patients of a whole variety of psychotherapies, since their prognosis is good under any circumstances.

Dependent Personality Disorder

Another group that can easily be confused with the avoidant personalities are the dependent personalities. The avoidant people, although shy, can often be quite self-sufficient. People with a dependent personality may be shy, but this is secondary to their lack of initiative and competitiveness and their avoidance of self-assertion. It is not clear whether the basic difficulty is an avoidance of self-assertion, which requires dependence on others to run interference, or a primary need for a supporting and nurturant person, which inhibits the development of self-assertion lest a growing independence weaken the essential ties.

One clue is the intense feeling of loneliness and the fear of possible abandonment and isolation, out of all proportion to the realities of the situation. This seems to indicate a primary desire for a dependent tie.

Unfortunately, this adaptation frequently leads to a leech-like, parasitic existence, in which the entire emotional and practical burden of these lives is placed on first a parent and then a spouse. Not infrequently, the attachment is maintained only because of the guilt of the supporting spouse, who becomes convinced—not without reason—that if he or she were to break up the relationship the partner would become desperately bereft and might commit suicide. Explicit and implicit blackmailing threats from the desperate dependent person are common.

The relationship of this syndrome to such other disorders as depression, separation anxiety, and agoraphobia—in combination with discouraging life circumstances—is not clear, and the syndrome seems to be a mixture. However, the response to structured and supportive psychotherapy may be good.

Panic Disorder, Generalized Anxiety State, Panic Phobia (Agoraphobia)

The attempt to explain inexplicable panic—especially repeated, apparently spontaneous, crippling panics—comprises much of the ornate edifice of psychoanalytic theory. As indicated in the example of Mary J. in the first chapter, we believe that this theory is largely irrelevant in the treatment of panic disorder.

People with this illness go through extraordinarily similar stages, from panic disorder to generalized anxiety state and then to panic phobia (often called agoraphobia). Discriminating among the stages of the overall illness is crucial, since different methods of treatment are appropriate at each stage; however, these distinctions have been affirmed only recently by Klein and his colleagues (Klein, 1981).

There are great variations from patient to patient in the features of this progressively unfolding condition. Some get only the panic attacks and never develop the generalized anxiety disorder, with its constant apprehensiveness and free-floating anxiety. Some patients develop a secondary generalized anxiety disorder but never develop the tertiary panic phobia, with its travel restrictions and avoidance of being alone. The disease is clearly more common in women.

During the panic attack, and episodically even without the panic attack, such patients often develop feelings of depersonalization and derealization. These are peculiar transient states in which they are dominated by feelings of strangeness, eeriness, and unreality about their surroundings or themselves. The environment is described as thin, insubstantial, flat, and as if it were made out of cardboard. The patients feel robot-like and mechanical, as if they were watching themselves act and not willing their own actions.

The cause of depersonalization and derealization is quite unclear. Such perceptual shifts are not limited to panic disorder but may also occur in the absence of panic or during schizophrenia or during a kind of epilepsy in which the brain's temporal lobes are affected. Unfortunately, in American psychiatry, such symptoms are frequently misdiagnosed as signs of an incipient psychosis and may lead to ineffective treatment with antipsychotic agents.

After patients have progressed to generalized anxiety disorder, they usually stop drawing a distinction between panic attacks and anxious feelings, complaining that they feel anxious all the time. The chronic anxiety prevents the patient from perceiving that his panic attacks may come and go and that he may have a bad spell for several weeks and then none at all for several months. During such panic-free periods, the generalized anticipatory anxiety and the phobic life pattern continue. The patient has developed avoidance conditioning, a phenomenon that has been well demonstrated in animals.

For example, a dog is placed in a cage with a low fence running down the middle. On one side of the cage is a grid that can be electrified. After the ringing of a bell, this section of grid is turned on and the shocked dog jumps about until by accident he jumps across the hurdle into the safe section. After a few repetitions, the dog automatically leaps the barrier on hearing the bell, and thus avoids getting shocked. Even if the electricity is turned off, the dog will still jump across the barrier when he hears the bell. By avoidance and fleeing, the dog thus loses the opportunity to learn whether the dangerous situation has changed. Panic phobia is somewhat analogous. The panics come and go, but in the meantime the patients have learned to avoid the consequences of panic by developing a host of avoidance procedures. Even when the panics stop, the avoidance procedures are not given up.

Patients sometimes do not realize the panics have not recurred for several years. When they finally realize that the panics are not occurring, they often attribute this to their avoidance of the situations that they think produce the panic, disregarding the fact that during the initial phase the panics occurred even under safe circumstances, such as staying at home. One is reminded of the person who constantly snapped his fingers to keep the tigers away. When a friend expostulated, "But there aren't any tigers around here," the triumphant reply was, "You see! It works."

In some patients the level of anticipatory anxiety slowly diminishes, and given encouragement, the patient attempts one "dangerous" venture after another. First he may walk from the house to the corner, then to a neighborhood grocery, and next to a crowded department store. Eventually, he may attend a movie or drive with a friend around the neighborhood. Some particularly fearful situations, such as the subway, may never be attempted.

During the phase when the panics have ceased, kindly consistent pressure on the patients and encouragement are helpful in getting them to try circumstances they consider dangerous or where they would feel helpless in case of a delay. Once they find that they can go into these situations without panic, a beneficial circle (the opposite of a vicious circle) is set up. Each success reduces the amount of anticipatory anxiety, and with each reduction in anticipatory anxiety the patient can extend his horizons.

Unfortunately, in the midst of such steady progress there may be a spontaneous recurrence of the panic attacks—such as in the case of Mary J.—which shatters the patient's hard-won gains and destroys morale. Some popular books on anxiety have emphasized that the only way to help such people is to convince them that the panic attack in itself is uncomfortable but not actually dangerous. These forms of therapy encourage the patient to float through the panic attack, trying to observe it as if he were a spectator rather than somebody suffused by terror. In a sense these therapies accentuate the depersonalizing aspect of the panic attack as a compensatory device. This treatment has considerable merit since it enables the patient to make a more adaptive response to the panics, so that life does not become completely constricted. A more radical approach is to block the panic attack itself—as in Mary J.'s final treatment—through a specific medication.

Such patients have traditionally been treated with analytically oriented psychotherapy or psychoanalysis, devoted to the exploration of unconscious sexual and aggressive impulses, with the phobically barred areas interpreted as symbolic of forbidden temptations—for example, walking the street equals streetwalking. Since the patients are desperately anxious to find some meaning in their inexplicable difficulties, a wide variety of interpretations for these symbols are produced by the patient-therapist duo and both may convince themselves that they have arrived at a deep understanding. Since the panic attacks occur episodically and a person may have a month-long series of panic attacks and then none for several years, even without treatment, it is natural for the patient and the therapist to share the comforting belief that the therapy has stopped the panics. Controlled evidence does not indicate that psychotherapy hastens the disappearance of panic attacks, however, or that the patient is any better off than he would have been if he had just waited it out. But psychotherapy during panic-free periods can help to move the patient out of the related avoidant situations.

Until recently, the only medications that seemed applicable to such states were sedative drugs, such as barbiturates and alcohol. Such agents do decrease anticipatory anxiety, and therefore the person with generalized anxiety disorder can be made more comfortable by them. But their continued use often leads to tolerance, so that larger quantities must be consumed for the same effect. Worse, they have no value for the treatment or prevention of the panic attack. Since the patient confuses the panic attack with anticipatory anxiety and finds that a drink is helpful for the anticipatory anxiety, it is reasonable for him to think that maybe three drinks would be helpful in treating the panic attack. This can lead to a steady upward spiral and to alcoholism or barbiturate addiction.

Recently, the class of medications that includes Valium and Librium (minor tranquilizers) has been used in this area with some advantage. They are effective anti-anxiety agents and are less sedative than alcohol and barbiturates. They are also not nearly as habituating. However, they too do not block panic attacks.

What does block panic attacks, researchers have been surprised to learn, is the class of drugs called antidepressants. After several weeks of administration of this medication, the panic attacks are almost always blocked and remain blocked during the period of drug administration. Further, if the drug is given for about six months, it can usually be discontinued without immediate resumption of the panic attacks. Since this is a recurring illness, the patients may develop panic attacks in the future. But renewed treatment rapidly halts the panic attacks without the common secondary anticipatory anxiety and tertiary phobic avoidant and dependent behavior.

During the period of panic blockage, any form of psychotherapy that raises the patient's morale and encourages her to try independent travel and to go into frightening situations will be effective in helping the person drop phobic restrictions. Although behavior therapy techniques have lately been highly acclaimed, it is not clear that behavior therapy is superior to *any* credible form of therapy that raises the patient's hopes and brings about new attempts at nonphobic behavior.

We have recently been experimenting with a form of group therapy in which patients, whose panic attacks are being controlled by medication, undergo four- to five-hour sessions in which they give each other assignments to carry out. This would probably be even better if carried out under the direction of a cured panic-phobic patient, a program we hope to try. The point is to demonstrate to the panic-free patients, as quickly as possible, that because of the medication they won't get panics in situations that they consider dangerous. Once they realize that they can enter such situations successfully, the restricting anticipatory anxiety may disappear, extinguished by success. The group process itself also seems to have a beneficial effect; agoraphobics are relieved to find kindred spirits and quickly share experiences and ways of coping with difficult situations (Zitrin et al., 1980).

So far, our group studies indicate that some patients do not have the courage to persist in the face of their massive anticipatory anxiety. Such patients require slower, more individual treatment.

Generalized Anxiety Disorder

Some patients have a generalized persistent anxiety without the panic attacks that characterize panic disorder. These patients act as if they are continually prepared to run, and display marked motor tension, autonomic hyperactivity, apprehensive expectation, and constant vigilance.

The motor tension is shown by complaints of being jittery, jumpy, tremulous, tense, and keyed up. Hyperactivity of the sympathetic and parasympathetic nervous systems—which control glandular function and the kind of muscles that occur in blood vessels, the gastrointestinal tract, and the heart—results in complaints of sweating, fast heartbeat, cold and clammy hands, dry mouth, tingling feelings, upset stomach, hot or cold spells, frequent urination or defecation, flushing, and sighing. Interestingly, these are exactly the symptoms produced by the chronic excessive use of caffeine-containing beverages such as coffee, tea, and cola drinks.

The patients act as if they are on sentry duty, are continually worrying that something bad is going to happen, and are on edge, impatient, and irritable. They may find it hard to keep their minds on tasks and have insomnia and fatigue on awakening.

The symptoms often develop during adolescence and are particularly exaggerated under conditions of possible social humiliation or embarrassment. If the anxiety is so great that the patients cannot attend dances or speak publicly, the avoidant pattern of behavior is referred to as a social phobia.

Psychotherapy is not particularly effective with anxiety of this kind, but the minor tranquilizers can be helpful.

Simple Phobia

Simple phobia is the term used for patients who have neither spontaneous panic attacks nor generalized anxiety disorder but pathologically avoid certain discrete objects, situations, or activities. Examples are fears of animals, particularly reptiles, insects, and rodents, or fears of high or enclosed places. Some can apparently occur on the basis of early experience, either direct (such as falling off a horse) or associated with parental instillation of fears (such as seeing one's mother avoiding large dogs). This condition also appears to be more frequent in women.

Such people understand that they are not in actual danger but nevertheless irrationally feel and act as if they were. A pussycat is avoided as if it were a ferocious escaped tiger. When suddenly exposed to the phobic situation, a phobic person becomes overwhelmingly fearful and may develop a panic superficially similar to the spontaneous attack of panic disorder.

People with phobias may be entirely at ease as long as they are in familiar circumstances where sudden confrontation with the phobic object is impossible. But they have distinct anticipatory anxiety about new situations. For instance, those with cat phobias will usually phone ahead to ask the host of a party whether he has a cat. If the host does have a cat, the person will explain, with chagrin, that he has this terrible peculiarity and doesn't want to put the host to any trouble but will simply be unable to come unless the cat is locked up. If the requested assurance is given, anxiety disappears.

Both supportive psychotherapy and behavior therapy are highly effective with simple phobia, removing the phobia in as many as 90 percent of treated patients. Group therapy in which patients with the same fear go into a real-life situation together to face the object of the phobia is particularly effective. Individual psychotherapy is equally effective but takes longer. Interestingly, antidepressant medication is entirely ineffective, indicating that spontaneous panics and simple phobic fears are quite different.

Compulsive Personality Disorder

A very common disorder (somewhat more common in men) is what is colloquially known as the uptight personality: the person who simply cannot relax, have a good time, and be irresponsible even in minor ways. Such people are overcontrolled and extraordinarily concerned with right and wrong, often as defined by the most narrow-minded social standards. Further, their standards are usually internalized manifestations of guilt rather than shame—that is, even in circumstances where repercussions are unlikely, there is no bending. They don't loosen up. They are also preoccupied with neatness, organization, and efficiency, but their effectiveness is subverted by an inappropriate focus on minor details and lack of ability to see the big picture. Their work often bogs down in indecisiveness and remains unfinished because of faulty priorities. They are victims of a type of paralyzing perfectionism.

The question of work style is an important one. A productive person seizes on the major issues, roughs them out sufficiently to get the work going, and refines and polishes the details once the basic job is underway. Since it is often impossible to predict what will arise, attempts to plan everything in advance can in some projects be an impeding waste of time. The compulsive personality's work style requires perfecting each detail, endlessly procrastinating and rechecking before moving on to the next detail, even though the major thrust of the activity is not moving.

Nonetheless, such people are very busy and industrious and are often known as workaholics, in that they gain their primary psychological rewards from routine work to the exclusion of both traditional hedonistic pleasures (sex, alcohol, eating, football) and the simple joys of personal relationships.

The compulsive personality is the special target for the now well-known Peter Principle, which asserts that everyone rises to his level of incompetence. Since each promotion brings new responsibilities, the worker finally ends up in a job that he can't do. Because compulsive personalities are good workers, they tend to rise in employment hierarchies. But, with growing importance, jobs demand a change from detail work to broad policy determination, and that is where the compulsive personality fails. This is a recognizable pattern in both corporate and government bureaucracies.

Another familiar and complicated aspect of the compulsive personality's social and personal difficulties is a strong authoritarian streak. They meticulously defer to their superiors and step harshly on subordinates. The more important the job they occupy, the more demoralizing is the effect of their rigid demands on their staff.

Compulsive personalities frequently recognize a certain thinness and lack of joy to their lives and often envy the self-indulgent freedom of the psychopath. If this is too threatening, they rigidly condemn all forms of personal freedom, especially those that seem to result in a good time.

There is a distinction, however, between compulsive traits and compulsive personality disorder. Many people are meticulous and somewhat unimaginative but enjoy their lives and relate well to others. The person with compulsive personality disorder is much too constricted for this and is handicapped both in personal relationships and at work.

Behavior therapy has reported some success with compulsive personalities. Many compulsive personalities also survive without severe discomfort, but some develop pathological depressive states or obsessive-compulsive disorders.

Obsessive-Compulsive Disorder

The term "obsession" is an inheritance from a more primitive stage of psychiatric thinking—a time when the strange behavior of the mentally disordered was believed to be due to demonic possession, retribution for sinful behavior. An extension of the theory of demonic possession seemingly accounted for the recurrent involuntary ideas, thoughts, images, or impulses that plagued some people. Such ideas seemed to invade the field of consciousness and to persist despite attempts to suppress them. Further, many of the thoughts were revolting or obscene, obviously Satanic. Such a person's soul seemed to be besieged by the devil.

Although the idea of demonic possession has lost its power (despite the popularity of *The Exorcist*), the experience of being captured by unwanted ideas is a real one. The most common forms of obsession are senseless and repetitive thoughts of doubt, violence, sex, and contamination. Self-doubt usually concerns the carrying out of necessary actions—for example, "Did I remove my keys from the ignition?" or "Did I leave the iron on?" Violent or sexual ideas might take such forms as "I may cut my child [or spouse] with a knife," or "The butcher must think I'm flirting with him." Although the obsessed person is afraid that she will do something extreme, she never actually does.

The person who is obsessively fearful of contamination may be continually tormented by the idea that she has dirt or feces on her hands. Frequently, she will develop a magic hand-washing ritual—a compulsion secondary to the obsession. She must wash her hands three times, or three times three times, or must wash them in a particular order or a particular way. It is important to note that the obsessed person remains clearly conscious of the irrationality of her obsessions. She does not really believe that there is dirt on her hands, but can't rid herself of the nagging doubt. A person compelled to go through associated repetitive acts may feel foolish and ashamed of the apparently senseless behavior.

In other variations, meaningless phrases, such as "alakazam," are repeated incessantly. Some compulsions apparently also occur without preliminary obsessive thoughts. People find that they must touch objects a ritual number of times or make sure that everything is lined up on their desks in a special way. If the compulsive action is deliberately omitted, tension rises and apprehension and anxiety become so uncomfortable that the ritual must once again be repeated. Continued attempts to resist usually lead only to a completely automatic performance of the ritual.

This illness is chronic and often starts in late childhood. Most patients' lives are not greatly disturbed by the symptoms, but some are prone to severe, agitated depressions, which at times can be alleviated by drug treatment. During the depressed state the obsessions and compulsions may multiply to a level that effectively paralyzes the person. They may spend most of their waking time washing their hands or taking protective measures. A patient may wash his hands with one piece of soap and then reason that if the dirt from his hands soiled the soap, perhaps some of it got back onto his hands from the newly dirty soap. He will then wash with a clean piece of soap, but the same logic will require still further washing, ad infinitum. When asked during this procedure whether he believes that his hands are clean, he will say that he thinks they are clean but that the possibility that they might still be dirty is overriding.

Obsessive-compulsive behavior is quite resistant to therapy. There is some indication that a specific form of behavior therapy known as response prevention may be more effective than ordinary psychotherapy. In this treatment the patient's compulsive activities are actively forbidden and blocked. The patient becomes more and more anxious; but the therapist is forceful and insistent. With time, the anxiety wanes, and after many repetitions, the compulsion is decreased markedly (Marks, 1975).

Explosive Personality Disorder

Explosive personality disorder involves a small and confusing group of people (usually male) who are prone to sudden discrete episodes of emotional upheaval, often accompanied by violence. They are distinguishable from those with antisocial personality disorder by the fact that the episodes are unexpected and out of character. Someone who has apparently been well controlled and retiring suddenly has an outburst of rage and turns into a sniper. Because such cases are rare, there are insufficient data to give a reliable description of their personality characteristics and development. On one side are the psychiatrists who claim that the rage episodes represent the upwelling of long-repressed aggressive and hostile impulses, and on the other are those who claim that the patients have brain damage, and that their aggressiveness is the outcome of an electrical brainstorm as in epilepsy. All that is known about them, really, is that their behavior is unpredictable and often dangerous. Preliminary experiments are exploring the possibility that lithium may be useful in this disorder.

Paranoid Personality Disorder

Some people are convinced of the general malevolence of mankind and develop marked suspiciousness, hypersensitivity, and mistrust. They are continually concerned about being taken advantage of or snubbed. To insure themselves against this, they incessantly review all personal interactions for evidence that they are not being criticized, injured, or exploited.

One might ask whether this behavior might not simply be the extreme of normal variation in suspiciousness and mistrust. But the paranoid personality regularly has other characteristics that cannot be simply understood as hypersensitivity. These people are envious and jealous and have an excessive need for self-sufficiency, to the point of egocentricity and exaggerated self-importance, showing hostile argumentativeness and a tendency to create mountains out of molehills. Although they are often ambitious, energetic, capable, and persuasive, and not infrequently rise to responsible positions, their personal relationships are conflict-laden, hypocritical, hypercritical, and blame-avoiding, with difficulty in accepting sensible compromise. They lack the ability to see a situation from another's point of view, and they do not have a full sense of reciprocal obligation.

These characteristics regularly result in disrupted friendships and vocational crises. At the extreme these persons may develop litigious preoccupations, so that they are constantly suing and testifying in court. They may suspect that actions that actually have no relevance to them are really being taken to harm them. Paranoid personalities regularly engage in self-fulfilling prophecies and vicious circles. Their behavior is so obnoxious and difficult that they engender retaliatory attitudes, which then confirm their predictions that others are out to get them.

Paranoid personality may be a milder version of paranoid schizophrenia, which will be described in the section on the schizophrenic illnesses. These persons do not bring themselves for treatment but are sometimes brought by family members or assigned by the courts. Psychotherapy is usually not effective, and drug therapy has usually been reserved for the more delusional cases.

Schizoid Personality Disorder

Just as the paranoid personality seems to be on a continuum with paranoid schizophrenia, so schizoid personality seems to be the precursor state of some chronic schizophrenias. Certain people, from earliest life, have difficulty in relating to family members or acquaintances. They seem to lack the capacity either to respond warmly or to evoke a warm response in other people. An absence of ordinary human responsiveness causes them to remain distant, estranged, and peculiar. When they attempt to relate socially, they are so imperceptive and blundering that they drive others away rather than bring them closer. Their social eccentricities can also make them scapegoats, so their original difficulty in socializing is hideously compounded by massive social rejection. They usually have only a few superficial acquaintances and no close friends. Not only are they unsatisfying companions for others, but they do not respond to attempts to bring them out of their shell unless these attempts are unusually persistent and well organized. In general, their ability to experience pleasure, and in particular the pleasure of social intercourse, is slight.

Schizoid children usually react disastrously to school because of their inability to perform either socially or academically. The other children ruthlessly exclude them. During adolescence they often become sexually preoccupied but do not have the skills necessary to date and court successfully. They are the classic loners and drifters—goal-less, seclusive, and vague. Marriage by males with this disorder is highly unusual. Female schizoid personalities, however, learn that one way to gain acceptance is through sexual compliance (a form of unskilled labor), and it is not as unusual for them to be involved socially and to marry. The marriages are almost always stormy and unsuccessful.

Over and above their social difficulties, schizoid people have very constricted interests. They may develop a monumental preoccupation with a very narrow hobby—for example, they may end up with the largest collection of trolley-car transfers in the world.

It is unclear what proportion of schizoid personalities go on to develop manifest chronic schizophrenia. Schizophrenics who have a history of early schizoid personality do conspicuously badly when they become ill. Their psychoses respond poorly to antipsychotic medications, and even after their psychoses have come under control, they become dependent and socially parasitic; almost never do they become functioning, independent citizens.

SCHIZOPHRENIC DISORDERS

Thus far, we have discussed psychological disorders that are in many ways exaggerations or variations of normal psychological processes. We ourselves may not have experienced profound anxiety or depression, but we have all experienced anxiety and depression. It requires no huge leap of empathy to participate in the experience of the affectively disturbed or extremely anxious.

The schizophrenias, however, range in severity from the incomprehensible madness of Bedlam to mild, persistent eccentricity. It is this element of difference, of foreignness, that led the German psychiatrist and philosopher Karl Jaspers to separate off certain forms of schizophrenic illness as true disease processes. He felt that the course of the illness did not obey ordinary laws of human psychology and that the imperviousness to empathy was both a diagnostic feature and the proof of an underlying disease.

The diversity of these disorders is clearly evident in the life histories of patients. Let us begin with a description translated from the work of Bénédict Morel, a French psychiatrist of the mid-nineteenth century, whose phrase *démence précoce*, latinized to "dementia praecox," eventually became the common label for that large, varied, and only partially treatable group of psychiatric disorders now known as the schizophrenias.

> My memories carry me back sadly to a case of heredity in a progressive form. . . . An unfortunate father consulted me one day about the mental status of his child, age thirteen or fourteen, in whom a violent hatred for the originator of his days had suddenly replaced the most tender feelings. . . . He was downhearted at being the smallest in his class, although he was always first in his composition and this without strain and almost without work. It was, so to speak, by intuition that he understood things and that everything was arranged in his memory and intelligence. He lost, insensibly, his cheerfulness, became somber, taciturn, and showed a tendency to isolation. . . . The state of melancholy depression of the child, his hatred for his father which extended to the idea of killing him, had another cause: his mother was a madwoman, his grandmother eccentric to the last degree. I ordered the interruption of the child's studies and his confinement in a hydro-therapeutic institution. . . . He grew considerably, but another phenomenon as disquieting as those mentioned above came to dominate the situation. The young patient progressively forgot everything he had learned; his intellectual faculties, formerly so brilliant, underwent a very disturbing period of stoppage. A sort of hebetude-like torpor replaced his former activity, and when I revisited him, I judged that the fatal transition to the state of *démence précoce* was in progress. This desperate prognosis is normally far from the minds of parents—as of doctors—who bestow their care on these children. Such is, nevertheless, the dire termination of hereditary madness.

For an illustration of what early onset of *démence précoce*, or schizophrenia, looks like in the twentieth century, consider the history of Susan.

Susan H.

Two months before her fifteenth birthday, Susan was brought to a psychiatrist by her concerned parents, who could no longer deny to themselves that her personality was changing. She had become increasingly withdrawn and was refusing to go to school. At home, giving no explanation, she ate only one meal a day and had lost 30 pounds of her original 120. She would not look her parents in the eye and became quite upset when they tried to establish eye contact. So far as they could gather, her only interest was the black arts. Previously a quiet, compassionate, sensitive child, she had threatened her sister with a knife when she ventured into her room. She had also begun to stay up very late and to sleep late in the morning.

Like so many children whose schizophrenic disorder begins in early adolescence, her developmental history was atypical. During pregnancy, her mother had had the mumps. During the first year of life, Susan's physiological functioning was irregular, without consistent sleep or bowel patterns. She slept well one day and poorly the next; constipation alternated with diarrhea. She walked and talked at an average age, but spoke very unclearly and required speech therapy until she was five years old. She was somewhat shy but not unusually so.

Susan was very attached to sameness. When she was one year old, her parents rented a mountain cabin. In her new surroundings Susan cried consecutively for forty-eight hours, until her exhausted parents gave up and returned home; back home, she stopped crying. As a preschooler, she became upset whenever her mother was out of sight and would only stay with a grandmother or aunt whom she knew very well. When she reached school age, it became apparent that she had serious academic problems. Although of normal intelligence, she was a mirror-image writer, had great difficulty distinguishing between *b*'s and *d*'s, and showed other familiar symptoms of dyslexia. Susan also had a very short attention span and was hyperactive, and reluctant to conform to the demands of the classroom.

Because of these persistent problems in school, the psychiatrist to whom she was brought at age fifteen put her on amphetamines, the drugs that often produce significant benefit in hyperactive, learning-disabled children. After two days of improvement, Susan became angry and disturbed, threatened to kill her parents, and began using obscene language at home. It is possible that this was a negative effect of the medication, since stimulant drugs are often toxic to psychotic patients.

When one of the antipsychotic drugs was substituted, Susan began to improve somewhat and lost some of her bizarre behavior. She became less interested in the black arts, returned to a normal sleep cycle, and began to eat. She still manifested extreme concern about others looking at her. The antipsychotic medication decreased the severity of her illness but did not return her to her previous level of functioning.

Because Susan's parents were having marital difficulties, the treating physician reasoned that these difficulties might have caused Susan's problems or, at least, be aggravating them. Susan's mother was a compulsive, perfectionistic housewife who spent her time irritably picking up after her children and husband, keeping a box score of her efforts, and attempting to extract the maximum amount of guilt from them. Other prominent psychological attributes were suspiciousness, hypochondriasis, and disorganization (for everything except the house). The mother's mother was an alcoholic and a brother had lived in a state hospital for twenty years, diagnosed as a paranoid schizophrenic. Susan's father was an introverted man who enjoyed his stamp collection, did not like family trouble, and wished his wife would leave him alone. Based on the observation of the familial friction, a two-pronged attack was initiated. The parents entered couple therapy, first individually and subsequently in a group. They talked, argued, expressed their feelings, struck bargains, took risks, but failed to change. For Susan, in addition to the medication, special placement was arranged to enable her to catch up academically and perhaps restore some of her self-esteem.

During the next year, life at first seemed smoother, but then Susan began to express unspecific fears about going to school. In the school setting she became increasingly panicky and her expressed thoughts became disorganized and impossible to follow. She began complaining about sounds and voices coming from the school television sets when they were not on. Among other strange ideas, she felt that if she wanted to be like someone in one respect she might become like that person in all respects—a concrete fear of being changed into someone else. Surprisingly, she began to write poetry —an unusual activity for someone with difficulties in learning to read and write. Here are some examples:

> All things must die and live at a single thought
> And being the way that life is
> While we were circling around each other
> Should we really expect to escape?

People who are around me
Need not know what lies they tell each other
For there is no truth in what they say
And while I think it over, is there any hope in truth?
Because I know that truth is lie.

The puddles stretching across the lot
Trying to recapture the pebbles
But the rocks rejected all its thoughts
And being annoyed
It took its boundaries
And pulled it across Heaven.

Fantasies seeking life
Like animals around death
Hoping death will come like darkness
And seeking the illusion.

While it is possible to point to disordered thought in these verses and to their symbolic expression of Susan's emotional state, they serve much more as poignant reminders of the sensitivities and assets that lie hidden in so many schizophrenics.

As her symptoms worsened, Susan was given larger doses of antipsychotic medication, yet her anxiety was paralyzing and she was withdrawn from school. The therapist hoped that gradual reintroduction into social situations with appropriate reinforcement and encouragement might help Susan, and she was placed in a day hospital, a facility serving psychotic patients who are not too ill to return home in the evenings. After approximately six months, Susan acclimated to this environment and it was possible to reduce her medication. An attempt to remove her from the protected situation, however, showed that no learning had taken place. When put into a sheltered workshop, Susan again began to complain to her therapist of hearing voices and of changing into other people and finding them changing into her. She also began to experience some difficulty in discriminating among her dreams, her hallucinatory experiences, and reality.

Somewhat unwillingly, because of possible toxic effects, the psychiatrist increased the dosage of antipsychotic medication, once again with mixed results. Her hallucinations, delusions, and confusion of self disappeared, but she remained anxious about leaving the house. She was apathetic, slept twelve hours a day, and only listened to her phonograph. She was an empty, unproductive, unhappy person, a burden to herself and her family.

Susan was in some respects similar to Morel's patient whose illness evolved into a "hebetude-like torpor." Apparently, the natural history of the disorder has not changed in the past century. Drug treatment *did* remove Susan's delusions and hallucinations, but did not change her lack of will (abulia), her apathy, or her social ineptitude. Medicine may well have kept her from being assaultive, bizarre, or unmanageable or from requiring custodial care, but it did not return her to full normal existence.

Susan's developmental history illustrates a chronic schizophrenic process that if not treated with drugs would probably have eventuated in the deteriorated dementia praecox described by Kraepelin. Without medicine, her speech (and presumably organization of thought) would have broken down completely, her behavior would have been dominated by anxiety and seemingly meaningless rituals, and she would have been completely preoccupied with frightening hallucinations and delusions. When antipsychotic drug dosage was reduced, overwhelming anxiety and hallucinations reappeared; medication suppressed but did not cure her illness.

By way of contrast, consider the case of Jack.

Jack F.

Jack was a skinny, frail sixteen-year-old brought to the hospital by the police. He had run into a private home, where he had pleaded in panic for permission to call the police because he thought he was being pursued by dogs. Jack was terribly frightened, but his speech and thought organization were excellent. He had no hallucinations, convictions of bodily change, or other schizophrenic symptomatology except for his elaborate delusional system about the dogs. He had discovered, he claimed, that dogs and cats were anthropologists from another planet who had taken on earth-like forms in order to pass among us. They had chosen the form of household pets since this provided an excellent means of entry into homes.

Jack's first awareness of this dangerous situation occurred when he observed a group of cats emerging from a culvert followed by a pack of dogs. He realized that the lead cat was none other than Darius, the ancient Persian king, and that the leader of the dogs was Petronius Arbiter, Nero's feast and orgy master. As he walked past the culvert, Jack realized with horror that several dogs were following him. The meaning of their pursuit instantly became clear: they knew that he knew.

Jack's childhood and adolescence had been typical of those of many schizophrenics. His promiscuous mother had abandoned him and his alcoholic father when Jack was two. He had been raised by his frequently absent father and his irritable, overprotective grandmother. A bright boy but gawky and poorly coordinated, he was shy and shunned the company of others; because he was an intellectual oddball and an athletic failure, his peers did not reach out to him. Jack consoled himself by spending all his free time in the city library, where he read widely and voraciously. He was particularly fond of Greek and Roman history and of science fiction. Otherwise, his life was bleak and pleasureless. His grandmother and father seemed unusually uninterested in him; their first visit to the hospital was approximately a week after his admission, and their subsequent visits were brief and infrequent.

In the hospital, Jack was treated with antipsychotic drugs in small doses and his disorganized agitation disappeared. But one day another patient's family brought that patient's beloved dog to the hospital and Jack reacted by immediately returning to his previous status. He concluded that the dogs had learned his whereabouts and were now hot on his trail. Later that day, Jack joined a group of patients for a visit to a nearby art museum. En route, a dog followed the group. Jack left the group long enough to compose a note, which he gave to the dog. The dog took it between his teeth, and Jack believed that he took it to Petronius Arbiter. Some surprised dog owner probably received a note that read: "I know that you know that I know. I have sworn secrecy and will never reveal your disguise. If I break my vow, you may deal with me as you will."

Shortly thereafter, Jack's antipsychotic medication was increased, his delusions disappeared, and he again became a shy, unhappy, lonely, displaced teenager. He was discharged to his dreary home, with the expectation that medication would be continued.

Since Jack, like most psychotics, did not believe that he was ill, and since his guardians were indifferent, his consumption of medication lapsed. At his last visit, his delusion showed signs of returning in a slightly altered form, with horses taking the place of dogs; in contending with his preoccupations, he was writing a science-fiction novel about horses from another planet. He had just finished reading *Gulliver's Travels,* one episode of which deals with horses of more than human intelligence. At the time Jack manifested no confusion of thought, however, and continued the warm relationship with the psychiatrist that had developed after he began taking the antipsychotic medication. Shortly thereafter, his family moved and his subsequent fate is not known.

Both Susan and Jack would be considered by virtually all psychiatrists to have manifested typical features of chronic schizophrenia.

Kraepelin initially identified dementia praecox by the typical life history of the disorder. Kraepelin thought that it began in adolescence or young adult life and progressed relentlessly to dementia, a deteriorated state. Other psychotic patients, in whom the illness often began later in life, did not deteriorate and sometimes even recovered. The deteriorative illness was characterized by striking symptoms, especially hallucinations and delusions. Hallucinations and delusions do sometimes occur in other psychiatric illnesses—in serious disorders of mood, in certain forms of brain injury, and as a result of some poisons and drugs—but overwhelmingly they are associated only with schizophrenia. Delusions and hallucinations are instances of positive symptoms, symptoms added on to normal psychological functioning. Schizophrenia is also characterized by several negative symptoms, an absence of or deficiency in normal psychological functioning.

Hallucinations are distortions of perception experienced as real by the percipient. They differ from perceptual distortions that the sufferer realizes are false. Some patients who have had a limb removed, for example, continue to feel sensation in a phantom limb, but they realize that the sensation is false. Hallucinations can occur in all senses, but auditory hallucinations are the most common. They may vary from whistlings and gurglings to inarticulate speaking, to distinct complex speech. A patient may locate them on the other side of walls, directly outside her ear, or inside her head. There may be one or many voices, and they may agree with or criticize the patient or argue among themselves.

The content of the hallucinations often reflects the patient's personal problems and cultural background. One study, for example, focused on schizophrenic women of the same racial background who lived in two adjoining but very different cultures. In one, a woman is scorned if she has no children, and in that culture hallucinated voices accused the patients of being barren, whether or not they had children. In the other culture, a woman is ostracized if she has been promiscuous, and the voices there accused the patients of being whores.

A distinguishing feature of schizophrenic hallucinations—as compared to those that may be produced in normals by psychedelic drugs—is that they carry an intense sense of belief and are not just interesting but irrelevant sensory experiences. In occasional instances, a patient's belief in their reality may be shaken and he may gain enough objectivity to realize that he is hallucinating.

In one case, an engineer was so vexed by voices coming from machinery, calling him a "Communist fag," that he was about to shoot the personnel manager. The psychiatrist who saw him asked how "they" managed to produce the voices, and the engineer replied that this had puzzled him but that he thought they probably had large parabolic mirrors which were able to focus the sound on his ear from a distance. He wondered if that was a crazy idea. It was pointed out to him that if there were large parabolic mirrors focused on his ear, when he moved his head slightly he would be unable to hear the focused sound. At that point his belief in the reality of his perceptions was shaken and he agreed to take antipsychotic medication.

Among the hallucinations in other senses are complex visions, or the taste of food or the smell of gas in the absence of a real stimulus. Patients may complain that others are having bowel movements in their rooms, for example, or pumping poisonous gas under the door.

A few patients experience hallucinations of the tactile sense. One thirteen-year-old boy, guilty about masturbation, informed the physician that when he touched the base of his brain (the roof of his mouth) with the tip of his tongue, he had simultaneous feelings in his genitalia and hands. In some complex way, masturbation (the simultaneous sensation in hands and genitalia) had apparently become symbolically linked to changes in his psychological experience. The recurrent but false belief that masturbation can drive one mad may have been involved.

Delusions are probably the most important positive symptoms found in many schizophrenics. A false belief maintained with utter conviction, a delusion may vary from the most trivial fragment of a thought to a complex and systematized belief structure. However, delusions are not a disturbance of sensory reception or intellectual function. They are disorders of inference.

For example, a young woman at the beginning of her first schizophrenic psychosis was walking down a street in a mild state of perplexity when she saw a stop sign. She immediately concluded that it was a command for her to stop moving in her current direction in life. Interpreting the command literally, she changed her path and came to a theater marquee that read "Tonight," with the name of the movie. This conveyed to her the need for immediate action before important steps were taken by unspecified powers "tonight." The question of why such signs should relate only to her was dismissed as unimportant.

An example of a more complex system involved a lawyer who gradually began to suspect from the newspapers and comments made by his employees that the FBI and the major world powers were interested in contacting him for top-secret operations concerning control of biological weapons. He derived data to support his conviction by reading portions of certain magazines with the kind of scrutiny employed by mystics who believe that major human problems can be solved by careful calculation and reworking of words and letters in the Bible. In accordance with the system, he evolved complex methods of communicating, employing color codes on his neckties and arranging his window shades in certain patterns. After several years, he believed that FBI agents were concealed behind his walls, monitoring his activities as the sole controller of the world's biological weaponry. His delusion came to a climax when he construed various signs as indicating that his supposed supervisors in the FBI had become displeased with him and would demand severe punishment unless he atoned for his crimes. His entrance into the hospital was precipitated by his act of penance—shooting himself in the foot, thereby amputating it. This is a characteristic paranoid delusion: grandiose beliefs concerning the patient's abilities, and associated beliefs that certain people, powers, or forces are bent on persecuting, injuring, or punishing him.

Bleuler, the Swiss psychiatrist who first used the term "schizophrenia," theorized that several psychological features were common to all patients who had been diagnosed as having dementia praecox. Unlike Kraepelin, who had defined dementia praecox on the basis of its onset and life course, Bleuler asserted that the disease could be defined by the presence of its typical attributes *whether or not* they occurred in the young and *whether or not* the illness resulted in dementia. His approach followed a pattern familiar in the history of medicine, attempting to define a disease by its primary symptoms and not by age of onset or eventual outcome.

Bleuler asserted that the symptoms occurred along a continuum from the very severe to the barely noticeable, and that there were many more mild cases of schizophrenia outside of institutions than there were serious cases in them. Bleuler's startling assertion is still being debated.

The symptoms by which Bleuler defined schizophrenia are the famous four "A's" that every psychiatric trainee is supposed to know by heart. Some of these are the negative symptoms to which we earlier referred—they involve an absence of some aspect of psychological functioning. The first is impairment of association. One of the characteristics of schizophrenics is a disorganization, a lack of coherence, a muddling of speech and presumably of thought. This looseness of association refers to the formal organization of thought, not to its content. Like the other characteristics, it ranges from an easily identified gross form to a subtle version that may confuse even the experienced clinician. A spontaneous essay by a patient of Bleuler's illustrates the gross form:

> At the time of the new moon, Venus stands in Egypt's August-sky and illuminates with her rays the commercial ports of Suez, Cairo and Alexandria. In this historically famous city of Calif, there is a museum of Sumerian monuments from Macedonia. There flourish plantain trees, bananas, corn cobs, oats, clover and barley; also figs, lemons, oranges and olives. Olive oil is an Arabian liquor-sauce which the Afghans, Moors and Moslems use in ostrich farming. The Indian plantain tree is the whiskey of the Parsees and Arabs. Barley, rice and sugar cane called artichoke, grow remarkably well in India. The Brahmins live as castes in Baluchistan. The Circassians occupy Manchuria and China. China is the Eldorado of the Pawnees. [Bleuler, 1950, p. 15]

At the other end of the spectrum is speech that is only confused, woolly, or vague. If the speaker is not retarded, attempting to evade cross-examination, attempting to appear profound, or obviously anxious and yet produces confusing effects, then the speaker may be manifesting subtle characteristics of schizophrenic speech. A rough clinical rule of thumb is that if you talk to a patient for ten or fifteen minutes and at the end of that time do not know what he has talked about or where his thought is going, there is a good chance that that person is schizophrenic.

The second "A" is affect—emotional response. Schizophrenics are said to have a flatness or blunting of affect and inappropriate affect. Flatness refers to an emotional coolness or indifference. As someone becomes schizophrenic, his loved ones may notice a gradual diminution in their sense of rapport with him. At first, these changes affect only the more subtle aspects of emotional life, but as the disease progresses, one may see inappropriate emotional responsiveness: the patient laughs when crying would be more appropriate, is angry when fear would be more appropriate, is indifferent when sorrow would be anticipated, and so forth.

One of the difficulties in attempting to understand the subjective life of the schizophrenic is that one can only learn about it from someone in whom the schizophrenic process has produced changes but not to a degree that prevents communication. The patient who is too well may not have experienced the typical changes, and the severely ill patient can no longer communicate accurately about them. However, some patients do reach an intermediate position in which they both experience and can report about significant subjective changes.

One adolescent girl reported that she felt as if she were in a telephone booth looking out and only able to communicate indirectly; she felt as if she were insulated from everything around her by a sheet of cotton wool. Early in the course of the disease or in very mild cases, this emotional blunting or perceptual distortion is often associated with the most exquisite personal sensitivity. A person who may be indifferent to the effects she produces in others may react violently to the most trivial or imagined slight. It is difficult to decide whether such individuals react the way they do because of massive egocentricity or because the indifference functions as a protective shell for extreme vulnerability.

The third "A" is autism, a withdrawing into one's own inner world. In a profoundly disturbed patient, the hospital ward may become Jerusalem, the other patients Romans and disciples of the schizophrenic Christ. These mental activities initially appear to differ only in degree and permanence from the fantasies and daydreams of the normal. With progressive illness, the fantasies assume the force of reality and become delusional. They are caricatures of daydreams of glory, power, and magnificence. In schizophrenic cases of intermediate severity, some patients will report more a pulling away from the world than a pulling into fantasy. One first mate in the merchant marine preferred to travel with a foreign-speaking crew because this prevented close contact and permitted him to maintain his distance. He also welcomed the long sea journeys despite (or because of) the forced separation from his wife. When the ship reached a port, he was glad to let his crew go ashore to brothels while he spent his time masturbating and advancing himself in mathematics.

Bleuler's fourth "A" is ambivalence—the simultaneous possession of intense, contradictory feelings. While all of us have some mixed feelings (we can feel angry at or envious of those we love, we can admire those we hate, and so forth), some schizophrenics experience contradictory feelings to an exaggerated degree. In extreme—and exceptional—instances, the patient may vacillate between puppy-like adoration and homicidal rage. A woman, for example, may experience a profound depression when hospitalized and removed from her children, only to be completely indifferent when they visit her. Of the four "A's," ambivalence is probably the least frequent, the least characteristic, and the least important.

A list of basic or primary attributes of schizophrenia depends on which authority you read. No supreme authority has pointed out ten thousand individuals and said, "They are all schizophrenics." If one had, it would be relatively simple to identify the traits these persons had in common and to list them as the basic attributes of the disorder. Our own basic list is subject to change without notice, but two other frequent attributes do deserve mention. The first is anhedonia—a diminished ability to experience pleasure, similar to that one sees in depression. Many schizophrenic people seem to have a lifelong limitation of the ability to get a kick out of ordinary diversions. The brighter and less sick ones are aware of the discrepancy between their perception of the world and that of other people. The schizophrenic may complain of apathy, indifference, and ennui, but he differs from the depressive in that depression often hurts—is emotionally painful—and is usually episodic rather than lifelong.

Some schizophrenic patients attempt to overcome these feelings by vigorously seeking intense experiences. They pile on stimuli like the jaded roué seeking debauchery, although the roué may once have had normal sensitivities, while the anhedonic person has not. In search of highs, anhedonic schizophrenics may pursue special drug experiences. The more intellectual may construct philosophies or religions to account for and solve their problems. Although such constructions can serve as rationalizations for a schizophrenic outlook, they may be widely accepted by others who are not necessarily schizophrenic. As we mentioned in connection with personality disorder, much intellectual, philosophical, and religious activity may be a compensation or rationalization for an intrinsic emotional disability. This may be true of his religion, her political views, and their philosophy; ours obviously derive from indisputable evidence and logic.

Another symptom seen in many schizophrenics involves abulia—disturbances of the will. Many lose their sense of initiative, of directed activity, of active concern with the outside world. Intellectual work that had been begun remains unfinished, files once kept neatly become chaotic, housekeeping languishes, and children are neglected. With abulia and anhedonia, there are six "A's," not four.

One of the "positive" symptoms that we have not yet mentioned is catatonia, peculiarities in movements. Catatonics may vacillate between repetitive, stereotyped movements, startling hyperactivity and excitement, and absolute motionlessness. Both stereotyped movements and motionless periods may have fairly clear-cut symbolic meaning. In their periods of motionlessness, some patients are apparently semistuporous, while others maintain full consciousness. In this state, some patients will maintain themselves in any position in which they are placed, no matter how awkward. The patient may hold her head inches off the pillow or balance herself uncomfortably on one foot for hours. For unknown reasons, the proportion of catatonics is decreasing all over the world—just as Freud's hysterics have mysteriously disappeared.

Finally—and we use the word only to mean that we will stop listing now and not that we have exhausted the possible symptoms of schizophrenia—some schizophrenics experience a blurring or dissolution of the boundaries of the self: the patient may feel that he is a part of others or that others are part of him, or that he and animals, God, other men, and nature are somehow one and the same. One notices immediately the parallels between this schizophrenic experience and the ecstatic union with the universe that is reported by some mystics and psychedelic-drug users.

This relatively extensive list, which comprises only a fraction of the psychological abnormalities that occur in schizophrenia, might seem to imply that the disorder always involves generalized deterioration in the functioning of the mind. But that is not so. One of the startling aspects of the disorder is that there are wide individual variations and that in some schizophrenics some psychological and intellectual functions are very well preserved. Space and time orientation, visual and auditory perception, memory, and special skills may be in remarkably good condition.

A catatonic adolescent maintained a rigidly fixed posture in front of the hospital-ward television set early one October, apparently oblivious to all that went on around him; on recovery, he commented on the high points in the just past World Series. A middle-aged schizophrenic, hospitalized for twenty years and convinced that he was a prophet of God and that dragon-like creatures were coming out of the walls, occasionally interrupted his agitated pacing to play a competent game of chess.

This juxtaposition of lunacy and sanity has led many to believe that the schizophrenic's madness is a learned reaction or even a put-on, and is only an adaptation over a core of sanity. Certainly, the schizophrenias appear different from madness produced by chemical, metabolic, or traumatic damage to the brain. The student on a bad LSD trip, the alcoholic with delirium tremens, the senile patient, and the patient with a stroke do not play a competent game of chess or reflect on subtleties of baseball strategy.

Not all the symptoms occur in any individual schizophrenic patient; and many of the symptoms can occur either in isolation or in complex combination with others. This variability tells us nothing about the schizophrenias. It certainly does not lead to the conclusion that the symptoms must be learned, since it is distressingly common for clearcut medical illnesses to appear in various guises. Rheumatic fever, a disorder whose cause is known and in which the mechanism of damage to the body is understood, can appear as a disease of the nervous system (Saint Vitus's dance), a disease of the heart (rheumatic heart disease), a disease of the joints, or a disease of the skin. Physicians were unable to recognize these different symptoms as manifestations of the same underlying disease until bacteriologists and anatomists discovered the common causes and tissue changes.

Because psychiatrists cannot yet identify changes in the functioning of the brain in the schizophrenias, they do not even know if there are several causes or only one for the disease(s). A satisfactory answer awaits elucidation of the suspected underlying biological abnormalities. Recent advances in measuring actual brain atrophy by the new CAT scanner, and decreases in regional blood flow by yet more esoteric machinery, clearly indicate that some schizophrenics have manifest brain dysfunctions.

The dazzling range of possible permutations and combinations of symptoms in schizophrenia has led to elaborate classification systems. These systems bear little relation to prognosis or treatment, and we will not add yet another. However, two major subdivisions are important: an acute form of schizophrenia, and a chronic or process form. It is possible that they have different genetic patterns and different biological alterations, and they do respond differently to treatment.

In chronic schizophrenia, only one subdivision seems worth distinguishing: paranoid schizophrenia. The word "paranoid" has crept into popular usage in an approximately accurate form. When we talk of paranoid schizophrenics, we are referring to a group of people who are preoccupied with delusions and hallucinations of persecution and who at first—unlike many other schizophrenics—may not show the peculiarities of unintelligible speech, emotional withdrawal, or changes in emotional life. As they become more seriously ill, paranoid schizophrenics become indistinguishable from other seriously ill schizophrenics. When the disorder is mild or in its earliest stages, paranoid schizophrenics are difficult to distinguish from those who suffer paranoid personality disorder, the group of exaggeratedly suspicious and untrusting people discussed earlier. Where schizophrenia ends and mere paranoia begins is often unclear.

One characteristic of paranoid schizophrenics and other paranoid people is that they frequently do get very angry and feel a need to retaliate—in contrast to other schizophrenics, who tend to be emotionally flat. When the judgment of paranoids is seriously impaired, they may become homicidal and dangerous. A number of political assassinations have seemingly been committed by paranoid people.

Acute Schizophrenia

The acute form of schizophrenia, as the name implies, tends to disappear with the passage of time with or without treatment, although treatment usually speeds the rate of recovery. It occurs in people who prior to their illness were psychologically and socially relatively well put together; tends during the illness to have some attributes of psychoses produced by chemicals and brain dysfunction, such as confusion; is often strongly colored by changes in mood, either depression or mania; and is often precipitated by a major psychological setback, such as the loss of a loved one or a profound disappointment.

Special aspects of acute schizophrenia that have been identified in the twentieth century were recognized as early as the seventeenth by an English physician, Thomas Willis. In *The London Practice of Physick* (1692), Willis noted the confusing relationship between melancholy (affective disorders) and madness (schizophrenia): "After Melancholy it remains for us to treat Madness which is so far ally'd to the other that these affects often change turns and each passes into the other." Nor did he fail to observe that madness produced by psychological stress was far more likely to be followed by recovery: "Madness raised on a sudden from some solemn evident cause, as from a vehement passion, is much safer than that invading by degrees."

Peter D.

Peter was a nineteen-year-old college student who was brought to the hospital by the police; they had found him wandering around, dazed and confused, in the early-morning hours. The police had at first assumed that he was drunk but on talking to him had decided that he was experiencing a "bad trip." When brought to the hospital, he was disoriented (knew his name, but not the time, the date, or the place), extraordinarily anxious and talkative, and reported incessant threatening voices that accused him of being a homosexual. The following day his college roommates informed the physicians that Peter had only taken marijuana (and only occasionally), and that they were relatively sure he had not taken any psychedelic drugs prior to his admission. They did report that he had involuntarily withdrawn from a passionate relationship.

With reports from the boy's parents, it was possible to piece together the relevant events in his life. Before coming to college, he had been an assiduous student, the president of the student council, and a member of his high-school baseball team. He was not extroverted but neither was he withdrawn or shut in. He had many male acquaintances and several good friends. He had dated several girls but had not been able to lose a feeling of chronic "ill ease" in their presence. His sexual experience had been very limited. At college, he had pursued his studies as usual and had begun to date casually.

Six months before his hospitalization, he had met "the woman of his dreams." His roommates described her as in the extreme upper percentile of good looks (in popular parlance, a "10"), seemingly sophisticated and poised, and sexually experienced. Peter's ardor had initially been returned, and as he spent more time with the young woman, his grades dropped somewhat, but not seriously. For reasons that are unclear—and how often they are—his lover and he had a parting of the ways. In successive weeks he began to eat and sleep less, complained of increasing depression and inability to concentrate, and appeared to his roommates to be preoccupied. On the day of admission, he had left his room in the morning and had failed to return. What had happened between the morning and the time of admission was unknown.

Peter was treated initially with large doses of antipsychotic drugs; over three or four days he became less agitated but lethargic, a familiar side effect of the medication. The dose was diminished, and the doctors noted that he was once again oriented, no longer experienced hallucinations, and was not confused. He still complained of depression, apathy, and an inability to mobilize himself. Within a few weeks, he was discharged from the hospital, still on medication, and continued to see a psychiatrist intermittently.

It became apparent that Peter had always been a conscientious, overachieving, self-punishing young man who never let himself go. The love affair was obviously a departure from his habitual style of life, and its termination was clearly linked to his symptomatology and the eventual schizophrenic psychosis. What is not clear is why Peter became psychotic in circumstances that would only depress or upset the average student.

Following the psychotic episode, Peter experienced extreme exhaustion and had only a hazy, dream-like memory of the psychosis itself—both typical phenomena of acute schizophrenia. His postpsychotic exhaustion was appreciably relieved by antidepressant drugs, which did not decrease his "normal" degree of unhappiness. Six months after his hospitalization, all medications had been discontinued, and Peter had returned to "normal." He was doing well academically, had several friends, and fortunately had loosened up somewhat in his pursuit of happiness, including women. Although he is doing well, his long-term fate remains to be seen.

Whether an illness such as Peter's can be produced in anyone by a severe enough stress or disappointment, or whether it can occur only in a person whose biology or previous life experience has rendered him vulnerable, is unclear. The subsequent history of such patients is difficult to predict, although patients who have suffered such illnesses have a greater than average chance of experiencing later episodes. Medication usually shortens the course of the illness. Psychotherapy can assist the patient in learning something about the precipitating factors, but its value is not established.

Chronic Schizophrenia

The natural history of chronic or process schizophrenias is considerably different. The mode of onset is more often gradual and insidious. A slow transformation of the personality seems to take place. Then, following a period of slow deterioration, the patient may experience acute flare-ups that result in hospitalization. As chronic schizophrenics become ill, they tend not to be confused and they have less of the vivid emotional coloring of the acute schizophrenic. Despite their lack of confusion, they may have persistent hallucinations and delusions.

Although drug therapy is helpful, the symptoms are often only reduced. Thought disorder, disorganization, impaired planning, poor judgment, irrationality, and peculiarity may all remain. Improvement is usually only partial. Discharge from the hospital is not synonymous with recovery. The patients' lives are generally characterized by enduring social incapacity and often by repeated hospitalizations.

Before their illness—if there is a before, for some evidence suggests that the illness is lifelong—many chronic schizophrenics have been deviant children. The preschizophrenic (usually male) child may alternatively be socially inept, isolated, friendless, a scapegoat, withdrawn, poorly coordinated, and anxiety-prone—or rebellious, rule-breaking, and initially indistinguishable from other juvenile delinquents.

In addition, between the extremes of the acute and the chronic schizophrenic states lie transitional forms. Some patients, not always considered really schizophrenic, have repeated acute episodes, each followed by "complete" recovery. In others, there is a residual defect in the form of social incompetence, fuzzy thinking, and reduced capacity for pleasure and planned effort, leading to accumulative impairment. Finally, after repeated acute episodes, some patients develop a chronic psychosis.

JILL L.

When Jill L. was sixteen and in her junior year at high school, the school authorities urged her parents to seek psychiatric help for her.

The parents contacted a psychologist, who diagnosed her as a paranoid schizophrenic and saw her several times a week for a total of 125 sessions.

Jill was obviously highly disturbed, doing miserably in school, and badgering her parents to allow her to quit. She was suspicious of her schoolmates, feeling that they were staring at her, talking about her, and laughing behind her back. She often started verbal and physical fights with them, as when she had a fight with a girl whom she accused of walking into her purposely. "I really ripped the sweater off her and told her if you ever do that again I'll kill you." She often contemplated suicide but "didn't have the guts" to go through with it. She refused to use public transportation, hated Negroes and Jews (although she herself was Jewish), and feared attack from behind. When in a group she felt that she actually shrank in size so that she was less conspicuous.

Jill withdrew increasingly from outside contact, and at the end of her junior year her parents allowed her to quit school. She stayed home and lived in her own world, where she fantasied that she was a beautiful eighteenth-century lady surrounded by servants and handsome men. She spent hours in front of a mirror, combing her hair and scrubbing her face, sometimes seeing the image of Elizabeth Taylor reflected in front of her and sometimes only a featureless face. Her only social contact was with a congenial married handyman, with whom she had almost daily sexual intercourse. Her therapist finally persuaded her to accept hospitalization about a year and a half after she had begun therapy.

Jill's motor development was average, although she was not completely toilet-trained until age four. Very early, she used foul language and cursed her parents. She was always irritable, abusive, sullen, withdrawn, and disobedient.

At age five she started school, which she hated immediately. She refused to have any interaction with the other children, feeling that they were staring at her. Her schoolwork was poor and she had to repeat fifth grade. In high school she attended a special class for slow learners.

When Jill was eight, her mother threatened her with hospitalization if she continued masturbating. Although her mother instructed her about menarche, she was frightened when it occurred at age eleven. She stopped masturbating at age thirteen, after reading that it was abnormal.

For a while she wore only old dungarees and refused to comb her hair, keeping it in curlers most of the time. She thought there was something wrong with her hair, nose, bosom, and height, picked at her face until it was a mass of lesions, and never went anywhere with her parents because she feared that she didn't look right. Petrified that she would get lost, she never went anywhere alone. At ages eight and thirteen, at the school's insistence, Jill had brief psychotherapeutic contacts, but neither she nor her parents remembered any details about them.

Jill felt completely rejected until age fourteen, when she went steady with a boy for a short time. Necking was their usual activity. Following their breakup, she met a young mechanic, whom she dated for three years. They usually went to a garage and had oral-genital sex but did not have coitus because the boy wanted to wait until they were married. She was extremely jealous and went into rages, hitting, clawing, and screaming if the boy so much as admired a girl on TV. She saw him as someone who would care for her as if she were an infant. As she pushed him toward engagement and marriage, he became frightened and finally abandoned her nine months before her hospitalization. Shortly after this, she started seeing the handyman, with whom she had daily intercourse. Jill was attracted to boys whom her parents considered socially inferior; she totally rejected Jewish boys of whom her parents approved.

In the hospital, Jill's appearance was bizarre. She had an attractive but vulpine face and was always unkempt and dirty, with her head enveloped in its garish halo of curlers. Her posture was stilted, with a conspicuous backward lean, so that her abdomen protruded. She wore skin-tight, off-the-shoulder blouses that inappropriately emphasized her flat-chestedness.

On interview, Jill was eager to relate her problems and instigated discussions of her sexual activity. Her nonstop monologues about herself were relevant and coherent, with angry, hostile, and depressed affect appropriate to her thought content.

When upset, Jill heard a male voice insulting her, which she thought perhaps was a combination of someone playing a trick and her imagination. Sometimes she yelled and cursed at strangers she thought were staring at her. Often when angry she clawed at her face with her nails.

Physical and neurological tests, including EEGs, were within normal limits. The examining resident thought her general intelligence above average, but on an IQ test her score was low normal. Her information level was low average, judgment and conceptual thinking were very poor, and simple arithmetic skill was completely deficient. On projective testing she functioned as an overt paranoid schizophrenic.

During the initial period of hospitalization, Jill, now age eighteen, became increasingly disturbed, withdrawn, paranoid, and hallucinatory. She refused to undress or bathe, insisting that others were staring at her, and asked to be placed in seclusion. She continued to see Elizabeth Taylor when she looked in the mirror. One day she leaned far out over a stairwell after "voices" told her to kill herself.

After six weeks of decline, she was given a substantial dose of antipsychotic medication. During the first two weeks on the drug, she looked affectively flat, like a zombie, wanted to be home, and spent almost the entire day sleeping. After an anti-Parkinson drug was added to block side effects, she suddenly appeared happy and alert, and said she felt reborn, alive, and better than ever before in her life. She took the curlers out of her hair, dressed neatly and attractively, and began to join in hospital activities, including the hospital high school, modern dance, and grooming classes. In group therapy, she expressed an eagerness to learn to interact with others. In individual psychotherapy, she was extremely passive and nonintrospective, and constantly begged to return home to her mother. Therapy was concrete and supportive.

After the first seven weeks of medication, her doctor complained that the medication was interfering with expressive psychotherapy and reduced the dosage several times. Two days after the last reduction, Jill was upset and withdrawn, extremely preoccupied with sexual thoughts, and complained about being in the hospital. The medication was immediately increased, but she remained distracted by sexual thoughts, requiring still higher dosage. Her therapist related her emotional setback to his impending vacation.

Because Jill continued depressed and apathetic, she was placed on an adjunctive antidepressant. Within forty-eight hours she seemed brighter and again enthusiastic about her activities. The dosage was difficult to regulate, however. With an increase, she became sexually provocative with patients and aides; but with a reduction, she became withdrawn, homesick, and lethargic. At an intermediate dosage she was alert and sociable but in two weeks began dressing grotesquely, like a femme fatale, requiring an increase in her antipsychotic medication.

As the hospitalization continued, Jill developed pride in her many new accomplishments, such as using a pay phone, riding an escalator, and especially earning her high-school diploma. But she still had a strong fear of traveling.

She was discharged after a year of hospitalization, much improved, on a daily drug regimen combining antipsychotic and antidepressant medications. She returned to her parents' home with plans to attend an after-care clinic, receive vocational guidance, and later live at a girls' residence.

For a year following discharge, Jill attended the after-care clinic. Three months after discharge, her medication was reduced. While she functioned fairly adequately, she could not look for a job and had considerable trouble with her parents, who objected to the "low element" she socialized with and worried about her promiscuity.

They felt all her problems would be solved if only she married "a nice Jewish boy."

Instead, she had an affair with an unstable, exploitative married man, twelve years her senior, and became pregnant. An abortion was arranged, but she became pregnant again. After her parents expedited the man's divorce, the couple married and lived with the L.s. When her husband left her after a few months, her parents persuaded her to place the child for adoption and divorce her husband.

Jill never got a job, found no real friends, and was primarily concerned with getting married. After two years of dating pickups, she fell in love with a porter, six years younger than herself, at a hotel where she was vacationing with her parents. They married ten months later and moved to a distant state, near the husband's family. Jill later described her second husband as sexually inexperienced but dominating; however, she liked having a jealous, masterful husband. Eventually they began to have physical fights, which in retrospect she felt were her fault. After a year, her husband became "sullen" and she came home.

Jill found living with her parents intolerable and frequently attacked her mother with fists and nails. Her father in turn beat her. Yet she was afraid to be far from her mother. She felt as if she had a hundred different personalities, heard people talking about her but realized these were hallucinations, and often screamed at people on the street. In this condition, Jill was rehospitalized seven years after her discharge.

On admission, she again looked bizarre, with heavy, clown-like makeup. Very depressed, hostile, and paranoid, she cut her wrists once and hid a knife in her clothing several times. She also threatened to kill other patients if they continued to talk about her. She was extremely seductive with all males. A small dose of antipsychotic medication helped calm her somewhat, but she could not be cared for in an open setting and after ten days was sent to a state hospital. She improved on antipsychotic medication and was discharged after a month, but was back in another four months after a repetition of her troubles at home. She was again placed on antipsychotic medication and released to her parents in two weeks.

One year later, her mother wrote requesting help. Jill was vegetating at home, leaving the house only with Mrs. L. Her mother wanted to place her in a permanent residence other than a state hospital, but all such placements were impossibly expensive.

In a follow-up phone interview eleven years after Jill's initial hospitalization, Mr. L. reported that Jill had not worked or been away from home in the past three years. She still took a daily moderate dose of medication but had received no other psychiatric care. Her symptoms were the same but more tolerable.

Jill L.'s history includes several typical aspects of chronic schizophrenia: a failing school career, the substitution of sexual activity for socialization, difficult marriages, the appearance of higher intelligence than that measured by structured tests, and grandiose compensatory delusions.

Our society has not yet developed the long-term care facilities that would provide such chronically limited patients with the structure they need to live at their optimum. The belief that such patients can be maintained in the community, or are receptive to special rehabilitative training that can enable them to rejoin the community to compete socially and economically, is simple wishful thinking. Dedicated hospital staffs can now use behavior therapy techniques to help social learning in patients (Paul and Lentz, 1977), but only a small fraction of such patients—about 10 percent—can function independently in the community without supervisory care. Chronic care facilities that are not simple custodial warehouses are indicated, in view of the uniformly poor adjustment these patients display outside such settings.

Many of the patients have circumscribed skills that can afford them both pleasure and productivity if their life is led within a structured setting. Such a setting, especially if it could be permissive about sexual relationships and at the same time ensure adequate contraception, could help the patients toward a fuller humanity than they can achieve living on their own. Too often, inherent problems prevent families from providing an optimal environment, and in many instances patients have no families able or willing to assist them.

Borderlands of Schizophrenia

Unlike the blood tests that warn of diabetic or even prediabetic conditions, there is no chemical test for schizophrenia(s) or its near relatives; nevertheless, accurate observers believe they can detect subtle signs of the illness. Many psychiatrists—rightly or wrongly—have been convinced that schizophrenia has a major genetic component. Among the relatives of schizophrenics, psychiatrists have observed a high proportion of unusual people, many of whose characteristics seem halfway between schizophrenic and normal. One chronic schizophrenic, for example, intermittently believed that various groups were persecuting and attempting to kill him. In periods of comparative recovery, he was described as eccentric, conscientious, depressed, and withdrawn, with feelings of inferiority and a strong capacity for fantasy. His three brothers were all competent but either withdrawn, depressed, or eager to "get away." Both parents had had episodes of paranoia and manifested depression and a variety of other symptoms.

The heterogeneous group of individuals who are believed by some to be biological—as well as familial—relatives of schizophrenics merges with the group described as having schizoid personality disorder. Called schizotypal, these people vary from the shy, timid, and unsociable to the callous, cold, harsh, and distant, from the quiet, empty, and intelligent to the sensitive and poetic or to the militant, rigid, and fanatic (political or religious). Intellectually, the class ranges from the scatterbrained to the imaginative or the pedantic. Obviously, lumping what may be minor personality variations with schizophrenia raises crucial questions of definition.

Another loosely defined category, a little further along the illness spectrum and also believed to be related to the schizophrenias, is variously called ambulatory schizophrenia, pseudoneurotic schizophrenia, or borderline schizophrenia. "Ambulatory" implies that such persons are walking around freely rather than being locked up in asylums. "Pseudoneurotic" calls attention to the fact that many such persons have passed as neurotic. "Borderline" refers to their supposed near relationship to the true schizophrenics. The attributes of borderlines are almost as numerous as the authors who have written about them.

Many so-called borderlines, we believe, have illnesses that are causally related to the affective disorders rather than to schizophrenia. There is increasing evidence that the large group of people called borderline is quite heterogeneous and that the word is applied to a mixed bag of psychiatric diseases. One of us (Klein) has done some research showing that drugs that help affective disorders—and which do not help or which actually worsen schizophrenia—help certain types of borderlines, those described in the section on personality disorders as emotionally unstable character disorders and hysteroid dysphorics.

Genetic evidence on borderline schizophrenics will be discussed in the chapter on nature and nurture. To avoid confusion, we will refer to the group of people apparently related genetically to schizophrenics as schizoid-eccentric or schizotypal and we will refer to the other group as affectively vulnerable.

Eva J.

Eva, a somewhat disheveled, thirty-year-old woman, was admitted to a psychiatric teaching hospital because of numerous undiagnosable complaints of aches and pains, fevers and malaise. The physicians initially wondered if her ailments were conversion reactions or if she was unusually hypochondriacal. She recounted her history at great length, but because her style of communication was extraordinarily fuzzy, it was extremely difficult to piece together a coherent story. Some of the facets of her life that did stand out clearly were typical of the characteristics sometimes said to be associated with borderline schizophrenics.

Eva's parents were European émigrés who had fled Hitler. She and her older brother were raised in a home with economic comforts, strict rules, and parental coldness. During grammar school and high school she had had a few friends and perhaps one or two confidantes. After high school she went to secretarial school, and then, eager to flee the parental nest, had found a job in a relatively distant city.

Away from her parents, her hitherto orderly life broke down. Her sexual life went from nonexistent to active, and then, over the next seven years, to frenetic. She sometimes slept with three men in one night, and interspersed her heterosexual adventures with homosexual ones. Concomitantly, her diligent work pattern broke down. She was absent frequently, performed her work inadequately, and was eventually fired. Between that time and her arrival at the hospital, she managed to exist on welfare, handouts, and occasional temporary jobs. During this period she associated with the intellectual and bohemian fringe of the city she lived in. She read widely and spent hours discussing existentialism with her cadre of associates.

Eva's history indicated that she had been chronically anhedonic. Nothing had given her much of a kick in life. Her sexual escapades—and some mild experimentation with drugs—appeared to be an effort to escape the pallid, dull gray of her existence. She had never known how to form relationships with people. She felt uncomfortable both by herself and when close to someone else unless that person acted as a parent. Sexually she was totally unresponsive, but sex did provide a sense of security and the feeling of being wanted. She found it comforting to be held, and her running from partner to partner was a pitiful effort to obtain someone to sleep (in the literal sense) with her for the whole night. Her fantasy life was vivid and raw. When asked about sexual fantasies, she replied with such examples as: "Do you mean things like walking on men's testicles with spiked heels?" Or "Like biting women's nipples?" She had never experienced anything remotely akin to hallucinations or delusions.

She was intellectually quick and when focused on a problem could produce neat, simple answers. She spent the next year, with frequent leaves of absence, in the hospital and its therapeutic community. She was in individual and group psychotherapy and had trials with many potent therapeutic drugs, but nothing helped. She rapidly became superficially friendly with a group of patients whose personalities were very similar to hers—perpetual graduate students—and all enjoyed a long stay, with little benefit, in this open, socially advanced, state-financed commune. Her sexual activities diminished somewhat (the hospital rendered them inconvenient), but her fuzzy thought and lack of life-goal-directedness persisted.

Finally, the staff had to recognize that she was not changing for the better and that there was no reason for hospitalization to continue. After she was discharged, her disorganized and gray life resumed, until a miracle occurred. Eva had the good fortune to meet an energetic woman in her fifties who collected somewhat younger waifs and out of the goodness of her heart or her own needs endeavored to straighten them out. She took Eva into her large Victorian home and began to act like a beneficent but strict mother. She insisted that Eva's blouses be starched and her skirts pressed, and she packed her a lunch and sent her off to look for a job. Because of her substantial secretarial skills, Eva had no difficulty in finding one. Supervised by her foster mother, she arrived early to work and did not leave at the stroke of five. She was one of the most disciplined of the employees in the office and was given several bonuses and a promotion. Her sexual life ceased entirely. In a remarkably short time, Eva went from being a sexually liberated, undirected member of the peripheral intelligentsia to being a typical, albeit sexually inhibited, white-collar worker.

The characteristics and course of Eva's life illustrate many of the qualities claimed to be typical of borderlines. The two most prominent are her anhedonia and the fuzzy nature of her speech. She sometimes used colorful metaphors and similes, but any richness in her speech was diluted by her inability to use reasonably clear-cut prose. (We are reminded of a perhaps apocryphal conversation between James Joyce and Carl Jung. When Joyce asked Jung what the difference was between the loose associational speech of his novels and the similar speech of Joyce's schizophrenic daughter, Jung reputedly replied, "You dive—she falls.")

Another typical feature of Eva's life was her problem with human closeness. Both independence and closeness (except with parental figures) were intolerable—a pattern one sees repeatedly in borderline schizophrenic relationships. In chronic schizophrenics, one sees not so much an intolerance of closeness but an overly clinging, parasitic relationship without feelings of closeness. When such a relationship ends—say, with the death of a parent—some schizophrenics often get worse. Unhappiness with both closeness and distance has been characterized by Burnham et al. as the "need-fear dilemma" (1969).

Eva's sexual life was also supposedly typical of borderline behavior—promiscuous sexuality, including bisexuality, without much pleasure. So many women are sexually unresponsive, however, that frigidity can hardly be said to be specifically characteristic of the anhedonia of borderline schizophrenics.

Two other characteristics are worth comment. The first is the neurotic—that is, hypochondriacal—symptomatology. Some borderline schizophrenics have shifting patterns of neurotic symptomatology, while "good neurotics" usually cling to their own brand—e.g., phobias, obsessions, or hysteria. The other is Eva's ready access to a raw fantasy life, which occurs in some hysterics and is said to be typical of borderlines.

Although many psychiatrists would agree that Eva was a true borderline schizophrenic, we are not certain; she may have been affectively vulnerable.

There is little doubt, however, about the second case history, which follows.

Kurt W.

Kurt was brought to the psychiatrist's office by his wife, who was seriously contemplating divorce. They were both twenty-eight and had been married for six years. She had trouble describing the problems in their relationship. The best she could come up with was that Kurt was distant and hard to contact emotionally; he and she often had great difficulties in communication.

It was easy for the psychiatrist to see the problems that Kurt's wife had described with such difficulty. Kurt was a relatively short, slight young man who fidgeted, stuttered, and appeared somewhat distracted. He had a sometimes bland, sometimes perplexed facial expression, interrupted periodically by what can best be described as a grimace.

His life story was interesting, but his way of phrasing it was odd. He felt that as a child he had been more than ordinarily sensitive, shy, and withdrawn. He had limited contact with his peers, although he had had one "friend." School had been difficult. He was dyslexic and had done poorly. He summed up his feelings as "an anti-sympathy" to school.

Kurt said that as an adult he had become more open, a bit thicker-skinned, and less shy, but he added, "I am still too close-fisted with strangers" (apparently meaning reserved). He still had little interest in other people, and although he believed his social facility had increased, he spoke very little in company, and all of the couple's friends were his wife's. He apparently did not tolerate being dominated: "If I have an opinion, I use it or I don't use it" (a sentence that begins by making sense but ends meaninglessly).

The couple's courtship had evolved largely through the woman's efforts. She had met Kurt in his father's business, where Kurt was learning the ropes. She was extraverted and fun-loving and felt that she complemented Kurt, whom at the time she perceived as attractively sensitive, bashful, and little-boyish. From a poor background, she saw Kurt as an economic opportunity. If it had not been for her social aggressiveness, they would not have married. She had anticipated that as they got to know each other better their communication would improve. It did not, and as she grew to know him better, she became aware of his thought disorder.

Intercourse was infrequent, and when Kurt was asked whether he thought his sex drive was low, he answered, "It is difficult to parallel one's self with another" (his meaning may be that two people's sex drives are usually different, but the expression has an interesting double meaning). Kurt suffered from premature ejaculation, which may have contributed to his wife's infrequent orgasms; describing this, Kurt said, "There wasn't so much to complain about before, but now we have been better able to find the tune."

Kurt's communication deficits are clearly revealed in the following dialogue with the interviewer, who was discussing the marriage:

K.: It would be completely different if it were up to me to decide.
I.: How?
K.: Yeh, I don't know, I can't explain it. I said to her: "You'll soon be looking like an old married woman."
I.: Does she?
K.: No, but she is too fat, but then on the other hand I am too slender, so that it's probably all right anyway.

Kurt's "neurotic" complaints were moderate and all were unknown to his wife. He had multiple fears—of atomic bombs, small spaces, heights, and dogs. In one undecipherable expression he seemed to be saying that the world was foreign and "irrelevant." He also had some counting rituals: he would take his pulse and count to multiples of 7, or he might count windowpanes on the street or tiles on the floor. He was hypochondriacal and had been sexually abstinent before marriage because of an overwhelming fear of venereal disease.

Kurt was bewildered that his wife was contemplating divorce. He totally lacked insight into his impaired abilities to communicate with and form relationships with others, and he thought himself very close to his wife. After a number of conjoint meetings, his wife decided without rancor that it would be best if they separated. The psychiatrist had the feeling that she had initiated the psychiatric consultation for confirmation of her quite accurate impressions, and in a sense in order to gain formal permission to separate. Kurt was surprised but not hurt by her decision. He showed almost no reaction to the separation and later divorce.

Kurt, unlike Eva, had a lifelong history of social non-involvement. In addition, he had a clear thought disorder, inappropriate affect, and flattening of his emotional life. However, he had had no gross psychotic symptoms, no delusions or hallucinations. Quite possibly, he will never have such symptoms. In him, the development of a schizophrenic illness appears to have become arrested. The adoption research that will be discussed later suggests that people like Kurt are almost certainly genetically related to chronic schizophrenics; we are much less certain about people like Eva.

Most borderline persons are also said to exhibit a lifelong diminished ability to experience pleasure. They sometimes derive intense pleasure from intellectual and artistic endeavors, however. Mild thought disorder is frequently but not invariably present, and some function as successful academicians, physicians, and lawyers.

Although the experiencing of pleasure is deficient, the experiencing of anticipated pain is usually heightened. Much of the behavior of borderlines seems motivated by the need to avoid anxiety. They often cling to people for fear of losing them or avoid people for fear of forming attachments that must inevitably end.

Their reduced ability to tolerate stress, often produced by the loss of someone they were dependent on or the failure to reach a goal, may produce disproportionately severe anxiety and depression. Although socially perceptive with regard to others' behavior, the borderline patient, like some patients with personality disorders, may be quite obtuse about the effect her behavior has on others. Often, particularly if bright, the borderline person has recognized the fact that she has been "different" all her life. At the severe end of the spectrum, a very few may have transient episodes of psychosis with delusions, hallucinations, and loss of feelings of reality.

The attributes that supposedly denote schizoids and borderline schizophrenics encompass a large portion of the idiosyncrasies of mankind. The rationale for diagnostically labeling such people depends on two observations: first, the increased frequency of schizoid-eccentric patients among the close relatives of schizophrenics, which has led to the supposition that these disorders are a minimal genetic expression of schizophrenia; second, the superficial similarity of borderlines to true schizophrenia, which has led to the debatable assumption that the two similar phenomena must share an underlying causal or basic relationship to each other. This inference is obviously open to serious question.

Unlike the acute and chronic schizophrenics, only a small fraction of borderline schizophrenics experience psychological decompensation sufficient to land them in mental hospitals. It is difficult to estimate how frequently borderline schizophrenics are seen in mental-health centers and by private psychiatrists. Some psychiatrists who are sensitized to these problems report that approximately half of their chronically disturbed patients fall into this category, asserting that a large segment of "severe neurotics" are really borderline schizophrenics.

There may be a tendency among psychiatrists to overdiagnose borderline schizophrenia because unconsciously they learn that it is a safe diagnosis to make. If the patient becomes psychotic, the psychiatrist's predictive skill has been demonstrated. If the patient fails to get better, the lack of improvement can be attributed to the fairly well documented fact that schizophrenics do not usually benefit from psychotherapy. If the patient does get better, this reflects favorably on the therapist's skill in treating a difficult patient. On the other hand, if the psychiatrist does not make a diagnosis of borderline schizophrenia, he is vulnerable on several counts. If a "neurotic" patient becomes psychotic or fails to recover, the psychiatrist will be blamed.

In an attempt to systematize the thinking of psychiatrists on the borderline conditions, Robert Spitzer and Jean Endicott conducted an opinion survey of members of the American Psychiatric Association (Spitzer, Endicott, and Gibbon, 1979). Psychiatrists were asked to select patients of theirs whom they considered borderline and to rate them on a number of characteristics thought to be present among borderline patients. They were also asked to rate one of their patients whom they did not consider borderline. Data on over 1,600 patients were analyzed statistically, and two groups of symptoms seemed to emerge. One group consisted of odd communication—i.e., speech that is tangential, digressive, vague, overelaborate, circumstantial, or metaphorical; ideas of reference—i.e., inappropriate connections, such as the conviction that any laughter you hear is directed at you; suspiciousness or paranoid ideation; recurrent illusions—i.e., feeling strongly that something is true even though you know it isn't, such as, "I felt as if my dead mother were in the room with me"; depersonalization or derealization; magical thinking—e.g., superstitiousness, clairvoyance, telepathy, the belief that others can feel your feelings; inadequate rapport in a face-to-face interaction; undue social anxiety or hypersensitivity to real or imagined criticism; and social isolation in which social contacts are limited to essential everyday tasks. This group of symptoms seems very close to the schizoid-eccentric or schizotypal borderline disorder described earlier as a likely relative of genetic schizophrenia.

The other group was characterized by identity disturbance, manifested by uncertainty about self-image, gender identity, long-term goals or career choice, friendship patterns, values, and loyalties; a pattern of unstable and intense personal relationships; impulsivity or unpredictability in potentially self-damaging areas, such as spending, sex, gambling, or drug or alcohol use; inappropriate intense anger or lack of control of anger; physically self-damaging acts, such as suicidal gestures or self-mutilation; affective instability with marked shifts from normal mood to depression, irritability, or anxiety usually lasting hours but rarely more than a few days; chronic feelings of emptiness or boredom; problems tolerating being alone; and underachievement in school and work. This cluster comes close to the "affectively vulnerable" borderline state we have described.

This study seems to substantiate clinical opinion by a complex statistical analysis, but it is subject to criticism in that the data that went into the analysis came from psychiatric opinions that were probably affected by common professional beliefs; the psychiatrists may have been feeding into the computer a kind of stereotype rather than a real pattern. A better test would be a study in which patients are rated by interviewers blind to both the purposes of the study and the diagnoses of the patients.

Another peculiarity of this analysis is that it shows that the two kinds of borderline states are not mutually exclusive. In comparison to normals, patients as a group are higher on both sets of symptoms.

The study is, thus, only the first in the series of studies that are necessary to bring clarity to this confusing area. Of greatest importance is determining whether characterizing patients as having one condition or another will improve our ability to make firm predictions regarding heredity, natural history, or responses to treatment, and will help identify causes. Until then, all such categories can be considered only tentative.

Antipsychotic Medication

The most dramatic results in the use of medication in schizophrenia occur with acute schizophrenics, patients with a good prognosis who are likely to recover spontaneously within weeks or months. During the active phase of their illness, these patients are often panicky, agitated, frenetically restless, delusional, and hallucinated. They often need and tolerate doses of antipsychotic drugs up to ten times the amount needed to ameliorate the symptoms of chronic schizophrenics. With the medication, the patients' agitation and delusions may be eliminated in a matter of a few days and the natural course of the illness aborted.

Antipsychotic medications also affect favorably other symptoms of acute schizophrenic patients, such as torpor, perplexity, and withdrawal. Like electroshock treatment for depression, they abbreviate and mitigate an illness in which spontaneous recovery might be a prolonged and agonizing process.

The use of antipsychotic agents has made it possible for hospitals to become havens rather than prisons. Before the introduction of the antipsychotics, excited patients often had to be treated with physical restraints such as straitjackets or solitary confinement in padded rooms, or given prolonged warm or cold sedating baths (hydrotherapy) to prevent exhaustion or harm to themselves or their nurses. The frenetic activity, sleeplessness, and loss of appetite of some acutely schizophrenic patients impaired their physical health and in some instances caused death. Acutely agitated, delusional patients would sometimes attempt to hurt others, mutilate themselves (cutting, burning, blinding, castrating), or commit suicide.

Antipsychotic drug treatment has not only largely eliminated these dangers but, by drastically shortening the duration of the illness, often permits the patient to return to the community after a hospitalization of weeks rather than months. In such instances, the psychiatrist must consider the possible deleterious effect of returning the patient so quickly to an environment that may have contributed to the eruption of the psychotic episode. Psychotherapy may play a role in the exploration of such issues.

Although antipsychotic medication cuts schizophrenic episodes short, it does not cure the illness. Unless the medication is continued for several months, the patient often relapses. In many instances, the medicine can be discontinued after several months and there is no immediate reappearance of schizophrenic symptoms. The question of long-term antipsychotic treatment is discussed in the section on chronic schizophrenia.

There are no extensive systematic studies of the usefulness of antipsychotic medication in borderline schizophrenia. As mentioned, affectively vulnerable borderlines (emotionally unstable character disorders and hysteroid dysphorics) seem to have patterns of responsiveness to drugs other than antipsychotics. There is some anecdotal clinical evidence that the schizoid-eccentric borderlines may benefit from medications when their chronic pattern has been interrupted by an emotional upset. When depressed, they sometimes respond to antidepressant medications—although they sometimes get worse—and when agitated, they are often calmed by antipsychotic drugs. In either event, the effects of medication are limited. Medication generally returns such patients to their previous state of being undepressed, unagitated, and eccentric; it does not eliminate the underlying problem.

In the treatment of the chronic psychotic, antipsychotic medication has in some respects produced vast changes and in other ways has been a disappointment. It has been most strikingly useful in eliminating the so-called positive symptoms. For example, often delusions and hallucinations abate and sometimes cease altogether. Agitation, assaultiveness, hyperactivity, and grossly confused thought often improve appreciably. In some instances, negative symptoms such as apathy and withdrawal are also lessened, suggesting that they stem from inhibitions rather than defects. A very few patients show dramatic improvement, but most tend to retain their negative symptoms. In a sense, the medication turns the chronic schizophrenic into a borderline schizophrenic.

Apathy, lack of will, lack of social judgment, inability to experience pleasure, mild confusion of thought, all tend to remain. Because the patently mad individual can be changed into a less disturbed person, the benefit to both society and the patient is considerable, but many problems persist. With medication, the back wards of state hospitals have been transformed from snake pits into fourth-class residential hotels. With the help of medication, many chronic schizophrenic patients can be discharged to the community, since they are no longer affronts to public decency, but their social functioning often remains marginal and parasitic rather than self-supporting. Patients returned to their families often still function socially at a lower level than before they became ill. At times the return to the family is a difficult, distressing experience for everyone.

With increased release of patients to the community, it soon became evident that to remain outside the hospital, most chronic schizophrenics require maintenance medication. However, many medications have annoying side effects—for example, greater susceptibility to sunburn, to a stuffy nose, and to uncomfortably low blood pressure. Further, many patients stop taking medication and relapse, resulting in recurrent cycles of hospitalization, medication, and discharge.

Recently, a technological improvement has come to the aid of the patient and the community in at least one respect. Some of the new chemical relatives of one of the medications, chlorpromazine, are so potent that it is now possible to inject the patient with an amount sufficient to be slowly released into the blood stream over the course of a month. Thus, monthly visits to a mental-health clinic can supply the chronic schizophrenic patient with the needed medication. However, many patients refuse to attend clinics.

Other problems have emerged. Twenty years after the introduction of antipsychotic drugs, it began to be apparent that those which were administered in large amounts on a long-term basis were producing unwanted effects. At first a few case reports appeared, then more instances of a neurological disorder called tardive dyskinesia. Afflicted patients begin to develop involuntary movements of the tongue, cheeks, mouth, and lips. These movements can be stopped by great effort, but as soon as the patient gives up his efforts at self-control, they recur.

Paradoxically, discontinuing the antipsychotic medication makes the movements worse; they can be temporarily stayed by increasing the dose. If the tardive dyskinesia again appears, medication must be increased still further, and so forth. The majority of patients escape tardive dyskinesia, but the disorder obviously constitutes a bind for both patient and physician. Without medication, many patients are doomed to a psychotic, institutionalized existence. With medication, patients run the risk of developing a major and at times incapacitating physical illness.

What psychiatrists have done is to temporize. Once symptoms are controlled, they tend to lower the dose of antipsychotic medication to the lowest level possible and to give frequent "drug holidays" to see if the psychotic process might have spontaneously disappeared. Recent work indicates that if tardive dyskinesia is diagnosed early it may not be irreversible.

The story is different for acute schizophrenic patients. After recovery, some continue to do well without medication. However, a recent study indicates that even the relapse rate among acute schizophrenics can be reduced by medication. Further research is required to distinguish patients who will benefit from the continuing use of medication and those who will not.

The so-called megavitamin therapy, which has had considerable publicity, has never been proven to work. On the basis of unconfirmed observations, some psychiatric researchers hypothesized that the supposed metabolic abnormalities in schizophrenia might be circumvented by treatment with large doses of vitamins. The initial vitamin tried was niacin, although other vitamins have been also been tried. The proponents of niacin therapy used doses of 2,000 to 30,000 mg. or more per day. The presumed mean daily requirement is 10–30 mg. per day. Controlled drug studies have failed to show that niacin shortens the hospital stay, produces quicker discharge, or diminishes schizophrenic symptoms. In the absence of positive evidence, megavitamin therapists have recommended still larger doses, combined with electroconvulsive therapy, antipsychotics, and fasting.

It may be that a small number of schizophrenic patients have improved while on large doses of vitamins. To document the effectiveness of the vitamins, however, would require measuring the condition of such rare patients while they were alternately shifted between megavitamin therapy and placebo therapy. This has not yet been done. Further, although water-soluble vitamins such as niacin are rapidly excreted from the body when given in excess, they may still produce some toxicity. Large doses of niacin given for long periods of time may produce reversible biochemical changes in the liver and in skin pigmentation. The fact that vitamins are natural, unlike the antipsychotics, is not an argument for their safety.

Thus, drug treatment of the schizophrenias has its limitations. For the acute schizophrenic, drug treatment offers appreciable benefit at an undetermined cost. At best, it will enable him or her to function almost entirely intact. Medication may also enable the chronic schizophrenic to live as a dependent borderline schizophrenic. Often, maintenance dosage can be low and interrupted, so the increased risk may be small.

We see in all the mental illnesses—disorders of mood, personality disorders, and the schizophrenias—evidence of the interweaving of various degrees of biological vulnerability and particular life experiences.

In addition to the obvious handicaps and interpersonal frictions produced by specific symptoms, many of the severe mental illnesses can also result in a chronic demoralization, which we shall discuss in Chapter 7. Further, mental illness can impel the patient unconsciously to adopt a desperate invalidism—an attempt to compensate for the illness, to derive some benefit from it, by inducing those close to him to increase their attentions out of pity or guilt. Despite improvement in the illness, the invalidism can linger because of the independent rewards it has brought the patient.

In the twentieth century there have been two great intellectual and therapeutic movements to attempt to counteract the compounded wretchedness produced by mental illness. One of them, comprising the accumulated versions of psychodynamic theory, is now undergoing reappraisal as its limitations become apparent. The second—the renewed interest in organic causation and treatment—is becoming more prominent.

CHAPTER 4

An Intellectual Turning Point: The Drug Discoveries

The syndromes described in the previous chapter have been a source of agony, frustration, fear, and bafflement to victims, healers, and society for millennia. In attempting to ameliorate and control the symptoms, various societies have tried punishment, torture, incantations, imprisonment, exotic potions, isolation, nonchalant acceptance, contempt, ridicule, pity, ostracism, surgery and other drastic physical approaches, exhortation, straitjackets, kindness, exorcism, hypnotism, and sedation. Occasionally, societies have followed bizarrely afflicted persons as leaders, or even worshipped them. Rarely have any of these procedures or attitudes benefited either the sufferers or society.

It is therefore not surprising that Freud's conceptualizations, though complex and startling, were eagerly adopted by some workers in the field of mental illness. Here at last was the answer—an explanation for the heretofore inexplicable.

Although a substantial portion of both psychiatrists and the general public remained unpersuaded by the tenets of Freudian theory, by the mid-twentieth century techniques emerging from psychodynamic theory dominated the treatment of the mentally ill. At the same time, large pockets of disappointment and disillusionment with the results had developed. Countless patients and families were bewildered, distraught, or indignant when months and years of treatment brought little or no change. Many practitioners, too, who kept mental or actual tallies of their own successes were jolted by the discrepancy between the glowing prospects forecast by their mentors and the frequent stalemates encountered in their offices.

When in the mid-fifties the news of dramatic changes wrought in severely ill patients by new medications began to spread, many psychiatrists suddenly saw tangible evidence consistent with their mounting doubts about psychogenic and psychodynamic theory. Since then, hospital practices, training programs, and journal contents have increasingly reflected an intellectual turning point. The field of psychiatry is in the process of changing direction.

Serendipity is "the faculty of making happy and unexpected discoveries by accident." Much scientific discovery depends upon an initial chance observation, which is then succeeded by systematic observation that results in the detection of patterns of occurrence, the formulation of general predictive statements, and the development of experimental tests of these beliefs.

What differentiates science from common sense and speculation is the testing of hypothetical generalizations to see if they hold true as postulated. A real scientific hypothesis leads with its chin. It *must* make predictions that are capable of disproof. Anyone can invent a theory to account for all hitherto observed facts (e.g., the Ptolemaic theory that the sun went around the earth); a good theory, however, makes predictions about things not yet observed, and the observation of those things may disprove it.

One sometimes sees statements labeled as scientific which do not seem to be susceptible to proof or disproof—such as the idea that every thought is completely determined by psychological processes. Such statements are actually not scientific at all. They can sometimes stimulate scientists to investigate testable proposals, but the initial statements themselves must be distinguished from science.

In well-developed sciences, such as physics, completely new phenomena can be predicted theoretically before being observed. The atomic bomb, for instance, was constructed on the basis of hypotheses stemming from theoretical chemistry and physics in conjunction with the observation of nuclear fission. In relatively undeveloped sciences, such as medicine, psychiatry, and brain physiology, striking new advances have always occurred on the basis of accidental observation. We know too little about how the brain functions to predict in advance new ways of treating emotionally sick people. The ways in which the new psychiatric drugs and other somatic treatments have been discovered indicate our continued need for good, surprising observations.

Malaria and Paresis

The first effective organic treatment for mental illness was the malaria treatment for general paresis (syphilis of the brain) introduced by Julius von Wagner-Jauregg (like Freud, a Viennese) in 1917. This daring treatment emerged from the observation that some psychotic patients improved dramatically when they had a sudden fever. Many attempts were made to produce a fever—for example, by means of typhoid vaccine. Eventually, malaria seemed a good possibility because it could be controlled by quinine.

Researchers hoped that all forms of psychosis could be cured with this treatment, but only brain syphilis responded. Schizophrenia and the affective psychoses remained untreatable. Yet, because paresis was responsible for a high proportion of the admissions to mental hospitals (almost a third in some localities), malaria treatment was a great advance and was used until penicillin was developed. Wagner-Jauregg is the only psychiatrist who has won the Nobel Prize, though the recent changes in psychiatry are nicely illustrated by the award of a Nobel Prize in 1970 to Julius Axelrod, a biochemist at the National Institute of Mental Health.

Insulin Coma

Physical treatment of the schizophrenias has a long but only recently distinguished history. In various times and places the mad have been bled, purged, rotated, submerged, partially poisoned, had their colons removed, and been given a pharmacopeia full of ineffective medicines. In the latter part of the nineteenth and the early part of the twentieth century, standard sedative drugs were employed in the treatment of schizophrenic patients. These drugs, such as the barbiturates and opiate narcotics, did quiet agitated patients but did not counteract the patient's psychotic symptoms. Further, the doses necessary to afford partial control were dangerously high, threatening severe physiological dysfunction or death.

In 1922 the hormone insulin was first used in the treatment of diabetes. Six years later, another Viennese physician, Manfred Sakel, found that the administration of insulin relieved the excitement seen in morphine withdrawal. The effect was not the result of any specific curative properties of insulin for morphine addiction but was simply the manifestation of decreased brain activity in response to lowered blood sugar.

Since some acutely ill schizophrenic patients are similarly excited,

Sakel reasoned that insulin might be of use in their treatment. He further believed that insulin was most effective when given in amounts that would result in a comatose state—a state of deep unconsciousness in which even reflex responses are absent. This treatment was laborious and also dangerous because prolonged coma might result in death. Patients in early stages of schizophrenia appeared to recover more rapidly and perhaps in a greater proportion than before, but some studies suggest that insulin treatment was no more effective than a placebo. The efficacy of this treatment will never be known, because it has been replaced by other, safer therapies.

Convulsive Therapy

A still clearer demonstration of the shaky basis on which psychiatric therapeutic advances are made was the incorrect belief held during the 1930s that schizophrenia and epilepsy were antagonistic diseases—that is, it was believed that anyone who had epilepsy couldn't get schizophrenia. The claim had been made that some mental patients who developed spontaneous epileptic fits improved. For these reasons, Ladislas von Meduna, a Hungarian psychiatrist, induced convulsions in schizophrenics by injecting the drug Metrazol. Such treatment is now generally considered effective only rarely in schizophrenics but, strange to say, of value for the severely depressed patient. These early observations led to the use of electricity, rather than an unreliable drug, to provoke epileptic-like fits. Electroconvulsive therapy (ECT), also called electroshock or shock therapy, is still an effective treatment for many depressive patients who do not respond to medication.

But the efficacy of electroconvulsive therapy in schizophrenia (as with insulin shock therapy) has not and probably never will be fully evaluated. Controlled studies by Philip May (1968) indicate that when used as a primary treatment its effectiveness is somewhere between that of ineffectual psychotherapy and that of effective antipsychotic drugs. Some schizophrenics, partially refractory to drugs, derive further benefit from electroshock therapy.

It is worth dwelling on the benefits and hazards of ECT because the technique has had a bad press in the last few years. Objections to ECT seem to come primarily from concern about side effects, but the idea has also been voiced that ECT is used as a punitive measure to control deviant behavior. The failure to recognize that ECT is a medical measure for the reversal of serious, often life-threatening, psychopathology goes hand in hand with the belief that aberrant behavior is really a sane response to an insane political and social system. According to this belief, since there is no mental illness, all treatment is only psychological or behavioral management, and ECT is a particularly punitive form of such management. Ken Kesey's *One Flew over the Cuckoo's Nest* epitomizes this point of view.

Concern about immediate and long-term side effects of ECT arose from several sources. During the 1940s, the violent convulsions produced were sometimes sufficient to break bones. This danger has now been eliminated by the use of drugs that markedly diminish the intensity of the muscular contractions. The other concerns were over psychological effects: the anxiety induced by the procedure, the amnesia that the patient experienced for varying periods of time following ECT, and the long-term possibility of changes in psychological functioning as a result of possible brain changes.

The anticipatory anxiety has been eliminated by the use of brief anesthesia. The patient is put to sleep, given a muscular relaxant, and only then administered electroshock therapy. It has been common for the patient having ECT treatment to develop amnesia for several weeks for events preceding the electroshock therapy. Recently, however, these effects on memory have been diminished by supplying current to only one side of the brain—the nondominant side (usually the right side in right-handed people). The dominant side mediates speech and language; the nondominant side seems related to the perception of nonlinguistic images. This unilateral shock treatment is thus not only of practical importance but also of considerable theoretical value in terms of brain function.

The most critical concern regarding ECT is whether the treatment produces damage to the brain. So far as is known, when ECT is used in moderate amounts (e.g., three times a week for several weeks), no such changes are produced. It is possible that overvigorous treatment with early forms of ECT in which insufficient oxygen was supplied may have produced some enduring, minor forms of brain damage, but clear-cut evidence is lacking.

No satisfactory explanation for the effectiveness of ECT, either physiological or psychological, has yet been advanced. It remains clearly useful for severe, vital depression and less clearly useful for schizophrenia.

In the case of ECT, an erroneous clinical observation led to an incorrect theory, which led to the development of a treatment for the wrong group of psychiatrically ill patients (schizophrenics) but eventually was of great value for patients with severe mood disorders. Certainly, this is not a neat progression whereby useful treatments are derived from our deep understanding of the nature of mental illness.

If anything, the reverse is often true, since treatments based on our primitive organic theories of illness often prove ineffective.

For example, von Meduna proposed a theory of neurotic illness suggesting that the inhalation of carbon dioxide, producing various degrees of unconsciousness, would be beneficial to anxious patients. He became convinced of its efficacy and presented his procedure as a great advance. But general experience, and some experimentation, showed that the treatment was of no value. One must be wary of applying doubtful theory to practical matters in areas where we are still extremely ignorant. This applies to both psychological and physiological theory. Tentative application under rigid self-critical experimental scrutiny makes sense. Unfortunately, there is nothing so upsetting as a beautiful theory ruined by a grubby fact; and the theoretically convinced often have difficulty recognizing factual failures.

Stimulants

The discovery of the stimulant drug amphetamine stemmed from an attempt to find a new treatment for asthma. A modern Chinese pharmacologist had noted that ancient Chinese medical tradition prescribed a certain plant for treatment of this disease. Chemical analysis of the plant and subsequent testing showed that a compound within it, ephedrine, was indeed effective with asthmatics. Interestingly, ephedrine is closely related chemically to adrenaline, the naturally occurring hormone released during stress and anxiety. In an attempt to find a synthetic substitute for ephedrine, amphetamine was produced in the early 1930s. Tests revealed that it was an appetite suppressant, a powerful antifatigue drug, and a mood elevator. Amphetamines have been used successfully in treating hyperactive children and are being tested with hyperactive adults; other uses of amphetamine will be discussed later.

Major Tranquilizers (Antipsychotic Medications)

In the 1950s, two new classes of drugs revolutionized the treatment of schizophrenia—reserpine and the phenothiazines. These drugs are referred to as major tranquilizers, neuroleptics, or, most accurately, antipsychotic medications.

The first class of drugs, embarrassingly enough, came from Western recognition of *Rauwolfia serpentina,* a plant used by physicians in India for centuries. Thirty years ago, extracts of this plant and its pure chemical constituents were used in the treatment of excited psychotic patients. Unlike sedatives, *reserpine* induced calmness without producing confusion, disorientation, or sleep. This led to a tremendous burst of activity as investigators combed through numerous types of plants in a search for active medications—a task that primitive peoples had probably done for us already. The only important natural psychoactive compounds we have discovered had been noticed by indigenous peoples long ago—for instance, psilocybin (found in the sacred mushrooms worshipped by Central American Indians), alcohol, and opium. Reserpine was almost immediately replaced by an even more effective class of drugs—the phenothiazine antipsychotics.

Reserpine has also played a serendipitous role in the expansion of knowledge of brain chemistry, which also will be described later.

The discovery of the *phenothiazines* was pure accident. Chlorpromazine, the first such agent, was synthesized by a French pharmaceutical firm in response to a request by surgeon H. M. Laborit for a better antihistamine to be used as a surgical premedication. Laborit noticed its ability to quiet patients without producing either sleep or the kind of intoxication that often occurs with sleeping-pill pre-operative medication, and called this to the attention of a team of French psychiatrists, Jean Delay and Pierre Deniker, as a possible agent for the treatment of agitated schizophrenic patients. Delay and Deniker, to their amazement, found that it not only sedated their patients but resulted in the disappearance of the patients' irrational beliefs and horrifying sensory experiences. These drugs became known as major tranquilizers, but this is an unfortunate term since they are often very useful in activating to normal behavior patients who are quiet, perplexed, slowed down, and difficult to motivate. Further, the term "major tranquilizers" has obscured the fact that they are antipsychotics and has led some people mistakenly to assume that they might be more powerful agents for mild anxiety.

Because agitated schizophrenics occupied almost half of the inpatient psychiatric beds and had proven refractory to most treatments, there was great interest in determining whether the drugs were as promising as they seemed. Within a few years, many studies throughout the world clearly demonstrated that the drugs were not simply superior sedatives but also had a markedly beneficial effect upon the strange perceptual and conceptual distortions of psychotic patients.

One of us (Klein) was working at the U.S. Public Health Service Narcotics Hospital in Lexington, Kentucky, in 1954, when chlorpromazine was first being investigated in the United States. Two vivid memories of this period haunt him.

At the time, it was thought that all medications probably acted by reducing anxiety. This was the common explanation then for addiction to morphine and for alcoholism. There were, however, obvious inconsistencies in the explanation, since addicts who have been taken off opiates for some weeks or alcoholics who have been dried out, do not appear unusually anxious and, as a matter of fact, often seem to be pleasant, friendly folks.

Since it was believed that morphine addicts were treating themselves for anxiety and that chlorpromazine's effectiveness with psychotics was due to a similar reduction of anxiety, researchers at the Lexington hospital thought chlorpromazine might work with morphine addicts. This idea was further supported by some animal experiments that seemed to indicate—if looked at from some distance, while standing on your head, with one eye closed—that morphine and chlorpromazine might have similar physiological effects. The researchers approached several of the morphine addicts who had been withdrawn from drugs and asked if they would participate in the evaluation of the effect of the new tranquilizer. The patients agreed and under close observation were injected with chlorpromazine. Instead of the expected burst of relief from anxiety, the patients lay around on their cots looking stoned. That was a good sign, however, because morphine or heroin injections produced the same effect. The hypothesis that chlorpromazine produced a euphoric relief of anxiety was soon shattered when Klein questioned one of the subjects.

"How's it going?" he said in his best nondirective fashion.

"Doc," replied the junkie, "I don't know what that shit is, but it'll never sell."

Of course, he was quite right. It never did sell on the street.

About a year later, Klein was placed in charge of a ward of World War I veterans who had had the unenviable lot of being hospitalized for some thirty consecutive years. They had been given excellent nursing care and had been exposed to a wide variety of group and vocational therapies. Nevertheless, they sat quietly all day on benches, staring blankly at the walls.

Klein and his colleagues had received a supply of chlorpromazine for experimental use and timidly placed a number of these chronically impaired patients on what we now know were microscopic doses, with little expectation that anything useful would happen. Some weeks later, one of the patients came up to Klein in the hall and said, "Doc, when am I getting out of here?" Like Rip Van Winkle awakening from his long sleep, the patient didn't know where he was, how he had gotten there, or what had happened for the past thirty years. He knew nothing about the Depression, World War II, penicillin, or the atomic bomb, He didn't know that he had been in a hospital or that he was in Kentucky. He had spent thirty years essentially out of contact with reality.

Shortly thereafter, to Klein's astonishment, another patient showed the same incredible reconstitution. The patients' outlook had been unbelievably changed, and so had Klein's. It isn't every day that one sees an authentic miracle.

Minor Tranquilizers

To confuse matters further, another group of compounds being developed and marketed at about the same time were also called tranquilizers, though they had entirely different effects. The first of these agents was the familiar Miltown, whose quieting effects, predictably, were first noted during a search for an antibiotic. This drug was soon followed by a new class of drugs called the benzodiazepines, of which the outstanding members are Librium and Valium. These agents were more effective than Miltown and less likely to produce drug dependence. They were fairly effective in the treatment of chronic, free-floating anxiety but of no value in the treatment of severe illnesses such as the psychoses. As we've indicated, the fact that they are called tranquilizers has caused them to be confused with antipsychotic agents such as chlorpromazine. Of late, the term "major tranquilizer" has been partially replaced by the term "antipsychotic" and the anti-anxiety compounds are often referred to as "minor tranquilizers."

The Search for Better Antipsychotics

Because of the tremendous demand for effective antipsychotic agents, the discovery of the phenothiazines was a golden opportunity for the pharmaceutical industry. Hoping that a modified version of chlorpromazine might be more effective and have fewer side effects (see Appendix), the industry's biochemists immediately began making all sorts of minor changes in the chemical structure of the drug.

There is as yet no good theory that relates the chemical structure of antipsychotic medications to their functioning, and thus all such experimentation with molecular structure must be done on a trial-and-error basis. The new chemicals are produced and then tested on animals. If no adverse reactions appear, and the animals show the desired physical responses, the agents are cautiously tried with normal human volunteers. If the drugs seem harmless or the degree of side effects is tolerable, one can then try them on a group of sick patients. Even if no better than the parent drug, a drug as good as the parent drug (often referred to as a "me too" drug) might give a pharmaceutical company a patentable entry into the profitable tranquilizer or antipsychotic market.

Despite twenty years of active work, however, the search for increased efficacy has been a failure. Dozens of drugs as effective as chlorpromazine have been synthesized, but none better. The related compounds often cause appreciably different side effects, and many of them are more potent per unit dose weight, but these qualities are not of great practical importance.

Occasionally, the industry has found drugs with altogether different beneficial effects than those expected. That was the way in which the antidepressants were discovered.

Antidepressants

Tricyclics. In the mid-1950s, a Swiss pharmaceutical firm made minor modifications in the chlorpromazine molecule and found that the new compound, Tofranil (imipramine), was well tolerated and seemed to affect animals in much the same way that chlorpromazine did. Hopeful that they might have produced another important antipsychotic, the firm arranged with a German psychiatrist, Roland Kuhn, to try the medication on a group of chronically ill schizophrenic patients. Kuhn reported that the medication seemed of little benefit for delusions and hallucinations. However, he noted astutely that a number of the patients who had also been severely depressed were less so after having imipramine. Kuhn then tried imipramine in psychiatric patients whose predominant symptoms consisted of depression and who were not out of contact with reality, and found that imipramine was indeed effective in the treatment of severe depression. Soon after, numerous drugs with a similar structure were also found to be effective antidepressants.

The extraordinary, baffling discovery that a drug similar to the major tranquilizers produced a normalization of mood in severely depressed patients again led to tremendous interest. Depressed patients made up a considerable part of the inpatient hospital population, and even more of the outpatient load of every general psychiatrist. There have been estimates that 20 percent of the general population may suffer at least one major depression during their lifetime. A substantial proportion of this group will suffer repeated depressions. Such patients have been difficult to treat, even though one can be reasonably confident that their depression will eventually disappear. Without drugs, spontaneous recovery can be very slow, and there is always the threat of suicide.

Although psychotherapy had not been demonstrated to be particularly effective in the treatment of severe depression, many psychiatrists were convinced that even severe depressions were due to psychological conflicts dating from infancy and childhood, often involving guilt and hostility. The efficacy of the antidepressants in reversing depressed mood called into question the reasonableness of attributing these illnesses to psychological conflicts.

Hitherto, the only fairly reliable method of treatment for severe depression had been electroconvulsive therapy. Although one would think that a convulsive treatment would probably be effective for physiological reasons, some psychiatrists theorized that the convulsion had a disorienting effect that temporarily overrode the psychological factors, or that electroconvulsive therapy was experienced by patients as justified punishment, which alleviated their guilt and therefore their depression. Although obviously nonsense, the theory about guilt was seriously propounded and uncritically accepted by many therapists, despite growing evidence that the behavior changes were in reaction to induced brain changes. In a 1958 study, for example, Max Fink and his colleagues compared patients who had been administered standard convulsive electroshock therapy while unconscious with patients who had been administered subconvulsive electroshock therapy, also while unconscious. Although both groups of patients had the same subjective experience, only the first group showed any substantial benefits. Changes in behavior were correlated with the extent of induced changes in brain activity, as measured by the electroencephalogram.

Evidence of this kind, plus the discovery of antidepressant effects of pills, which are hardly punitive, and which scientific tests showed could not be attributed to suggestion, finally undermined the monopolistic hold on American psychiatry of theories of psychological causation.

Monoamine oxidase (MAO) inhibitors. The MAO inhibitors were also first tried in chronic schizophrenics, after reports that the antibiotic iproniazid, tested unsuccessfully in the treatment of tuberculosis, caused high spirits among depressed tubercular patients. By a process of trial and error, the drug was first used on schizophrenics and then on depressives. Its initial success as an antidepressant met a setback when it was found to be associated with occasional liver damage.

Pharmacologists discovered that the drug inhibited the brain enzyme monoamine oxidase, and began the search for a less harmful drug with this effect. (In Chapter 6, we will review how this effect was understood to benefit depression.)

Many such drugs, some useful and many worthless, have now been found and tested. One of them, the popular medication Parnate, was first developed in an attempt to perfect a new form of nose drops. Since many drugs that inhibit MAO are ineffective antidepressants, theories about the influence of this enzyme in depression are highly tentative.

Lithium

The value of lithium was also discovered by accident. This chemical element is closely related to sodium and potassium, which are the most common metals occurring in the body's cells and fluids, as components of dissolved salts. The close similarity of lithium to sodium accounted for its first use in medicine. Excessive sodium intake in the form of common table salt (sodium chloride) is harmful in certain forms of high blood pressure and heart disease. In the 1940s, an attempt was made to use lithium chloride as a similar-tasting, presumably harmless substitute for salt for people with these diseases. However, lithium is toxic in large amounts and thus constituted a very poor salt substitute, especially for people with impaired heart and kidney function. That first attempt left many doctors fearful of using lithium as medication.

Later in the 1940s, while experimenting on the effects of the urine of manic patients on animals, John Cade administered lithium to guinea pigs in an attempt to reduce the toxic effects of the urea. He noticed that the guinea pigs were quieted by lithium, and in a remarkable inductive leap, lithium was tried as a sedative in excited psychiatric patients. This is probably one more example of coming to the right conclusion for the wrong reasons. It is quite possible that the guinea pigs weren't tranquilized by the lithium but had received an overdose and were immobilized by nausea or weakness.

Carefully regulated within narrow limits because of its toxicity, lithium quieted manic patients in one to three weeks. The effect was not simply that of ordinary sedation but also frequently seemed to normalize the patients—reducing their excitement, slowing their overactive thinking, and decreasing their impulsivity, all without putting them to sleep. In succeeding years, systematic trials were conducted with lithium in the treatment of mania, and it was found to be approximately as effective as the antipsychotic drugs in moderate mania, without many of the unpleasant side effects.

Buoyed by their success with lithium and aware that manic illnesses frequently recur, researchers decided to administer it not only when the patient was suffering from the illness but also after she had recovered. Remarkably, the recurrence of manic illnesses was greatly reduced. Lithium had not only reduced the symptoms but had prevented them from returning. This was an exciting discovery because heretofore no drug had succeeded in preventing the recurrence of psychiatric illness. Since then, it has been consistently found that antipsychotics prevent the recurrence of schizophrenic episodes. Similarly, the continued administration of antidepressant medication during periods in which the patient is symptom-free may also prevent or reduce the frequency of attacks of depressive illness.

In the course of these studies, it was found that lithium produced yet another important unpredicted effect. In manic patients who also suffered from depressive periods—patients with bipolar mood disorders—lithium reduced the frequency of recurrent depressive attacks as well as manic episodes. It acted as a mood stabilizer in both directions, preventing low as well as high swings.

Preliminary experimental information indicates that lithium is also sometimes useful in preventing recurrent unipolar depressions—that is, in patients who have never been manic. Since these are far more common than bipolar disorders, its effectiveness here would be of great importance.

The full scope of lithium's usefulness remains to be determined. Preliminary evidence indicates that it may be useful in the explosive personalities who have periodic outbreaks of violent behavior—for example, controlled studies of lithium use with violent prisoners show some decrease in outbursts of temper and rage. As discussed earlier, it may also be an effective treatment for emotionally unstable character disorders.

Risks versus Benefits of Drug Treatment

Since psychotherapeutic drugs can sometimes have serious side effects, and overdose of some agents is potentially lethal, the question arises whether the benefits outweigh the risks. One way in which such a question can be answered is by the assessment of the relative mortality and morbidity associated with antidepressants and depressive disorders. Since there is little systematic data, such an assessment must be an educated guess; nonetheless, it is illuminating (Klein et al., 1980, pp. 409–11).

One estimate holds that 15 percent of persons with primary affective disorder (such as depression) die by suicide. An extension of this estimate in terms of the usual course of the illness leads to the conjecture that there may be ten thousand suicides for every million untreated episodes of the illness.

In contrast, deaths from antidepressant medication vary roughly from around twenty or thirty to around 170 per million episodes of the illness. Although these figures are gross approximations, it is obvious that the mortality from untreated affective disease vastly exceeds that from drug administration. Similarly, drug treatment often reduces the length of depressive episodes from many months (eight to seventeen) to six to eight weeks. There is no evidence concerning the utility of psychotherapy in the prevention of suicide. For individuals with serious depression, therefore, psychotherapy might not only be ineffectual but may prevent the patient from obtaining effective treatment for a dangerous disease.

Many treatments that are often considered useful when first used eventually prove worthless or even harmful. For that reason, it would be a mistake simply to accept a testimonial that any particular therapy is effective. Of course, this applies to all treatments. During the past thirty years, a well-defined method for assessing the efficacy of medications has been developed. The point is to show that all alternative explanations for the apparent effectiveness do not hold true, and therefore the benefits must be due to the effects of a specific drug. What alternative possibilities are there?

Sick people often get better even when given ineffective treatment. Why should this be so? The two major reasons are spontaneous recovery and the anti-demoralizing benefits of being in a hope-stimulating treatment situation. It is common knowledge that many illnesses are self-limited and certainly many psychiatric illnesses wax and wane. If you simply took a group of sick people and gave them all a pill, some would be bound to get better over a period of time. Could one attribute this improvement to the medication? Certainly not, because they might have gotten better anyway.

The reasonable procedure is to divide the patients into two groups; one gets the treatment and the other does not. In this way, you can control for the effects of spontaneous recovery, since the group that doesn't get any specific treatment will furnish a standard for what can be expected in the way of spontaneous recovery. If the treatment is useful, the treated group should have a clearly higher recovery or improvement rate.

Patients may, however, respond positively to the mere belief that they are receiving treatment. If we gave pills to one group, but not to the other, the group that received the pills might do better simply because they think they are getting help, without any actual specific benefit from the medication. Modern medication research has dealt with this problem, seeing to it that both groups receive everything, except the specific treatment, in an identical way. Both groups should get the same amount of attention and both groups should receive pills. If there is a standard medication and the question is whether a new medication is superior, then one group should receive the standard medication and the other the new medication, in identical form. If there is no well-demonstrated standard medication and the question is whether the new medication can improve over the spontaneous-improvement rate, then one group should get an inactive identical-appearing pill (referred to as a placebo) and the other group should get the experimental medication.

There are two additional scientific requirements to make sure the treatment is properly tested. One is that the two groups do not differ substantially from each other. If it were up to the doctor to choose which persons would go into which group, and the doctor believed that the new drug was likely to be helpful, he might then assign the sickest patients to the drug-treatment group and the most healthy patients to the placebo-treatment group. Under these circumstances, there would be a bias against showing that the drug was effective. Patients must be assigned to each group by a random process.

Since the effect of the drug will be evaluated both by the patient and by an evaluator, if either knew whether the patient was receiving a real drug or a placebo, his perceptions and reports might well be affected. Neither the patient nor the evaluator can know whether the patient is receiving an experimental medication, a standard medication, or a placebo. This procedure is referred to as double-blinding.

To sum up, the standard form of new-drug evaluation entails a controlled, double-blind study in which placebos or standard medication are assigned at random. Under these circumstances, if the actively treated patients do considerably better than the others, one can be almost positive that the benefit was due to the specific pharmacological effects of the drug and not to spontaneous recovery or the suggestive effects of being in treatment. If the study is then repeated several times with substantially the same result, one can be sure, as sure as one can be of anything, that the medication is specifically effective.

In any one study, unexpected chance fluctuations can produce startling data that lead to incorrect inferences. A single study should at best be considered stimulating and warrant further work, rather than definitive in any way. In one recent study, for instance, cognitive therapy was found superior to medication in the treatment of a scantily defined group of depressives. Numerous aspects of the study aroused skepticism, among them a strikingly low improvement rate in the pharmacotherapy group. Even if this study had been entirely convincing, however, the basis of scientific advance remains demonstration of the facts by repeated study.

What can be said about the value of the antipsychotic, antidepressant, anti-anxiety medication referred to in this book? During the past thirty years, thousands of studies have shown beyond any doubt the specific benefits of these agents. Most of the residual doubt does not concern whether they are effective but precisely what classes of patients will be helped. For instance, in a typical trial of an antidepressant it may be shown that 30 percent of the patients get better on a placebo but 70 percent get better on the medication. Although the medication has clearly been shown to be useful, further questions must be dealt with: Why did some of the patients not respond to the medication? Might they be suffering from an entirely different disease that only superficially resembles that of the other patients? Are they perhaps metabolizing the medicine in a different way, so that it is destroyed more quickly? Do the unresponsive patients have unusual sensitivities that may block the beneficial effects of the medication? Can we tell in advance who will benefit from this medication and who will not? Another group of questions revolves around the patients who got better on placebos. If we could predict who would get better on placebos, perhaps we could avoid drug treatment altogether for such people. Unfortunately, attempts to predict this have not been successful.

There have been an enormous number of studies of drug effectiveness. In a recent examination of the evidence with regard to a particular type of antidepressant, all the studies published from 1958 to 1972 that used a placebo control group, random assignment, and blind evaluations were summarized. There were ninety-three such studies, and in two-thirds of them the drugs were clearly effective. In no study was a placebo superior to drugs. It is not surprising, however, that drugs were not superior to placebos in all studies, because a variety of factors can cloud drug effectiveness even when it exists. Many of the earlier studies undoubtedly included poorly defined mixed groups, including patients who may not have required drug treatment but who were demoralized, unhappy, etc.

Studies may have demonstrated that psychiatric drugs are better than a placebo, but are they *much* better? It is conceivable that they are only slightly better, and therefore not really worth the bother and expense. A number of comparisons of psychiatric drugs with other standard drugs—such as antibiotics, antihypertensives, and drugs for the relief of various physical discomforts—show that psychiatric drugs work at a level of effectiveness quite comparable to and in some cases superior to usual medication.

It should be emphasized that drug-therapy studies have been the most extensive and most scientific of all examinations of the effects of therapies in psychiatry. Until recently, the various psychosocial therapies had been established entirely on the basis of clinical anecdote, without comparative studies of any sort and usually without any follow-up studies. More recently, there have been a number of comparisons of various forms of psychosocial treatment against no treatment at all. These studies often showed what seemed to be some benefit from the psychosocial treatment. It should be noted, however, that there was nothing analogous to a psychosocial placebo, so it remains entirely obscure whether the patients did better because of the specific effects of the treatment or because of the mere fact that they were in treatment.

Recently, some studies of psychosocial treatment have compared various forms of psychotherapy. If it was shown that one form of psychotherapy was clearly better than another, then you could make a fair inference that something beneficial was going on, over and beyond the mere fact of being in treatment. Both forms of psychotherapy would have to be believable to the patient and stir the patients' hopes, of course. But there are very few studies of this sort and, in fact, almost all such studies have not shown any distinctions between supposedly different psychotherapies. In Chapter 8, we will discuss in more detail the question of establishing the efficacy of psychotherapy. Here we simply wish to make the point that among the range of psychiatric treatments the drug therapies have the most solid scientific basis.

Drug Effects That Mimic Mental Illness

At approximately the same time that the powerful antipsychotic and antidepressant drugs were discovered, still another chemical family, the psychedelics, made their eventful appearance. Because of the role these agents have played in the social phenomena of the past twenty years, it may be difficult for some readers to understand the intellectual excitement with which they were greeted. First, they *seemed* to mimic accurately the symptoms seen in some schizophrenias. Their ingestion produced a rich pathological fare, including paranoid feelings, hallucinations, and sometimes delusions; but most important, in many instances—and in this they were different from previously known drugs

—the changes did not produce other gross disturbances of consciousness, such as not knowing where you were.

The production of psychosis by drugs was not new. Many drugs known for centuries produced psychosis, but with a clouding of consciousness. Such drugs—alcohol, ether, the barbiturates, and atropine, to name but a few—might produce hallucinations, delusions, and altered perception but simultaneously also caused confusion and disorientation. Atropine, an extract of deadly nightshade, has been employed at least since the Middle Ages for its psychedelic properties. At that time, it was used by witches' covens, perhaps because it sometimes produces the illusion of flying. Don Juan—the Yaqui Indian mystic described by Carlos Castaneda—also employed loco weed, which contains atropine, in order to produce the sensation of flying. But LSD and its relatives seemed to be able to imitate madness and yet leave the subject with sufficient clear consciousness to report with some reliability on the experience.

The second interesting attribute of this class of drugs is that many of them are effective in incredibly minuscule amounts. For example, a quart of vodka contains approximately 500 grams (i.e., about 16 ounces by weight) of 100 percent alcohol. This amount—if it didn't kill one—would produce a monumental drunk. By comparison, only 100 micrograms ($1/300,000$ of an ounce) of LSD are enough to produce spectacular effects. LSD, in other words, is approximately two and a half million times as potent as alcohol.

High potency was important because for years psychiatrists had toyed with the idea that mental derangement might be the result of the body's production of self-intoxicating substances. Obviously, the amounts of such substances couldn't be very large or they would have been readily detectable. Any self-poisoning would have to be caused by quantities so small as to elude measurement. The observation that tiny amounts of psychedelic agents could produce psychosis was, thus, encouraging to those who believed in auto-intoxication.

The third exciting feature of the psychedelics was that some seemed very similar chemically to substances occurring naturally in the body. Mescaline, the chemically active ingredient in peyote, the cactus button, bears a very close resemblance to norepinephrine (noradrenaline), a natural chemical in the brain. LSD has some close resemblances to serotonin, another compound active in the brain. It is general biological knowledge that manufactured partial copies of body chemicals sometimes mimic and sometimes prevent the effects of the substances they resemble.

Putting these three facts together, it was possible to hypothesize that the schizophrenic forms auto-intoxicants, that such intoxicants need be present in only minute amounts, and that they exaggerate or block the effects of brain chemicals necessary for normal functioning.

Two factual flies soon appeared in the theoretical ointment. First, psychiatrists observed that the symptoms of LSD intoxication did not fully mimic the symptoms of schizophrenia. Following LSD administration, the subject might experience intense visual perceptions, but they were not at all similar to the typical hallucinations of schizophrenia, which are almost always auditory, not visual. In addition, the advantageous clear consciousness also meant that the drugs did not induce the characteristically incoherent schizophrenic thought disorder, emotional withdrawal, and changed interpersonal behavior, although they did produce moments of delusional conviction.

Second, like alcohol abusers and heroin addicts, LSD users developed tolerance. A subject who takes LSD daily will become intoxicated for the first several days but toward the end of the week will have no drug response. This dealt a mortal blow to an auto-intoxication theory that depended on an LSD-like substance. Even if one's body was mistakenly manufacturing such a substance at a fast rate, it could not continuously poison the mind.

These difficulties, together with the fact that there is a faddish quality about the popularity of particular psychiatric theories, seemed to result in a decline of research interest in psychedelic agents. They are still, however, compounds with fascinating effects, and legitimate scientific experimentation would undoubtedly not have diminished as much as it did had it not been for governmental pressures provoked largely by reactions to the so-called counterculture. LSD was suddenly classified as a dangerous drug, and showing scientific interest in experimenting with LSD or similar compounds became professionally indiscreet. Hence there was comparatively little scientific protest when government officials made research on psychedelic drugs difficult. It was easier to ban new agents—whose chronic toxic properties are open to debate—than to eliminate the use of alcohol or tobacco. (The former is addicting in about 10 percent of users and is probably physiologically harmful to many of the non-addicts. The latter is now labeled as possibly harmful to your health. That is correct, and an absurdly inadequate statement of the possible risk.)

At about the time the psychedelic drugs were being introduced, a paradoxical discovery was made. Reserpine, one of the first antipsychotic drugs used with schizophrenics, was found to produce symptoms of mental disturbance in others. When reserpine was first used, it was confirmed that—as Indian physicians had maintained—it lowered blood pressure, and that it could do so in smaller doses than were necessary in treatment of psychosis. It became widely used as the first really effective agent in the treatment of hypertension, but approximately 5 percent of psychiatrically healthy individuals who had it developed vital depression, often of severe proportions. Such depressions often persisted after the drug was stopped and could be terminated only by electroshock treatment.

Two obvious questions arose. First, why did only some people become depressed with reserpine? One hypothesis—which has never been tested—is that only those persons who had a genetically transmitted predisposition to develop depression became ill. This could easily be tested by examining the family histories of those who did and did not become depressed when being administered reserpine. Those who became depressed would presumably have had close relatives (parents, brothers, sisters, or grandparents) who had developed spontaneous severe depression.

A second question was: What was reserpine doing to brain chemistry which might be related to depressions? When reserpine was administered to animals, it profoundly depleted the brain of the chemicals serotonin, dopamine, and norepinephrine—all known as monoamines. Nerve cells that used these chemicals to transmit impulses were rendered nonfunctional. It was reasoned that groups of nerve cells using one or more of these chemicals were necessary for the maintenance of normal mood, and that absence of these chemicals and the consequent failure of the nerve groups to function resulted in depression. This theory has generated a large body of experiments during the past twenty-five years, and we will speak of it in detail in Chapter 6.

One additional chemically produced mental illness is amphetamine psychosis. Since the end of World War II, amphetamines have been increasingly abused. These drugs, variously known as "ups," "meth," Dexedrine, and "speed," were first taken by mouth and then injected into veins for more pronounced effects. Abusers develop tolerance for them and must take increasingly larger doses. As amphetamine addicts—"speed freaks"—began to take larger and larger doses, a startling clinical phenomenon was noticed. Some abusers developed psychotic episodes virtually indistinguishable from some forms of schizophrenia. Unlike LSD psychoses, amphetamine psychoses tended to produce auditory, not visual, hallucinations, and paranoid hyperalertness. At times they were mistaken for paranoid schizophrenia, in which auditory hallucinations and delusions of grandiosity or persecution are prominent. By screening the urine of newly admitted patients for amphetamines, some hospitals have found that as many as 50 percent of the patients diagnosed as schizophrenic were really suffering from amphetamine psychosis.

From an experimental standpoint, this was a very useful discovery. Amphetamine was then administered to animals for the purpose of exploring its chemical effects in the brain. Prominent among its many effects was increasing activity in the portions of the brain that utilized dopamine and norepinephrine as their clinical messengers or neurotransmitters—a result that fits together with the reserpine findings.

The obvious next question was: If phenothiazines relieved the symptoms of schizophrenia, what would their effects be on amphetamine psychosis in man and amphetamine toxicity in animals? The ready answer was that they relieved psychosis in man and prevented the toxic effect of amphetamines in animals. From a knowledge of what amphetamine did to chemical transmitters and from the observation that phenothiazines blocked the effect of amphetamines, it was a reasonable hunch that phenothiazines blocked the action of dopamine or norepinephrine. The hunch was correct; its consequences will be elaborated in Chapter 6.

All three of the substances discussed here have thus yielded important scientific knowledge, and two of them are useful therapeutic agents. Yet in one way or another they create social problems—the use of new therapeutic substances with possible serious side effects, and the possibility of drug abuse. Society should weigh the possible advantages and disadvantages in deciding how such chemicals are to be used. Such rational social consideration is conspicuously absent.

In the case of many of the psychedelic drugs, chronic toxicity from mild to moderate use has never been clearly shown. Comparatively small amounts of LSD produce vivid ideas and the return of long-blurred impressions and memories. Further, findings made since large-scale psychedelic research stopped continue to point to rich research possibilities. First, some forms of animal tissue possess the requisite enzymes for changing normal bodily constituents into psychedelic agents. This was initially discovered in the rabbit lung, and subsequently within the human brain. Second, it has been discovered that the phenomenon of tolerance might *not* occur with *all* psychedelic agents. Some seem to produce psychological abnormalities continuously. Thus, the way has been reopened for the auto-intoxication theory.

Still other *possible* benefits of LSD are of a different kind. Twenty years ago, when scientific experimentation with LSD was both popular and sanctioned, some psychiatrists found that small amounts might not only speed up the process of psychological therapy but might make it possible when other approaches had failed, as with chronic alcoholism.

About the only research continuing with LSD consists of its administration to the dying. The data are not controlled, but there is a strong suggestion that in some persons LSD produces a change that enables them to accept their inevitable fate more philosophically. Early scientific experimentation with these drugs was relatively nondiscriminatory and in many instances they were given to persons—such as borderline psychotics—for whom they were harmful rather than helpful. But drugs may have different effects on different people, and the same drug may have different effects depending on its dosage.

The experimental use of the amphetamines has faced sociopolitical problems similar to those facing experimentation with LSD. Because of the increased abuse of amphetamines, an anti-amphetamine movement has developed both within and outside of the medical community. The hippies claimed that "speed kills," and they were partially right. When taken in doses hundreds of times larger than recommended, amphetamines, like alcohol, may well produce permanent brain damage. The medical profession, through the Department of Justice, acted to prevent such abuse by instituting the same prescription rules for amphetamines as apply to morphine.

The social revulsion against amphetamines has led to the unwarranted assertion by some doctors that tolerance always occurs and that abuse is always likely, even when administration is medically prescribed and supervised. We have seen many patients for whom the chronic moderate use of amphetamines has been extremely rewarding —for example, the hyperactives mentioned earlier—improving their ability to act in an energetic, focused fashion. Moreover, some do not seem to develop tolerance but maintain a heightened effectiveness and improved mood on continued daily doses. Additional research is necessary rather than a blanket prohibition.

CHAPTER 5

Nature, Nurture, and Psychiatric Disorders

Our belief that mental illnesses arise frequently and sometimes exclusively from biological malfunctioning of the brain stems in large part from studies of genetic patterns of mental illness. Although the classic aspects of human genetics are well known, we will review them briefly to set the stage for the material that follows. When the mother's egg cell, containing twenty-three different chromosomes, is fertilized by the father's sperm cell, also containing twenty-three different chromosomes, a new cell, or zygote, with twenty-three *pairs* of chromosomes is formed; each chromosome carries genes that are responsible for controlling the development of the offspring. As the zygote divides and further cell divisions occur, the specialized cells that will form the various parts of the body appear, developing by processes that are still very poorly understood.

An important aspect of genetics that tends to be forgotten is that only *some* inherited characteristics are manifested no matter where the individual was raised. The black child who inherits the right (or wrong) number of genes for sickle-cell anemia will suffer from the disease under all ordinary terrestrial conditions. But for many characteristics, what we inherit are predispositions for the development of certain attributes, depending on the environment. For example, some plants that are genetically identical grow to be trees in the tropics, bushes in temperate climates, and ground-hugging cover in the Arctic.

The importance of environment is illustrated even more cogently by experiments that subject animals to environments that they would never encounter in nature. In a classic example, when fertilized eggs of a particular species of fish are raised in a solution with too many magnesium ions in it, the fish develop one eye in the middle of their foreheads instead of their normal quota of two. What they inherited was a tendency to develop two eyes under most circumstances. But, given these sufficiently deviant conditions, the developmental mechanism was led astray.

Good human examples of the principle that heredity and environment (nature and nurture) are not either/or propositions are provided by the anemias. Some persons inherit a genetic defect that causes their red blood cells to rupture if they eat fava beans (an important food staple in parts of southern Europe) or are exposed, for example, to antimalarial drugs, sulfa drugs, and phenacetin (in many over-the-counter pain relievers), which didn't exist during the early evolution of man but were produced in the last fifty years. If such people do not eat fava beans or are not exposed to these chemicals, their predisposition to developing the anemia is not discovered. The genetic disorder sickle-cell anemia also responds to environmental *change:* high altitude aggravates the symptoms because of the diminished oxygen supply.

Nature and nurture interact not only in disease but also in normal development. An individual may inherit genes that would under normal circumstances make him tall. If he is raised under conditions of starvation, his growth may be stunted. It takes no great leap of the imagination to believe that such accomplishments as high musical and intellectual performance depend not only on inherited talents but also on the opportunity for training early in life.

In psychiatry, an example of a genetic predisposition that seems to produce the disease regardless of the environment is Huntington's chorea. This disorder becomes apparent in middle life and is characterized by intellectual deterioration, psychosis, and abnormalities of muscular function. It is conceivable that someday someone will come along with a medication that could be given to the pregnant mother in order to produce a fetal environment that would block the possibility that the child would later suffer from Huntington's chorea. If so, the normal-looking offspring, carrying the Huntington's chorea gene but not developing the disease, would be indistinguishable from the majority who do not inherit it.

A concept used in genetics that we believe is very important in understanding psychiatric illness is the idea of a phenocopy, which we mentioned briefly earlier. The term refers to instances in which nongenetic causes can produce the same effect as heredity. For example, a common, purely environmental cause of anemia—insufficient iron in the diet—in the past was indistinguishable clinically from some of the hereditary anemias. Affected patients showed pallor, fast heartbeat, and a decreased ability to tolerate exercise. Iron-deficiency anemia would be a phenocopy of sickle-cell anemia if one had no recourse to laboratory techniques. With the aid of a microscope, one finds that the red blood cells of people with sickle-cell anemia have a different shape from those of the other anemias. Similarly, techniques for measuring the amount of iron in the blood and microscopic examination of the blood enable one to recognize iron-deficiency anemias.

Many other conditions can occur as phenocopies. Acheiropody, a rare, genetically transmitted disorder in humans, is characterized by the complete absence of hands and feet. A very similar condition, phocomelia, characterized by shortened limbs with a flipper-like appearance, frequently and tragically resulted from the use of the drug thalidomide as sleeping medication in pregnant women. The relevance of the phenocopy notion to psychological illness resides in the confusion produced by disorders that have the same symptoms but may be produced by diverse causes, some genetic and some perhaps not. Further, in mental as in physical illness, influential environmental experience may include biological as well as psychological factors.

One final important point must be made about genetics. The process by which an inherited characteristic combines with the requisite environment to produce a particular disease can be exceedingly complex. This can be illustrated by a kind of breast cancer in mice. It had been known for many years that in certain inbred strains of mice the females had a very high rate of breast cancer. If high-risk baby mice were immediately separated from their mothers at birth and raised on the milk of mice from a strain in which cancer was uncommon, they did not develop the disease in later life. However, mice from other strains nursed on the milk from breast-cancer-prone mouse mothers also did not develop breast cancer. Thus, both the cancer-carrying genes and the "cancer" milk were required. Continuing investigation produced strong circumstantial evidence that such mother mice secreted cancer-producing viruses in their milk, and that the viruses infected their genetically susceptible daughters.

But the picture was even more complicated. If baby female mice from the cancer-carrying strain were fed their mother's milk but also had their ovaries removed before they reached sexual maturity, they did *not* subsequently develop cancer. Thus, if a female mouse was to develop breast cancer in later life, apparently (1) she had to have particular genes; (2) she had to be exposed to the cancer-producing virus in the milk; (3) she had to reach sexual maturity (presumably in order to secrete pertinent hormones). The fact that such complex chains may be necessary, if genes are to produce a given outcome, should be borne in mind as we continue the discussion of genetics and psychiatry.

Although numerous factors have been arraigned as possible causes of psychiatric illnesses—for example, infection, birth injury, culture, social class, genetic factors, and experience within the family—until recently none had been convicted. During the past several decades, genetic factors and psychological experience within the family have been the chief suspects. Both are consistent with the ancient observation that mental illness tends to run in families.

A reference of sufficient pedantic utility may be found in a quotation from Thomas Willis, the seventeenth-century doctor mentioned earlier: "It is a common observation, that men born of parents that are sometimes wont to be mad will be obnoxious to the same disease: And that often they have lived prudently and soberly about 30 or 40 years, yet afterward without any occasion or evident cause will fall mad." This observation has been made repeatedly since; only its interpretation has occasioned dispute.

Family Studies of Schizophrenia

When in the early decades of this century the Kraepelinian school of psychiatry searched for quantitative evidence that dementia praecox (schizophrenia) was hereditary, the investigators studied the frequency of the disorder among the parents, siblings, and children of their patients. These early workers diagnosed family members on an all-or-none basis: relatives were either schizophrenic or not. There was no question of gradations of illness. Using these criteria, they found that approximately 4 percent of the parents and about 8 percent of the siblings of schizophrenics had been diagnosed as schizophrenic; about 10 percent of the children of couples in whom one parent was schizophrenic were themselves schizophrenic.

The early researchers in schizophrenia hoped by this sort of nose-counting to be able to determine the mechanism of genetic transmission. This is a standard technique in human, animal, and plant genetics. One studies the frequency of certain patterns in genealogical hierarchies and can with mathematical formulas induce the so-called genetic mechanism: whether one or many genes are involved, whether the genes interact, whether they multiply or diminish one another's effect, and so forth. Such analyses perform a double duty in that some kinds of patterns imply that the traits involved are almost certainly genetically produced. The early psychiatric geneticists—and those who followed—were not this lucky. No clear pattern emerged.

In succeeding decades, psychiatrists studying genetics introduced the idea that schizophrenia might not be an all-or-none phenomenon. Early psychiatrists had used the phrase "hereditary taint" to describe relatives who were not paragons of mental health. Such relatives did exist in abundance in the families of psychiatrically ill patients, but their frequency was about as great in the families of normals; human perfection is the exception rather than the rule. What psychiatrists next did, led by the German psychiatrist Ernst Kretschmer, was to describe certain forms of abnormalities seen with greater frequency in the relatives of schizophrenic patients. Kretschmer noticed that families of schizophrenics seemed to have greater numbers of people who were unsociable, quiet, reserved, serious, eccentric, timid, shy, sensitive, nervous, supersensitive, or callous, or were adherents of extreme religious or political groups. The description matches that of one of the borderline groups identified later by Spitzer and his colleagues; Kretschmer used the term "schizoid" for people with these characteristics.

As a reminder of the flavor of the schizophrenic's family, let us refer back to the borderline family mentioned in Chapter 3. The schizophrenic patient was quiet, eccentric, conscientious, and depressed, with chronic feelings of inferiority and a strong capacity for fantasy. One brother was stormy, depressed, passionate, restless, eager to escape; another brother was conscientious, shy, good at business; yet another brother was quiet, serious, logical, unsocial, and eager to escape. The patient's father was paranoid, eccentric, anxious, misanthropic, and depressed; a paternal aunt was unsociable and extraordinarily excitable. His mother had had a brief, schizophrenia-like illness during a period when she was an alcoholic; at other times she was sensitive, humorless, pedantic, depressed, and obsessed with the family's hallmark, a desire to escape. (A desire to escape obviously might have realistic as well as genetic origins.)

Another German psychiatric geneticist, Franz Kallmann, used the term "schizoidia" to describe personality syndromes similar to those identified by Kretschmer. Kallmann listed "autistic introversion, emotional inadequacy, sudden surges of temperament and inappropriate motor response to emotional stimuli, and ... bigotry, pietism, avarice, superstition, suspicion, obstinacy or crankiness" (1938, p. 103).

It can readily be seen that such characteristics might be hard to agree on; there might be considerable disagreement among psychiatrists examining the same person whether to identify him as schizoid or not.

Yet, looking at schizophrenic families this way, Kallmann found that approximately half of the offspring of schizophrenic parents were either schizophrenic or fell in the flexible category of schizoidia. With this broadened definition, the risk of psychological abnormality in the offspring rises from about 10 to about 50 percent. One can readily see how attempts to examine the genetic mechanisms must necessarily flounder until the boundaries of an illness are defined accurately enough to indicate whether or not particular kinds of patients should be included.

Not only did most European psychiatrists assume that the schizophrenias were hereditary, but European psychoanalysts believed the disorder to be untreatable psychotherapeutically. Their American cousins did not share this belief. In the 1930s, a number of innovative American psychiatrists, such as Harry Stack Sullivan and Frieda Fromm-Reichmann, attempted to treat schizophrenia by psychotherapy. In the early 1940s, some of them began to observe the parents of schizophrenics, and like the Europeans, they found that in many instances schizophrenics came from very odd families. However, using the same kinds of data, they came to directly opposite conclusions. They asserted that schizophrenia runs in families for the same reason that speaking English, Swahili, or Chinese runs in families—that is, the children react on the basis of some kind of learning involving the parents. If a household speaks Chinese, the probability that a child in that household will speak it is virtually 100 percent, and speaking Chinese is psychologically, not genetically, transmitted. Contrariwise, if someone has red hair—a genetically transmitted characteristic—the probability that her child will likewise have red hair is rather low. As these psychiatrists pointed out, the frequency with which a characteristic runs in a family tells us little about nature and nurture.

Several very plausible processes were advanced to explain the psychological transmission of schizophrenia. First, psychiatrists have long observed a rare form of illness named folie à deux, in which one of a pair of psychologically close persons (most frequently mother and daughter, sisters, or husband and wife) becomes psychotic and transmits his or her illness to the other. Usually the illness is paranoia: suspicions and delusions are easily transmittable. When the pair is separated, one member remains ill and the other recovers. This both demonstrates which of them is autonomously ill and proves that even very severe illness can appear contagious. Now, if folie à deux can occur between two adults over a short period of time, one argument ran, what must be the effect on a child of being surrounded by madness or oddness for years? If, without consciously trying, parents can bring up their children to have particular ethnic prejudices or attitudes toward sex, why can't they unconsciously bring them up to be schizophrenic?

Second, there was the issue of communication. One of the characteristics of schizophrenics is that they talk, and seem to think, in a disorganized fashion. Some of the parents of schizophrenics were also found to display abnormalities of thinking. Although not displaying gross confusion of thought, they tended to communicate in a way that was obscure, mystifying, and illogical. What would be more natural than that the child of such a parent learned to communicate in the same way?

Similarly, clinicians found that some of the schizophrenics' parents, particularly mothers, tended to be cold and withdrawn. It seemed reasonable to postulate that a child of such a parent might withdraw within himself and keep his own counsel. If carried to an extreme, such behavior might become autistic.

Some investigators thought that schizophrenics' parents gave simultaneous confusing commands; their tone of voice would suggest one thing and the content of their speech another, putting the child in what was called a double bind. In a typical instance, a mother would say, "Come to Mother, darling," but would have a look of distaste on her face. Animals who receive contradictory messages—that is, who are simultaneously rewarded and punished for doing the same thing—behave in a stereotyped, senseless, repetitive fashion that might be seen as psychotic.

Finally, these observations overlapped a fascinating but short-lived "discovery" that was never actually established. For a while, it was thought that persons placed in sensory isolation would begin to hallucinate and undergo other psychotic experiences. In preliminary experiments, people who were, for example, blindfolded, ear-plugged, and laid down on a couch of cotton wool, or who were suspended in a tub of warm water with an oxygen mask, underwent most unusual psychological experiences, such as the conviction of death and rebirth.

Things seemed to fit together with extraordinary neatness. The case for the psychological origin of the schizophrenias appealingly hypothesized that parental coldness, rejection, and confused communication would lead to social isolation and withdrawal, and that social isolation, like sensory isolation, would produce hallucinations.

But this tidy theory ignored a few clinical facts. For instance, most schizophrenics were not disoriented, poorly communicating, isolated people prior to the onset of psychosis. Further, although statistically one does find greater proportions of schizophrenic-like characteristics in the parents of schizophrenics, one also often finds adequate communication and child-rearing in the immediate families of schizophrenics. Finally, the most puzzling aspect of the psychogenic hypothesis was that, even in a family environment that was noticeably odd, not all the children developed schizophrenia.

Twins; Adoption Studies

Let us restate the nature-nurture controversy briefly. Both the psychological and biological camps observed and agreed that insanity ran in families. Each interpreted the observation differently. Both paid lip-service to the other's position, the environmentalists acknowledging that biological predisposition might be necessary, and the geneticists giving trivial obeisance to the importance of experience. The situation was at an impasse. The available information was completely ambiguous and revealed only the prejudices of the investigator rather than the nature of the real world.

Unlike many other psychiatric disputes—which have borne an embarrassingly close resemblance to theological ones—the question debated was of vital importance. If schizophrenia was indeed caused by deviant psychological experience, its prevention would necessitate changing parents' behavior or moving children away from schizophrenia-producing environments. If schizophrenia was genetically transmitted, however, little help could be expected from changes in child-rearing practices.

Both in Europe and in the United States, it occurred to investigators that the study of schizophrenia in twins might yield convincing findings. The proposed research was designed to capitalize on the facts that monozygotic, or identical, twins come from the same fertilized egg and are genetic carbon copies of each other, while dizygotic, or fraternal, twins arise from two fertilized eggs and, except for their shared embryonic nursery, are biologically no more alike than any other pair of siblings. Researchers hypothesized that if schizophrenia was an entirely genetic disorder, then if one member of a monozygotic twin pair had the disorder, his or her twin must necessarily have it also. Correspondingly, they predicted that if a dizygotic twin was schizophrenic, the other twin's risk only equaled that of an ordinary (i.e., nontwin) sibling.

Both in Europe and in the United States, the second part of the hypothesis was confirmed: if one member of a dizygotic twin pair had schizophrenia, the risk in the twin was only approximately equal to that of any other siblings. The hypothesis was not fully borne out, however, in regard to monozygotic twins, since only approximately half of the pairs were concordant—that is, in only half of the instances in which one member was schizophrenic was the twin also schizophrenic.

To complicate matters, it was found that the nonschizophrenic identical (monozygotic) twins of schizophrenics did show a much greater incidence of abnormal psychological functioning resembling schizoidia. If these schizoid twins are counted as concordant, the rates increase from 50 to 80 or 90 percent in most studies, but not in all. It is still problematic, therefore, as to why these twins are not true schizophrenics. Why should one member of the pair be severely, incapacitatingly ill while the other is either healthy or only schizoid?

Those who believed that schizophrenia was psychologically determined provided still another hypothesis, derived from the commonly observed special, intense relationship that frequently exists between monozygotic twins. They are often dressed and treated alike, singled out as unique by parents, relatives, and the community, and identify strongly with each other. Accordingly, the researchers reasoned that some part of the psychological abnormalities in identical twins might simply be transmitted by unusually intense contagion. Schizophrenia was held to be psychologically caused by a blurring of the boundaries of the self. Therefore, identical twinship itself might be subversive of mental health and independence, regardless of family background. However, actual testing of the hypothesis that identical twins run a greater risk of becoming schizophrenic than fraternal twins, or the population at large, quickly dispensed with that theory. Identical twins are no more likely than anyone else to develop schizophrenia.

But surely the fact that one identical twin develops schizophrenia and the other does not clearly proves that psychological factors play a role. Not necessarily. It does prove that nongenetic factors are important. Other diseases in twins illustrate analogous phenomena. In a number of disorders believed to be entirely biological in origin, identical twins are not one hundred percent concordant. Club foot, an abnormality that results from fetal maldevelopment, is concordant in only 32 percent of identical twins. Rickets, usually the product of vitamin D deficiency, is concordant in only 68 percent of twin pairs, although both presumably are raised on the same diet. That all genetically identical twins, triplets, or quadruplets are not biologically identical is exemplified by the armadillo, a remarkable beast. For reasons unknown, it always reproduces as identical quadruplets. Nevertheless, at birth, brain weight varies among members of the quartet by more than 60 percent, and brain amino acids—some of which are related to chemical transmitters in the brain—vary fivefold. One explanation may be that the intrauterine environment varies slightly for each of the genetically identical armadillo fetuses, and the result is non-identical identical quadruplets. What the researcher is faced with in situations of this kind, however—both in armadillos and in human identical twins—is a huge gap in knowledge that remains to be filled.

A final example suggests another possibility. The kind of diabetes that occurs in the young, juvenile diabetes, has large genetic contributants, but only about half of identical twin pairs are concordant for the disease. Some evidence suggests that juvenile diabetes may be produced by viral infection—presumably only in genetically susceptible people. The same thing may be happening in schizophrenia. Some forms of schizophrenia may be viral diseases produced in people with the inherited capacity for catching the illness. In discordant pairs, one schizophrenic or diabetic twin may be severely infected, while the other is infected mildly or not at all. This theory, too, leaves the ultimate source of the variability unexplained.

In the 1950s and 1960s, twin research on schizophrenics was the subject of virulent infighting between those favoring nature and those favoring nurture as the cause of schizophrenia. Undoubtedly, the dramatic changes wrought by the antipsychotic drugs played a role in the heightened controversy. By the mid-1960s, however, another research technique—the adoption study—began to provide clarifying data.

A number of researchers simultaneously hit upon a rather simpleminded but hitherto unexplored technique that, it was hoped, would permit final resolution of the bitter nature-nurture controversy: the study of adopted people.

Adoption is in a sense a natural experiment. The adopted person is unique, having two sets of parents. One gives the adoptee genes, and the other provides the familial environment. Thus, by inspecting illness in the biological parents, in the adopting parents, and in the adoptee, we can begin to separate out the effects of nature and nurture.

The technique had already been used in the thirties and forties to study the effects of nature and nurture on intelligence and alcoholism, with mixed results. The idea of using it to study schizophrenia simultaneously occurred to several researchers, including one of us (Wender), in the early 1960s. The question whether there is any genetic component to the chronic schizophrenias can be answered by examining adults who were born to schizophrenic parents and were adopted away at an early age. The time of adoption is obviously of great importance. If a child was adopted at the age of one week, exposure to the schizophrenic parent was limited. Contrariwise, if he was adopted at age eighteen, a considerable amount of psychological damage conceivably could have been done. For purposes of comparison, a control group is also needed: adopted persons who are similar to the experimental group in all respects but one. For each person born to a schizophrenic and reared by normal adopted parents, it is necessary to find a person the same age and sex who was born of psychiatrically normal parents and who was placed in a socially similar adoptive home at the same age.

If the genetic predisposition(s) to schizophrenia will manifest itself under a wide variety of family environments, then one would expect that children born to schizophrenic parents and adopted by nonschizophrenic parents would be more likely to be schizophrenic in adult life than the adopted-away children born to nonschizophrenic parents. Comparing adoptees with adoptees should cancel out the possibly deleterious psychological effects of adoption itself. One of the scientifically aesthetic characteristics of such an experiment is that the nature and the nurture theories each make an explicit prediction that is open to direct confirmation or refutation. Furthermore, refinements can be introduced in this experiment in order to answer more questions.

Two groups of researchers were able to locate the people necessary to implement this plan. One group was headed by a young psychiatrist in Oregon, Leonard Heston (see Heston, 1966), and the other consisted of a team of American and Danish investigators (David Rosenthal, Seymour Kety, Paul Wender, Fini Schulsinger, and Joseph Welner; see Rosenthal et al., 1971; Kety et al., 1971)* who launched a collaborative program of studying adoptees in Denmark. We will describe the Danish work in detail, but Heston's studies have produced similar findings. Heston investigated two groups of adopted adults. One had been born of psychotic mothers, the other had not. Heston found a statistically significant increase not only of schizophrenia but of sociopathic personalities among the offspring of schizophrenics. The offspring of nonhospitalized mothers were in a state of reasonably good psychological health, both relatively and absolutely. (The latter is of interest because as children these people had frequently been shuffled from foster home to foster home, which is held in some circles to be irrevocably damaging to one's personality.)

In Denmark, the existence of extensive and exquisitely detailed files permitted the location of the individuals the researchers wished to

*Brought together by an American psychologist, Sarnoff Mednick.

study. To give some idea of the magnitude of the administrative problems of the study, the investigators first had to obtain the names of adopted persons, then obtain the names of their biological parents from the adoption records, then see which of the biological parents had been hospitalized for medical illness and particularly schizophrenia, and then find and interview the now adult adoptees.

By means of the Danish records, the requisite two groups of adopted persons were studied: adults who had been born of schizophrenic parents (usually so diagnosed after the birth of the child whom they gave away), and a control group of adoptees of the same age and sex, born of nonschizophrenic parents, who had been placed in similar adoptive homes at a comparable period after their birth. Through this study the first hypothesis was confirmed: adoptees born of schizophrenic parents and reared by nonschizophrenic parents are indeed more likely to be schizophrenic than adoptees born of nonschizophrenics and reared by nonschizophrenics. Related studies done since have had similar results. The exact percentages varied from study to study, but in general 10 or 20 percent of the adopted children of schizophrenics developed schizophrenia (or around 45 percent if both parents were schizophrenic), while none or very few of the adopted children of nonschizophrenics developed schizophrenia (Kessler, 1975). Clearly, *some* forms of schizophrenia have a genetic component.

The reason for the continued use of the word "some" despite the encouraging results of the adoption studies can be illustrated by the case of retardation. We have clear evidence that some forms of reduced intelligence are genetic in origin and that others are the result of brain damage or fetal maldevelopment. Some forms of reduced intelligence *may* be the result of severe social neglect or environmental impoverishment, such as that which produces malnutrition. If we studied the adopted-away offspring of retarded people, we would find that their children, even though raised in adequate homes, would be more likely to be retarded than adopted-away offspring of nonretarded people. But we would probably also find some retarded children among the adopted-away offspring of normal parents—victims of nongenetic mongolism, infection, or brain damage (and some of the retarded children among the offspring of retardates might also be manifesting such nongenetic retardation, or combined forms). Similarly, this investigation can only show us that statistically *some* forms of schizophrenia are genetic in origin, but it cannot rule out other possibilities. Nevertheless, the genetic findings are far from trivial.

A second question that was tested by the adoption studies was: What is the fate of children born to schizophrenics and reared by these same schizophrenic parents? Do these people become sicker than adoptees born to schizophrenics and raised by normals? (This is not the perfect experiment of children born to schizophrenic parents and adopted by schizophrenics, because such monumentally unfortunate people—born to, adopted away from, and then raised by schizophrenics—are uncommon.) Does deviant rearing aggravate psychological difficulties in those who carry the genes now demonstrated to be "bad"?

The answer is *no*. So far as psychiatric diagnosis is concerned, they run no greater risk of becoming schizophrenic than those seemingly more fortunate individuals who have been raised in normal homes. However, this study has not yet examined the social adjustment of the two groups. It is conceivable that the adoptees, raised by normals, are making better life adaptations than the children raised by their schizophrenic parents, and might be better able to adjust themselves to normal social and cultural demands.

A final question concerned the fate of children born to nonschizophrenics but reared by schizophrenic adopting parents. If such children developed schizophrenia at a greater rate than similar children adopted by normal parents, we would have evidence that schizophrenia—perhaps indistinguishable from the genetic kind and therefore a phenocopy—could be produced solely by psychological experience. This study was particularly difficult because adoption agencies do their best to place their infant charges with normal parents; only an unusual kind of schizophrenic—whom the adoption agency cannot detect—would receive a child for adoption. Such schizophrenic parents might become ill only later in life, long after having adopted a child, or they might be able to conceal their illness from prying adoption-agency eyes. So the group of adopting schizophrenic parents is different from the group of schizophrenic parents who have their own children. Thus, the question of what would happen if children born of normal parents were placed in the homes of typical schizophrenics cannot be answered.

Still, the data—which are straightforward and fairly easy to interpret—do tell us something about the effects of subtle forms of parental madness on the developing child. Children born to nonschizophrenic parents and raised by schizophrenic adopting parents turn out no sicker than adoptees born of nonschizophrenics and raised by nonschizophrenics (even though they tended to complain to our investigators along these lines: "Doctor, you can't believe what a crazy home I was raised in"). In this situation, then, environmental factors alone did not produce schizophrenia, and the psychologically produced phenocopy for schizophrenia was not documented.

To return to the adoptees born of schizophrenics but raised by normals, a further aspect of genetic inheritance that was investigated was the kind of schizophrenia developed by those that did manifest it. From these studies it appears that among biological children of schizophrenic parents one is more likely to find not only typical severe schizophrenia but also people with the schizoid-eccentric characteristics often labeled as borderline. These are the schizotypal people rather than the affectively vulnerable borderlines, who perhaps should be classified with mood disorders rather than schizophrenia. Thus, there is empirical confirmation that a great many people called borderline, with personality characteristics resembling those of true schizophrenia, are indeed genetically related to patients with the illnesses described by Kraepelin and Bleuler.

Adoption studies have also been done on the acute schizophrenias, which seem to be triggered by psychological stress and which seem to have a high likelihood of recovery. Few acute schizophrenics who fit the research design could be located, however, and the statistics are inconclusive. Acute schizophrenias may well be related to bipolar affective disorder, which clearly has genetic components, but for the moment the decision about acute schizophrenia is a Scotch verdict: neither guilty nor not guilty; insufficient evidence.

The critical question of what fraction of schizophrenias is genetically produced and what fraction is produced by other forces is difficult to answer accurately. If one starts with a group of schizophrenic adults who had been adopted in early infancy and asks how many of these people have schizophrenic illness anywhere in their closely related biological families (parents, brothers, sisters), one gets an answer that sets *only* a lower limit to the frequency of genetic schizophrenia and its relatives. This lower limit is about 50 percent. The true fraction may be much higher.

Phenocopies of Schizophrenia

We strongly suspect that other biological forces besides genes can produce schizophrenia—that is, that there are nongenetic phenocopies for schizophrenia, or phenocopies that result from the interaction of other kinds of genetic susceptibilities and environmental factors. In a recent review of the role of nongenetic biological risk factors in schizophrenia, Seymour Kety and Dennis Kinney presented the current evidence implicating such factors as obstetrical complications, season of birth, prenatal stress, infectious processes, and dietary factors.

Several studies have found that obstetrical complications increase the risk for the schizophrenias, interacting with genetic influence. Prolonged labor is the complication most consistently associated with increased risk for schizophrenia, suggesting oxygen-deprivation as a possible cause.

Over twenty studies during the past four decades have shown a consistent 5 to 15 percent increase in schizophrenic births during the winter and spring months in comparison with the general population. The phenomenon has been reported in North America, Western Europe, Japan, the Philippines, South Africa, and Australia, and for the most part is more striking in geographic areas where the seasonal variation is more pronounced. Researchers have postulated that the increase may be associated with greater susceptibility to infectious diseases during those times of the year, to greater prevalence of viruses at such times, or to a greater tendency to hemorrhage in newborns, especially if agricultural produce supplying vitamins C and K is not available.

Association of prenatal stress with brain and behavior problems in the offspring has been shown in both animal and human studies; in particular, one study showed a greater incidence of schizophrenia among children whose fathers had died during the mother's pregnancy but a normal incidence among children whose fathers died during the child's first year of life.

The viral theory of schizophrenia continues to have some prominence, and it has been proposed that the increased incidence of the illness in lower socioeconomic groups may be related to greater susceptibility to infectious processes as a result of environmental deficiencies.

In the area of dietary factors, Linus Pauling's vitamin-deficiency theory has not yet been confirmed, but there is a suggestive correlation between schizophrenia and a digestive disorder (celiac disease), and between schizophrenia and high wheat and rye consumption. Schizophrenia patients on gluten-free diets in two clinical trials have shown greater improvement than the control patients. Further, Ireland, which reports three times more schizophrenia than England and Wales, also has a considerably higher prevalence of celiac disease.

In addition to the factors discussed by Kety, studies of psychosis in children (not necessarily related to adult schizophrenia) indicate that a large fraction of such children have either symptoms or past histories suggesting damage to the brain. A study of soldiers who suffered wartime brain injuries found that twenty years later the men developed schizophrenia at five times the rate of soldiers who escaped such injury. Unless one assumes that schizophrenics stick their heads out of foxholes at five times the rate of their fellows, one must conclude that brain injury can somehow be involved in the development of schizophrenia. Relatively straightforward investigations that might have a bearing on this conclusion have not yet been carried out. One could compare persons who are the only schizophrenics in large families (and thus presumably suffer their difficulties on the basis of brain damage rather than genetics) with schizophrenics who come from families with many schizophrenic members. Differences in symptoms and response to treatment in the two groups might help to differentiate types of schizophrenia.

Despite the clinical literature, we do not have any scientifically confirmed examples of phenocopies of schizophrenia that are solely due to social or psychological influences. Although it is possible that psychological or social influences might affect the form of the symptoms, at present there is no reason whatsoever for believing that psychological forces can cause chronic schizophrenia.

Disorders of Mood

In describing disorders of mood earlier, we pointed out that depression could be the outcome of several distinct processes—for example, it can have biological components, as in vital depression; it can result from reactions to life events, as in nonvital, "neurotic depression" or enduring maladjustment; and it can be a symptom of other mental disorders, as in the anhedonia of borderline schizophrenics, the depression of adults who were hyperactive as children, and the depression seen in hysteroid dysphoria. Depression is thus an excellent example of the phenocopy principle—a number of superficially similar disorders with different underlying causes.

Vital depression. As we have said, the causes of affective illnesses have been the subject of considerable debate. The evidence that vital depressions are often genetic in origin and biochemically produced comes from the same types of data that demonstrate that the schizophrenias frequently have a genetic origin. First, relatives of a patient with vital depression are more likely to have similar disorders than the population at large. The closer the relationship, the greater the probability of vital depression. As in the schizophrenias, this increased probability reaches its maximum in the case of identical twins: if one identical twin has bipolar illness, the likelihood that his co-twin will suffer from the same illness is between 50 and 80 percent. In comparison, the risk of depressive illness in the siblings of a bipolar patient or in the other member of a set of non-identical twins is approximately 10 percent.

Although borderline depression—or, to use the phrase we have used previously, affective vulnerability—has not been studied as intensively as borderline schizophrenia, the relatives of vital depressives tend to be more likely than the population at large to have mild depressions; because they have fewer symptoms, they are less likely to be treated and thus less likely to be noticed among the relatives of the more seriously ill depressives. The same kinds of objections to the conclusions from family and twin studies in the schizophrenias have also been raised about the affective illnesses—namely, the transmission within families may be the result of psychological and social factors rather than genetic ones.

Here again, psychiatric researchers have begun to use adoption studies to try to separate the effects of nature and nurture. The research is in an early stage, but one study completed in Belgium deals with bipolar affective disorder (see Mendlewicz and Rainer, 1977). The investigators examined biological and adopting parents of adopted adults who had been diagnosed as manic-depressives, and three comparison groups: (1) the parents of non-adopted adult manic-depressives; (2) the biological parents of adults with polio; (3) the biological and adoptive parents of normal adoptees. The families of non-adopted bipolar patients were studied to see if they showed the anticipated increase of bipolar illness. The polio patients' parents were studied to see if a serious disease in the children produced psychological depression in their parents. Finally, the biological and adoptive parents of the healthy adoptees were compared with the biological and adoptive parents of the ill adoptees.

The investigators found that the biological parents of the adopted adults with bipolar illness had as much psychiatric illness as the biological parents who had reared their own manic-depressive offspring. The adoptive parents of the adult manic-depressives had no more psychiatric illness than either the adoptive parents of the normal adoptees or the biological parents of the adult polio patients. In most non-adoption family studies of bipolar patients, an increase is found not only in bipolar illness in relatives but in the more common unipolar illness as well; in this study, most of the ill biological parents of the adopted manic-depressives were not manic-depressives but unipolar depressives.

In another recent study, adoptees with affectively ill biological parents were found to have a higher prevalence of depression than adoptees with normal biological parents or biological parents with other psychiatric conditions (Cadoret, 1978).

Nonvital depression. There has been a great deal of speculation concerning the role of early-life experience in the generation of neurotic depression and depressive character. Theoretically, one could design a scientific experiment, but in practice it would be almost impossible to carry out. Because much of the theory involves alternate ways of raising children, most such experimentation would require intolerable control of people's lives.

In examining the data to which we are limited, we must look for firm evidence that the proposed antecedents of depression actually do occur more often in the background of depressed people. Even this is not sufficient, however, because, as with schizophrenia, the abnormal child-rearing practices might be a manifestation of a genetic disorder in the parents which has been inherited by the children.

A further difficulty about psychological theories is that they derive from accounts of development given by depressive patients. These patients will describe a variety of their experiences in childhood and adolescence, but the reliability of such narratives is open to question. First, as with all historical accounts, they are subject to the post hoc propter hoc fallacy: after the fact, therefore because of the fact. For example, "I was rejected by my mother [true] and that is why I drink too much [not necessarily true]." There are countless possible explanations for the drinking here, and a particularly plausible one is that the abnormal parenting and the alcoholism are different expressions of the same genetically transmitted biological abnormality. Rejection may not have been a precipitating cause at all.

Another reason for caution regarding patients' accounts is that psychiatrists never learn what truly went on in the patient's early life but only what the patient perceived. Everyone perceives inaccurately, and abnormal people perceive abnormally. It is possible that the factors leading to the illness were present when the patient was a child, and so he erroneously perceived what was taking place in his life. The depressed patient, for example, may report that his parents did not pay much attention to him. But if he was already anhedonic as a child, the reported lack of caring might be his perception of parents providing ordinary care for excessive needs.

Still another source of error is the fact that children are not merely passive receptors of experience. Children generate reactions in their parents. As every parent knows, the child is frequently blissfully unaware of her role in parental responses. Child psychiatrists frequently see hyperkinetic children who act in an offensive manner but are totally unaware of the impact of their behavior. They habitually report that their parents are too punitive, but do not recognize that they have triggered their parents' actions. Further, if a parent has indeed dealt with the child harshly, he may have done so because of the hot temper associated with his own hyperactivity, or because such children frequently try the patience of a saint, or because of a combination of these factors. When hyperkinetic children experience emotional problems in later life, it is difficult to determine the major causes, which might well be biological disabilities or residues from parental treatment or simply events. Clearly, it is more likely that the irritable adult will attribute his temper to being mistreated as a child than to his biological constitution.

Another and very large source of error is the fact that most clinicians are not aware of the frequency for normal people of deviant life experience. Research shows that a very large fraction of the healthy population has been subjected to deviant child-rearing practices. The number of people exposed to abnormal childhood experience is far greater than the number of people who develop difficulty in later life. Only a small fraction of those who have experienced unusual parenting subsequently develop psychological problems. It is even possible that only people who are already vulnerable may react to unusual life experiences with subsequent problems (see Wender, 1967).

Finally, with hindsight one can almost always achieve a plausible explanation for why things had to work out as they did. Freud himself was fully aware of this. In discussing the case of a young woman who had developed homosexual interests, Freud examined many details of her past life and constructed what he regarded as a plausible explanation for the course of her development. He realized, however, that looking backward, it is easier to construct an explanation than to predict the course of events. He stated:

> But at this point we become aware of a state of things which also confronts us in many other instances in which light has been thrown by psycho-analysis on a mental process. So long as we trace the development from its final outcome backwards, the chain of events appears continuous, and we feel we have gained an insight which is completely satisfactory or even exhaustive. But if we proceed the reverse way, if we start from the premises inferred from the analysis and try to follow these up to the final result, then we no longer get the impression of an inevitable sequence of events which could not have been otherwise. We notice at once that there might have been

another result, and that we might have been just as well able to understand and explain the latter. The synthesis is thus not so satisfactory as the analysis; in other words, from a knowledge of the premises we could not have foretold the nature of the result.

It is very easy to account for this disturbing state of affairs. Even supposing that we have a complete knowledge of the aetiological factors that decide a given result, nevertheless what we know about them is only their quality, and not their relative strength. Some of them are suppressed by others because they are too weak, and they therefore do not affect the final result. But we never know beforehand which of the determining factors will prove the weaker or the stronger. We only say at the end that those which succeeded must have been the stronger. Hence the chain of causation can always be recognized with certainty if we follow the line of analysis, whereas to predict it along the line of synthesis is impossible. [1920, pp. 167–68]

Many philosophers assert that a theory that can only explain the past but cannot predict the future is not really a scientific theory at all but simply an elaborate set of rationalizations.

Keeping this long list of generally neglected cautions in mind, we now proceed to the psychological theories relating early-life experience and subsequent depressive personalities, and to the evidence supporting them. The early theorists—primarily psychoanalytic—constructed their theories to explain phenomena now subdivided into biological (vital or endogenous) and neurotic depressions. The fact that much of their theorizing about neurotic depression was based on observations of endogenous depression adds to the difficulties of evaluating the accuracy and significance of their work.

A special sensitivity to deprivation of affection, to frustration, and to loss may predispose some individuals to neurotic depressive reactions. Many neurotic depressives give histories of unusual sensitivity to slights and wounds, which produce not only a fall in mood but also a fall in self-esteem—a transition from "I am not happy" to "I am no good." The fragility of the neurotic's self-esteem is as characteristic as the instability of his sense of well-being. The depressive feels—to a greater extent than the rest of us do—that he is of value only insofar as he is loved and is able to achieve his aims. Many theorists have attributed the depressive's sensitivity to loss of affection to his early childhood upbringing. The evidence for this, however, is largely retrospective clinical data of unknown reliability.

To further substantiate this clinical hypothesis, certain old studies, impressive but incorrectly believed to be conclusive, are cited over and over. Among these are studies in which the emotional development of infants in understaffed, primitive adoption homes with no warm, continuing contact was observed. The studies clearly showed that the infants suffered profoundly from these conditions, but the suffering is difficult to interpret, since the infants also suffered from sensory privation and absence of human contact (as contrasted with the postulated causal factor, absence of loving contact). No adequate medical analysis was conducted for anemia, malnutrition, parasites, etc. In addition, there was no follow-up on the fate of these children. More recent surveys of maternal deprivation do indicate that prolonged deprivation of infants of psychological and social stimulation may be somewhat harmful (see Rutter, 1972), but antisocial personality rather than depression seems a more frequent consequence.

Also cited frequently are the famous experiments by Harry Harlow (1958) in which rhesus monkeys were raised without mothers, with deleterious effects on later psychological and social adaptation. More recently, work by Martin L. Reite with infant pigtail monkeys indicates that the animals become depressed and also suffer physiological changes when experimentally separated from their mothers. The inference sometimes drawn from studies of this kind, however, is that a psychologically absent mother is equivalent to a physically absent mother.

For us compulsive purists who require evidence with the force of a blow on the head, this remains to be proven. Further, it is inferred that any long-term psychological effects of this kind cannot be helped by later environmental experience, an assumption contradicted by later Harlow work (Suomi and Harlow, 1972). Thus, although these drastic experiments clearly demonstrate that social experience plays a critical role in some monkey (and probably human) development, very little can be concluded from them about relationships between the usual range of child-rearing variations and later pathology.

Another psychological factor believed to predispose to neurotic depression is the strength of the conscience. We observed in discussing the syndrome of biological depression that guilt, although a common accompaniment to depression in the Western world, may not be an intrinsic part of the ailment. Within our culture, however, guilt frequently does precede depression. Examples abound. Not too many decades ago, it was common for a religious boy to believe that masturbation was sinful (a belief still current in some orthodox religions). Since masturbation is irresistible to most adolescents, they "abused" themselves frequently anyway. It was a secret pleasure and a great pain. Depression was unavoidable. The belief that virginity is a woman's greatest asset provides another example. When a young woman succumbed in a fit of youthful passion, chronic feelings of transgression, sinfulness, guilt, and depression could not be avoided, often even after a happy marriage to an accepting husband.

Certainly, conscience and guilt are instilled in the bosom of the family. The values instilled, and therefore the transgressions that will later engender guilt, vary as a function of the family and of the culture to which it belongs. Even so, guilt does not seem to be simply the result of upbringing. In describing the personality disorders, we mentioned the possibility that individuals differ in their susceptibility to developing guilt, so that given the same family background, different children manifest greater or lesser degrees of conscience.

The goals that an individual feels he must strive for in life represent another psychological factor believed to be related to the development of neurotic depression. These ego ideals—values, achievements, attainments, and good behavior—are programmed into the young child. One set of parents may somehow convey to a child the idea that people who get C's on their report cards are good people; another set may get across the idea that only people who get A's are good people. Upon receiving a B in school, the former child would be delighted, whereas the latter would consider himself a failure. A child rigidly indoctrinated into excessively self-demanding values is in many instances doomed to a life full of feelings of failure. To the extent that a sense of failure contributes to low self-esteem and self-depreciation, such a person will be far more likely to become depressed in later life.

This is a possible psychological cause of depression that is difficult to quarrel with. William James, speaking with his psychological hat on, observed that happiness was proportional to the quotient of success over pretensions: greater happiness could be attained not only by an increase in the numerator, success, but also by a decrease in the denominator, pretensions. The fat man may have his happiness increased not only by losing weight (increasing the numerator) but by deciding that obesity is not so terrible (decreasing the denominator). One often achieves happiness not by "getting there" but by deciding "Why am I knocking myself out to do it?"

Many psychotherapists believe that—along with such childhood determinants—certain personality characteristics, presumably also acquired during childhood, bring on or maintain the depressive state. Such therapists emphasize: (1) an inability to express one's needs; (2) an inability to express aggression (to be appropriately self-assertive and self-defensive when necessary); (3) excessive anger (perhaps innate) not balanced or leavened by sufficient loving feelings. The inability to express reasonable needs is seen as a continuing source of disappointment and frustration. An inability to express aggression and excessive anger ostensibly result in both cases in the anger being turned on oneself. According to these theories, anger must be expressed, and if it is not expressed toward others, it is, somewhat paradoxically, directed against oneself. Thus, many therapists encourage self-assertiveness.

Although this may be valuable, it is debatable whether an inability to express personal needs and anger is restricted to depressives or necessarily causes depression. Further, recent observations have shown the theory to be factually wrong with reference to vital depression, which casts doubt on it in nonvital depression. Vital depressives express more anger toward others when they are depressed than when they recover.

Interpretation of the importance of life experiences of the kinds discussed above is complicated by the fact that psychiatrists generally do not describe the characteristics of their patients fully enough, providing only brief vignettes. Reading the psychiatric literature, one cannot determine which kinds of neurotic depressive symptoms go with which sorts of deviant experiences. It may be, for example, that the described psychologically formative experiences do indeed generate mild depressive disorders but do not explain more severe depressive illness. Psychiatric clinical experience is often suggestive but insufficient for the drawing of tidy conclusions.

In some patients, however, the influence of experiences on depression seems very clear, even though at first the patients themselves may be unable to recognize the relationship. Many people are locked into intolerable circumstances, such as a difficult marriage, inadequate living conditions, or a job that they detest, but are unable to admit it to themselves. They may have told themselves, or they may have been told by relatives, that theirs is the perfect spouse, that they always wanted to be a farmer or a doctor, or that they always wanted to live in a small town. They believe that to admit to themselves that a mistake has been made would be to acknowledge failure, ineptitude, or self-deception, or to be forced to disagree with the opinions of those they respect or have been taught to honor. They find it less painful—at least in the short run—to repress or deny an awareness of the reality of their situation.

In depressions of this kind, psychological therapies are often extremely effective. If the patient can be helped to develop the courage to face changeable life circumstances as the source of psychological pain, he or she can often alter those circumstances and evolve a more satisfactory life. The case histories of Carole G. and Rebecca S., presented in Chapter 3, illustrate depression of this kind.

Suicide. Like alcoholism and demoralization, suicide is a final common manifestation of many different causes. Psychologically healthy people may commit suicide after a reasoned decision to deal in this way with a painful, progressive, incapacitating illness. Immature and histrionic people may slash their wrists with safety razors to attract the attention of loved ones and may inadvertently kill themselves. Schizophrenics, depressives, and alcoholics have a markedly high suicide rate. Since these disorders are to some extent genetic, one would assume that some forms of suicide have genetic components. More direct evidence is available. In one of the adoption studies of schizophrenia discussed, the investigators discovered an increased frequency of suicide and accidental death among the biological relatives of adopted schizophrenics. A similar finding occurred in a study of the biological relatives of adopted depressed people: the biological relatives, with whom the depressed people had not been raised, had a noticeably increased risk of committing suicide.

The Danish adoption study with which Paul Wender was associated also investigated the biological and adoptive relatives of adoptees who had committed suicide, comparing the number of suicides in that group with the number of suicides among the biological and adoptive relatives of adult adoptees who were still alive. There was a markedly increased risk of suicide among the biological relatives of the suicides as contrasted with the adoptive relatives of the suicides and also as contrasted with the biological and adoptive relatives of the living adoptees.

The idea that one's urge to commit suicide may have biological rather than psychological or existential causes—that is, that one might be rationalizing bad feelings engendered by biological abnormalities—might help a potential suicide to hang on to life. Most depressives rationalize their depressions. They are analogous to metaphysicians, whose task in life is "to find bad reasons for what they believe on instinct." Knowing that they may be justifying remediable biological impulses to suicide might prevent some depressives from acting.

The Unnamed Quartet

Four of the personality disorders—antisocial personality, alcoholism, childhood hyperactivity, and one that we have not yet discussed—constitute a family of diseases. They not only occur on a genetic basis but can be produced by brain injury and possibly by upbringing.

Because the same outcome may stem from differing sources, they too illustrate the phenocopy principle.

Briquet's Syndrome, the illness that we have not yet discussed, is a hysterical disorder in which the patient (usually female; it is estimated to occur in 1 or 2 percent of women) complains of multiple physical difficulties over a period of years. These difficulties, which usually cannot be linked to underlying physical disease, include headache, numbness, tingling, palpitations, shortness of breath, pain during sexual intercourse, painful joints, and a painful abdomen. Because of continuing complaints, the patients often convince their eventually desperate physicians that they may have real physical diseases and thus need exploratory surgery. As a result, many Briquet's patients have undergone multiple surgical explorations and their abdomens are as scarred as a battlefield.

Psychiatric researchers at Washington University in St. Louis noticed a tendency for antisocial personality, alcoholism, Briquet's Syndrome, and hyperactivity to cluster in families. On the basis of clinical observations, they noted that the close relatives of a patient with one of these disorders not only were more likely than the population at large to have that disorder but also were more likely to have one of the three other disorders. They tested their clinical hunches by more precise counting of the frequency of the four disorders and documented their hypothesis. For example, starting with men convicted of felonies —most of whom were antisocial personalities—they found an increased frequency of alcoholism and antisocial personality in close male relatives and a probable increase in Briquet's Syndrome among the close female relatives. Half of the felon antisocial personalities were alcoholics as well. A comparable study of female felons showed that most were antisocial personalities and that about half were alcoholic and hysteric. About half of the close male relatives of these women were alcoholic and a third were antisocial personalities. Of their female relatives, about one-fifth were alcoholic and one-third had Briquet's Syndrome. The same sorts of findings occur when one studies the close relatives of women with Briquet's Syndrome or of hyperactive children. The clustering of these disorders has led us to call them the Unnamed Quartet.

For all of the Unnamed Quartet except Briquet's Syndrome, adoption studies have also been done in an effort to parcel out possible genetic and psychological causes. There is also suggestive information on possible sources of phenocopies.

Antisocial personality. To an even greater extent than with schizophrenia, the observation that antisocial personalities run in families has been attributed to environmental, not genetic factors. The parents of antisocial personalities are inclined to be neglectful, harsh, and unloving. Those who believe the disorder is psychologically transmitted have reasoned that the children learn to "do as Caesar does, not as Caesar says." That is, they do not learn to inhibit their angry impulses but learn to inflict them on those who are smaller or weaker than they are. Nonetheless, the possibility was suggested by psychologically obtuse psychiatric geneticists that the admittedly unpleasant behavior in the parents might be a manifestation of a disease that they were genetically transmitting to the child, rather than the cause of the behavior in the child. Once again, adoption studies were tried.

Fini Schulsinger (1972) compared four groups: biological and adoptive relatives of adopted adults who had been diagnosed as psychopathic, and biological and adoptive relatives of adopted nonpsychopaths. Schulsinger found an increase in psychopathy only among the biological relatives of the adopted psychopaths. In other words, the study showed evidence only for the operation of genetic factors.

There is also increasing evidence that a phenocopy of antisocial personality may be based on brain dysfunction. Electroencephalograms of antisocial personalities indicate a high incidence of abnormal brain waves, their psychological tests yield a high incidence of performance resembling that of patients with known brain damage, and their medical histories suggest a greater than expected history of difficulties during pregnancy and delivery.

Another phenocopy is probably produced by unusual childhood experience. During the 1940s, a number of psychiatrists observed that there seemed to be increased frequency of psychiatric disorder—primarily of an antisocial type—in children who had been raised in foundling homes or orphanages (see summaries in Rutter, 1972). The aspects of the children's upbringing that seemed to play a role in the development of the problems was the absence of a consistent mothering figure and of sensory stimulation. Although hygienic, the homes were often sterile and barren. The staffs may have been sufficient, but the children were shuffled from one surrogate mother to another so as to comply with administrative regulations. They lacked what most children have, an ever-present, caring adult. How valid these findings are is unknown and in fact they may be spurious, but they have a human appeal that makes one hope there is never an opportunity to test them. Because of these observations, however, child-care agencies have tried to ensure that no children are exposed to a comparable experience. Instead of placing children in institutions, an attempt is made to place them with foster or adoptive parents who will provide continuous care as quickly as possible.

Alcoholism. Alcoholism involves obvious environmental factors in that alcohol must be available and a culture must not effectively prohibit it in order for alcoholism to occur. The availability of alcohol is limited in traditional Moslem cultures, and religious strictures often function as effective inhibitors among Baptists, Mormons, and various other denominations.

But, as we noted, alcoholism is also often associated with psychiatric syndromes that have genetic components, such as antisocial personalities, some schizophrenias, and bipolar affective disorders. Thus, some forms of alcoholism appear to be genetic because they are associated with disorders that are genetic in origin. However, even for many alcoholics who are free of other psychiatric illness, alcoholism runs in the family.

Genetic data are available on alcoholism in a half-sibling study and an adoption study. In the first, Marc Schuckit and his co-workers (1972) used a clever strategy to disentangle the roles of nature and nurture, examining the half brothers of alcoholics. Some of the half brothers shared an alcoholic biological parent, and some did not. Similarly, some were raised with the alcoholic parent, while others were raised with a non-alcoholic stepparent. Schuckit found that only genetic relatedness made a difference—that is, half brothers showed increased alcoholism if they shared an alcoholic parent with the alcoholic siblings, whether or not they were raised by the alcoholic parent.

The same findings were obtained from an adoption study. Donald Goodwin and his colleagues in Denmark (1974) studied three groups of men: the adopted whose biological fathers were not alcoholics, the adopted whose biological fathers were alcoholics, and the non-adopted sons of alcoholic fathers. Moderate drinking and heavy drinking were equally frequent in all three groups, but the rate of alcoholism —defined in terms of concrete problems such as blackouts, hospitalization because of alcohol abuse, and job impairment—was far greater among the adoptees whose biological fathers were alcoholic. The rate, which was four times the rate in the comparison groups, was the same as that for non-adopted offspring of alcoholics who were raised by their alcoholic fathers—that is, the alcoholic environment did not increase the rate. The adoption studies also showed a genetic linkage with hyperactivity.

Again, these studies do not demonstrate that all alcoholism is genetic; only that some forms are.

Finally, if social factors decrease the likelihood that some people will become alcoholics, such factors probably can also increase that risk. As pointed out in Chapter 3, we are probably seeing here an interaction of biological predisposition and social influence. Individual differences may be necessary for the person to go from the stage of social user through the stages of abuser, alcohol dependent, and alcohol-addicted. Individual psychodynamic factors could of course conceivably play a role, but the discouraging responses to psychotherapy do not support any consistent trends.

Hyperactivity. The story with regard to hyperactivity is similar, but an important adoption study used a different strategy. Dennis Cantwell (1975) investigated the frequency of psychiatric illness in three groups of parents: (1) those who had adopted a child who subsequently manifested hyperactivity; (2) those who had reared their own hyperactive child; (3) a comparison group of parents of normal children. The adoptive parents of hyperactive children were not different from the parents of the normal children, while the natural parents of the hyperactive children had an increased frequency of all forms of the Quartet, including histories of hyperactivity when they themselves had been children.

There are also several phenocopies for hyperactivity. Hyperactivity on a large scale was first described as a consequence of brain damage. The worldwide epidemic, following World War I, of the exceedingly virulent Spanish flu frequently produced brain infections in adults and children. When they recovered from the illness, many children showed a profound behavioral change. In case reports of the early 1920s, the descriptions of the "post-encephalitic behavior disorders" sound remarkably similar to current descriptions of hyperactivity. Furthermore, hyperactivity has been linked to other sources of brain injuries, including difficulties of pregnancy and delivery, prematurity, and lead poisoning. In addition, the children alluded to in the discussion of antisocial personality who were raised in extremely deprived environments such as institutions may develop problems similar to or indistinguishable from hyperactivity. Finally, there is an increased probability that mothers who drink during pregnancy will give birth to children with "fetal alcohol syndrome"; such children are retarded, mildly abnormal in their appearance, and may have problems of hyperactivity.

A possible relative: criminality. "Criminality" is a legal term, not a psychiatric one. However, since many criminals are antisocial personalities and many antisocial personalities are criminals, and since there is evidence that antisocial personality has contributing genetic factors, one would anticipate that there are also genetic factors in criminality. This hypothesis flies in the face of conventional liberal and egalitarian beliefs, which attribute criminality to impoverished environments and pathological upbringing. Obviously, the question is not one of either/or but, rather, of the extent to which genetic and environmental factors play a role in producing criminality.

Adoption studies on criminality have been done in Denmark, Sweden, and the United States. The Danish study compared adult adoptees on the basis of whether their biological or adoptive fathers had been legally identified as criminals. The study revealed *both* genetic and environmental components. Adoptees showed an increased frequency of criminality if their biological fathers had been criminal and a further increase if their adoptive fathers also had been criminal. A recent Swedish study came up with some different results. In this study, criminality alone in an adoptee's biological father did not increase the probability that he would be a criminal, but the combination of criminality and alcoholism in the biological father increased criminality or alcoholism or both in the offspring.

These data are of critical social importance, and further studies should be undertaken. Apparently, genetic factors do play some role in some forms of criminality. Obviously, genetic data on crime constitute only a small contribution to a vast social picture in which the influence of deprivation, social contagion, and disaffiliation with the dominant society must be considered. The extent to which the effects of any predisposition to "criminal behavior" might be lessened or increased by a particular kind of upbringing and social surroundings is of vital importance to society. Slums may foster crime, but not all slum dwellers are criminals; the relative roles of organic and social deterrence here are unknown. Finally, because the word "criminal" includes an enormous range of transgressions, further adoption studies must also investigate the role of genetics in different kinds of "crime." We are a lot more concerned with crimes of violence than with speeding tickets.

Genetics and Mental Illness: Evolutionary and Ethical Questions

Two important issues remain to be discussed—the evolutionary question of why mental illnesses are so common, and the ethical problems raised by new knowledge about and treatment of mental illness. Instead of considering the possible implications of these issues for all genetically produced mental illnesses, we will use the most severe, schizophrenia, as an example.

In the light of the theory of evolution, the persistence of deviant, incapacitating hereditary characteristics that seem associated with reduced reproduction is puzzling. If a biological characteristic presents an obvious disadvantage, we assume that it tends to die out with time. Slow-moving zebras will be caught by lions and the zebra family will tend to become speedier—or disappear. Presumably, the human species developed as it did because only the strongest and smartest of our anthropoid ancestors could escape predatory animals and find good hunting grounds and edible plants. It is surprising when evolution tolerates persistent hereditary deficits.

Yet the schizophrenic male is much less likely than the nonschizophrenic to marry, or, if unmarried, to have the drive and social finesse necessary to produce illegitimate children. How, then, can we account for the continued occurrence of schizophrenia? The same question may be asked concerning the large proportion of the population that suffers from physical disorders, such as diabetes, which are genetically transmitted and shorten the life span.

First, the disorder may not affect the individual before he has reproduced. Consider hardening of the arteries and high blood pressure. If these characteristics are associated with an ambitious and successful person who does not die of the disorder until the age of seventy, the disorder might tend to be perpetuated. Presumably, his vigor would be transmitted genetically to his children, and his financial success would further favor their survival. Thus, the genetic disadvantages of predisposition to late-onset circulatory disorders would have no evolutionary import.

A second mechanism by which disease-producing characteristics may survive in the population is a high rate of mutation, the alteration of the genes so that new traits appear. It may be induced by, among other things, radiation and exposure to various chemicals. Mutation, however, is relatively uncommon, and if a disorder interferes seriously with breeding, a gene cannot mutate fast enough to keep from being bred out.

A third explanation for the persistence of detrimental characteristics is that possession of a fraction of a hereditary disorder may be beneficial to the individual. For each genetically determined characteristic, each person receives at least one gene from his mother and one from his father. These may be identical—homozygous; or different—heterozygous. An example of benefit from a partial genetic share occurs in sickle-cell anemia. The disorder, which evolved in malarial Africa, affects one structure of the hemoglobin molecule in the red blood cell. Possession of a double dose—a homozygous state—of the genetic material tends to shorten the life span by producing sickle-cell anemia.

However, possession of a single dose—the heterozygous state—may render that person less susceptible to malaria and does not cause anemia. Heterozygotes are far more common than homozygotes. If heterozygotes breed, they do increase the number of ill homozygotes, but they also increase, and much more rapidly, the number of malaria-resistant heterozygotes.

Schizophrenia affords no obvious advantages to the individual, and flagrantly schizophrenic persons do not breed at a rate rapid enough to maintain their own level in the population. In days past, when severe schizophrenics were incarcerated and removed from the breeding pool, one would have expected the frequency of schizophrenia in the population to have diminished even more rapidly than by simple lack of success at the mating game. Is it possible that possession of a little bit of schizophrenia is advantageous in a manner analogous to possession of half of the gene pair for sickle-cell anemia? There are many more mildly afflicted individuals than seriously afflicted ones; perhaps the milder schizophrenias have some adaptational advantage.

On the positive side of the ledger, it has been argued that madness and genius are "oft allied." Perhaps a small quantity of schizophrenia tends to be associated with intellectual and creative abilities that confer some advantages on the carrier. We know of no definitive studies, though, of either the diagnoses or fertility of geniuses (to cite an illustration of the variable fertility of geniuses—an illustration *not* related to schizophrenia: Bach had twenty children, Newton none).

It could be speculated, also, that those with a small amount of the illness might be more fertile. If so, it would only take one rooster in the barnyard to sire a lot of chickens. Certainly, many borderline schizophrenic women are promiscuous and may have borne disproportionate numbers of children and thus compensate, in replenishing the schizophrenic gene pool, for the poor reproductive performance of schizophrenic men.

Still another formulation is that schizophrenia is an expression of a genetic phenomenon called polymorphic balance. The greater the variety a species possesses—even when that variety includes poorly functioning individuals—the more it is able to adapt to differing demands and changing environments; hypothetically, the increased adaptability enables the species to survive longer as a species, even though that species-wide adaptability seems to have paradoxical origins in less adaptable individuals. This formulation, like the preceding ones, provides no definitive answer to the question of why the incidence of schizophrenia seems to have been relatively constant.

With improved treatment of schizophrenics, however, the possibility now arises that their reproduction rate will increase. As noted above, hospitalized schizophrenics reproduce themselves at a much lower rate than their nonschizophrenic fellows. With the increased use of antipsychotic medication, many of these people have been released from state hospitals, with a consequent increase in the likelihood that they will have children. Whereas, formerly, chronic schizophrenics bred at about one third to one half the rate of the rest of the population, they may now have achieved parity (Burr et al., 1979). According to incidence data on children of schizophrenics, approximately 10 percent will become chronically schizophrenic, and perhaps another 40 percent will have schizophrenia-like conditions.

We do not have enough information to answer the ethical questions that come to mind, but it is not too early to consider them. Since it is not possible to predict the consequences of the mating of schizophrenics, whose welfare should be of first importance? That of the schizophrenic parent who wants children? That of the half of the schizophrenics' offspring who seem entirely normal? That of the 10 percent of the schizophrenics' offspring who may look forward to seventy-odd years of misery? That of the 40 percent of the offspring whose lives can vary from distancing oddness to creative advantage? It is illegal for parents to brutalize their children. If their judgment is impaired, should they be allowed to decide questions of this kind?

These are ethical and political, not scientific questions, but society requires facts for informed decisions. The ethical philosopher cannot meaningfully cogitate until the geneticists and psychiatrists provide him with the facts. In the meantime, patients, families, physicians, hospitals, clinics, and the community should realize that voluntary genetic counseling is already available (Brady and Brodie, 1978).

A recent study by the National Institute of Mental Health suggests that such counseling not only might affect decisions about marriage and childbearing but also might enable couples who are planning or involved in a marriage in which one partner (or both) is mentally ill to understand more clearly the nature of the problems that may arise (Targum et al., in press). In a small NIMH study that bears extension to a larger sample, nineteen manic-depressive patients and their healthy spouses were given questionnaires to learn their opinions about the etiology, familial risk, and chronic burden of manic-depressive illness, and their attitudes about marriage and childbearing. In the responses to the questionnaire, 10 (53%) of the healthy spouses but only one (5%) of the patients said they would not have married if they had known more about the illness before marriage; 9 (47%) of the healthy spouses but only one (5%) of the patients said they would not have had children if they had known about the genetic risks. Of the sixteen families with children, seven (44%) had children with some form of psychiatric illness; five (31%) had children with bipolar (manic-depressive) or unipolar (depressive) illness.

The strategy of studying adopted persons has begun to answer age-old questions of nature and nurture. So far, the technique has been applied to study of the schizophrenias, the mood disorders, and the Unnamed Quartet of personality disorders. But, in fact, the technique can be used to examine any aspect of psychiatric illness or even normal personality.

One point has been made repeatedly: the fact that some instances of any disorder are genetic does not prove that all are. More important, what is not genetic is not necessarily psychological. Individuals experience many biological vagaries in the course of their existence that may affect psychological function.

Psychiatric illnesses that are genetically transmitted must have biological substrates. How these are mediated—through faulty chemistry, through a predisposition to viral infections or abnormal immune reactions, or through other abnormalities as yet unsuspected—remains to be discovered. However, from observation of the highly specific responses some illnesses show to therapeutic chemicals, and from the knowledge now available of what these chemicals do to brain functions, it is possible to make increasingly sophisticated guesses as to the abnormal chemistry that may underlie these illnesses.

Of what practical relevance are these findings to the lay person? First, they emphasize something all of us do—or should—realize: that one must choose one's biological parents with exquisite care. We are, however, not privileged to take part in making this basic, and possibly most important, decision of our lives. Second, we should exercise great care in choosing the person with whom we plan to have children. Many of us have witnessed the unhappiness of the twice-married parent raising children conceived in a first impulsive, youthful marriage. Some parents raise the offspring of an alcoholic or antisocial or schizophrenic spouse in a new, wholesome environment only to find to their horror that the ex-spouse's psychological deficits are unfolding relentlessly in the child. This has been scientifically documented in the case of individuals whose mothers married twice, and one of the mates was alcoholic. Increased alcoholism was found only among those offspring whose biological fathers had difficulties with alcohol (i.e., the chance of being alcoholic was higher if the biological fathers were alcoholic, even though the mother remarried when the offspring were young and they were brought up in a non-alcoholic household). To make matters worse, mental disorders sometimes seem to skip generations. One of us remembers poignantly the anger and grief of a mother of a schizophrenic who said about her husband: "I knew that half his family was mentally disturbed but that he wasn't [a correct diagnosis on both scores]. If I knew then what I know now, I never would have had his children." Though these are disturbing matters about which all of us do not like to think, the consequences for self-protection are obvious.

CHAPTER 6

The New Biology of the Mind and Its Psychological Implications

A major insight into the underlying mechanisms of mental illness comes from the recent expansion of knowledge of brain physiology and chemistry, which has been accumulating exponentially during the last twenty years. These tantalizing new inroads into a vast, hitherto unknown area are already enabling us to see patterns in much of what had formerly been mysterious. Of special importance in the field of psychiatry are the conjectures concerning how nervous transmission may occur within the brain. The part of the brain that governs sensing, thinking, and feeling consists of at least 10 trillion (10,000 billion) cells. Each cell consists of a round body, microscopic in size, which contains much of the chemical machinery, and an extension, the axon (or wire) connecting the cell, in an incredibly complex manner, to hundreds or even thousands of other cells. The diameter of the axon is microscopic, but its length may be inches to feet. Coordinated brain activity is produced by the conduction or transmission of electrical impulses (discharge, or "firing") from one nerve cell to another by means of the axon. This process takes place, not only by simple electrical conduction, as with two copper wires that are touching each other, but, surprisingly, by chemical means.

Available evidence allows the following hypothesis about how chemical conduction from one cell to another may take place. When the first cell is stimulated, an electrical impulse travels the length of its axon and at the end discharges or releases a very small packet of chemicals known as neurotransmitters. When the neurotransmitters are released, they drift rapidly across an extremely small space—the synaptic cleft—between the axon and the adjoining nerve cell, either stimulating that nerve cell, causing it in turn to fire, or inhibiting it, diminishing its ability to respond to stimulation by other nerve cells. Obviously, if the neurotransmitter remained in contact with the second cell indefinitely, its action would continue indefinitely. Such prolonged action appears to be prevented in several ways. In one, the cell releasing the neurotransmitter can be compared to a wet sponge. When it fires, it squeezes and releases fluid; when it stops firing, it reexpands and reabsorbs the released fluid. In this way, the cell continues to use its supply of neurotransmitters over and over again in an economical manner. Among the other ways in which indefinite firing of the second cell can be prevented is chemical breakdown of the neurotransmitter by substances that exist for this purpose in the synaptic cleft.

This system of nervous transmission can obviously be affected by a number of factors. First, synthesis of the neurotransmitter by the first cell could be diminished. Second, the ability of the first cell to release the neurotransmitter might be impaired. Third, if the sensitivity of the second cell to the released compound was decreased, the second cell would fire less actively. Fourth, if some mechanism interfered with the re-uptake ability of the first cell, the concentration of the neurotransmitter outside the cell would remain high, with an increased tendency for the second cell either to be fired or to be inhibited. Drugs with powerful effects on mood and behavior may operate on these mechanisms.

In the last decade, researchers have also learned that there are a number of different neurotransmitters. In certain sectors of the brain, substance A may be released, affecting particular kinds of nerve cells, while in other areas it may be substance B, and so on. It is not clear whether each nerve cell releases only one sort of neurotransmitter or whether some cells release a mixture. Chemicals that affect the synthesis or release of particular neurotransmitters will affect only those parts of the brain in which those neurotransmitters occur. If they amplify A's activity, they will increase the activity of that portion of the brain. If they inhibit A's activity, they will decrease activity there. Moreover, even if a drug excites one part of the brain, the overall effect may be one of inhibition. If you stimulate a brake, you don't go faster; if you cut off power to the brakes in a car going downhill, you accelerate (or excite) the car.

Heretofore, researchers could stimulate specific parts of the brain only by inserting electrodes through the skull into those very areas. This procedure has been used for diagnostic and therapeutic purposes but it is of course difficult and sometimes dangerous. Such differential stimulation of the brain can now be done in many instances solely by chemical means. In a general way, we have made the first crude connection between chemistry and the mind.

This knowledge of chemistry helps us to understand the three major forms of genetically produced mental illness: the disorders of mood, several personality disorders (hysteroid dysphoria and the Unnamed Quartet), and the schizophrenias; in other words, how chemistry is related to sadness, badness, and madness.

Biopsychology in Disorders of Mood

As indicated earlier, we believe that the diminished experiencing of pleasure is the critical aspect of depression. Vital depressives are not merely sad or disappointed: they do not anticipate pleasure or pursue it, and even when they are in situations most people would regard as enjoyable, they fail to feel pleasure. Some kinds of neurotic depressives do not *seek* consummatory pleasure, but enjoy it if it is presented to them. They may not want to go to the party, but have a good time when they get there. In the manic, the pursuit of pleasure seems greatly exaggerated, so that ordinary sensible precautions are ignored.

The fact that, in some disorders, *only* the joys of the chase are lost, while in others the joys of *both* the chase *and* the feast are lost, leads us to believe that both the joys and their causes are distinct and separate. Clinically, we find that stimulant drugs, such as the amphetamines, impart a burst of energy and optimism. They sometimes relieve the symptoms of demoralization, increasing the joy of the pursuit. In vital depressives, stimulant drugs do not restore the joys of either anticipation or consumption. The implication is that there are brain centers regulating energy, self-evaluation, and appetitive, goal-directed activity, and that amphetamines activate them only in patients without a vital depression. A further implication is that antidepressant medications must affect brain centers concerned with the enjoyment of the feast.

Moreover, depressed people eat or sleep too much or too little and usually have no sex drive, whereas manics are often hypersexual. The monoamines or biogenic amines are intimately involved with the regulation of these processes, but our knowledge of them is incomplete and only tantalizing. Appetite appears to be regulated by an appestat that tells the individual when he should start and stop eating. Amphetamines turn down the appestat and thus facilitate weight loss. Direct application of various biogenic amines to the portion of the brain thought to contain the appestat will similarly affect an animal's tendency to eat. Some biogenic amines foster and others inhibit the tendency to sleep. The amphetamines, which increase the activity of adrenaline-like substances, keep people awake. These substances are thought to act in a portion of the brain called the reticular activating system, whose function is to regulate wakefulness. Finally, chemicals that decrease the amount of one of the biogenic amines, serotonin, in the brain apparently turn male rats into Don Juans. When used to treat certain illnesses, these chemicals seem dramatically to increase the sex drive. Preliminary studies also indicate that the agents also increase the sexuality of nondiseased persons. (Unfortunately, the substance in question is rather toxic and cannot be routinely used to restimulate flagging desires.)

The hypotheses about how these mechanisms work have also drawn upon findings from reserpine research. As mentioned, reserpine produced severe depression in some patients to whom it was administered in the treatment of hypertension. Experimental work with animals revealed that reserpine profoundly depleted the brain of three chemicals belonging to the family of monoamines. Two of the chemicals are very close relatives of adrenaline. The antituberculosis drug iproniazid, which produced euphoria in some patients, was found to increase the brain content of these biogenic amines (monoamines) by interfering with the chemical-breakdown process that ordinarily prevents the accumulation of excess amounts of these substances in nerve cells—that is, by inhibiting the enzyme monoamine oxidase. The conclusion tentatively reached was that the biogenic amines are concerned with the control of mood, and that a deficiency of such amines—as induced by reserpine—produces depression; an excess—as induced by iproniazid—produces a state of being high, excited or manic.

This was a tenable but crude hypothesis. The major trouble with it is that most people are not depressed by reserpine or elated by antidepressants. These drugs seem therefore, to be acting in a way that to some degree must depend on the preexisting health of the mood center involved.

These observations have coalesced with earlier discoveries. In the 1950s, investigators had found that electrical stimulation of parts of the brain could be interpreted as producing pleasure in animals; at least, animals would work very hard to obtain electrical stimulation of certain portions of the brain (and would work equally hard to avoid such stimulation in other portions). Limited experimentation with humans undergoing neurosurgery indicated that electrical stimulation of comparable areas of the human brain was associated with a feeling of generalized well-being, which patients sometimes characterized as having sexual overtones. Of extreme interest was the fact that these pleasure centers correspond roughly to the anatomical areas of the brain containing high concentrations of the biogenic amines. This was further circumstantial evidence that areas containing biogenic amines were concerned with the regulation of pleasurable experience.

Experiments with animals revealed that chemicals that depleted nerve cells of biogenic amines decreased the tendency of the animals to respond to electrical stimulation of such parts of the brain. That meant that these chemicals had to be present in order for the electrical stimulation to generate pleasure. Interestingly, stimulants such as amphetamine increased the tendency of animals to respond to such electrical stimulation of the brain. Antidepressants reinforced the effects of amphetamine but, curiously, were not effective on their own. Moreover, animals became socially inactive when given drugs that diminished the brain's ability to produce biogenic amines—in other words, they manifested one of the symptoms of depression.

As a result of these and similar findings, some neurochemists and psychiatrists evolved the biogenic amine theory of depression. This theory proposes that serious depression occurs because of an underactivity of nerve cells—some of which are intimately connected with the experience of pleasure—whose neurotransmitters are the biogenic amines. The theory loosely hypothesizes that such underactivity might be due to deficient production of the neurotransmitters, excessive breakdown of the neurotransmitter before it is released, inability to release the neurotransmitter, or a decreased response sensitivity of the stimulated cell. In its most simple formulations, the theory pictured mania as the reverse side of the coin, with too much of the critical biogenic amines available. Research is currently being done to try to determine if this theory is correct and which processes are involved if so.

The theory also prompted investigation of the actions of the tricyclic antidepressants. These agents immediately block re-uptake of the neurotransmitter by the releasing cell, which may leave an excess of the neurotransmitter available to compensate for a postulated deficiency. Unfortunately for this theory, the re-uptake blockade occurs immediately, whereas beneficial effects on mood are delayed for several weeks.

The biogenic amine theory also offered an explanation of the actions of drugs such as amphetamines and cocaine in producing euphoria in normal individuals. The amphetamines were found to have many functions: they cause the release of biogenic amines, prevent their reuptake, and, like iproniazid, prevent their breakdown within the cells that synthesize them. Cocaine was found to cause similar actions.

Peculiarly, neither amphetamine nor cocaine has any value in the treatment of vital depressions. Animal experimentation revealed that both drugs gradually lost their ability to stimulate when administered repeatedly, which corresponds to the experience of addicts. Recent studies indicate that nerve cells may act like thermostats, tending to keep the rate of their firing constant. When chemicals such as amphetamines are given, the cell tends to release more neurotransmitter at first, but then the thermostat goes into action. The cell compensates by making less neurotransmitter, so that the overall rate of release is returned to normal. Thus, chemicals such as amphetamines and cocaine can only temporarily trick the brain, until it compensates for their actions. This may be one reason why these drugs are of no practical use in vital depressions and why normal people develop tolerance to them. On occasion they temporarily produce improvement, but then the brain cleverly reverts to normal.

The differences in the actions of stimulants and antidepressants on both normal individuals and patients with vital depression are difficult to understand. The antidepressant drugs will usually relieve depression in vital depressives but will *not* produce euphoria in persons who are not depressed. Accordingly, they are not abusable or habit-forming drugs. Their action may be roughly compared to that of aspirin, which lowers temperature when a fever is present but does not produce an abnormally low temperature when the temperature is normal.

Another remarkable property of these drugs is that vital depressives do *not* become tolerant to them. When they work, the depressed patient does not need to take larger and larger doses to obtain the same effect. Perhaps they actually temporarily repair a defective "thermostat." This would account for their lack of effect on normal persons and their profound effect on persons with depressive states. All this is hard to account for by a simple biogenic amine theory.

These explanations, if valid, only indicate that electrical or chemical stimulation of certain portions of the brain is associated with an increased ability to experience pleasure. *Why* such activity in the brain is paralleled by a *subjective* experience epitomizes one of the fundamental unanswered questions of science: the origin of consciousness.

Three familiar and interrelated psychological attributes seem to play an especially large part in depression: self-esteem, separation anxiety, and aggression. What possible interrelationships exist between physiological components of mood disorders and these attributes?

Self-esteem, as pointed out earlier, is closely tied to mood. Vital depressives have low self-esteem. They are self-critical, demean their accomplishments, believe they are unattractive, and think they are unloved and unlovable. The reverse is true in mania. Manic patients are grandiose, overevaluating their abilities and reacting with surprise when others do not regard them as favorably as they regard themselves. When depression or mania gets better spontaneously or is successfully treated, the disorder of self-esteem is also normalized. When the manic is successfully treated with lithium, his overevaluation disappears.

Drugs can also affect self-esteem in normal persons. In addition to producing euphoria, amphetamines increase feelings of self-worth and the worth of one's products. When amphetamines wear off, however, there is often a rebound of depression, typically accompanied by a feeling of below-normal self-esteem. The transient drug-produced euphoria is very evident when college students use these drugs when they write papers at the last minute. While influenced by the drug they frequently believe they are composing masterpieces. The morning after, their brains somewhat depleted of biogenic amines, they often reappraise their product—perhaps overcritically—and perceive it as considerably less worthy.

Self-esteem is probably another example of the phenocopy. As noted in Chapter 5, the psychodynamic explanation of the development of self-esteem is that it is a product of the infant's relations with others. If his parents value and love him, if others esteem him, presumably he believes that he is worthwhile. The developing child learns that he is good or bad in the same way that he learns racial and religious prejudice, political preferences, and ethnic loyalty. Self-esteem is believed to be stamped in early in development and to persist, as do prejudices, in the face of contrary evidence.

The individual's real characteristics may also influence the judgment of others and thus his or her self-esteem. If the person is unattractive, clumsy, or stupid, it is unlikely that she will receive unbounded admiration and love. In a sense, attributes that she cannot control indirectly generate her feelings of self-esteem. Since some of the characteristics mentioned are genetic in origin, one gets a complex chain of events in which biology may endow someone with unfortunate attributes, leading to perceptions of that individual by others as undesirable; in turn, she realistically learns to regard herself as undesirable.

An interesting aspect of the development of self-esteem is that there seem to be critical periods. This was shown in a clever study by psychiatrist Albert Stunkard in which relatively svelte adults who had been fat in childhood, adolescence, or early adulthood were questioned regarding their attractiveness. Whatever weight they had lost as adults, those who had been fat in childhood and adolescence—especially adolescence—tended to continue to perceive themselves as physically undesirable. The persistence of negative body image did not characterize those who gained and lost weight as adults.

It is also entirely possible that many persons with feelings of diminished worth—seemingly neurotic or inexplicable in origin—suffer from undetected vital depression. The question may be answered through the administration of antidepressants. As we saw in the case history of William M., if medication that usually only sedates normal persons increases self-esteem in a given individual, we can be relatively certain that the feelings of low self-esteem were the product of faulty chemistry rather than the learned residues of unfortunate early personal experience.

Thus, the possibility of biologically based self-esteem—and mood in general—seems to us to have evolutionary utility. Optimism and pessimism and one's feelings about oneself are useful temporary guides in dealing with a fluctuating environment that provides patches of danger or sustenance. If one is subject to a series of defeats, it pays to adopt a conservative game plan of sitting back and waiting and letting others take the risks. Such waiting would be fostered by a pessimistic outlook. Similarly, if one is raking in the chips of life, it pays to adopt an expansive risk-taking approach, and thus maximize access to scarce resources.

A second but not as widely recognized attribute that seems closely tied to depression is *separation anxiety,* which has been studied in depth by Donald Klein. When Klein began to study patients with agoraphobias, he noted that when younger, they had often suffered from overpowering homesickness or school phobia. School phobia is a psychological disorder defined by a child's extreme reluctance to go to school, but it can extend to camp or even to sleep-overs at a friend's house. Earlier studies of the disorder had led psychiatrists to believe that it stemmed from parent-child interactions. They postulated that the mother covertly supported the child's wish to stay at home, or communicated to the child her anxiety about the child's going to school, or formed such an intense relationship with the child that he became anxious whenever he left his mother.

These explanations were in line with the psychological observation that school-phobic children had anxieties about their parents and not about the school. They feared that when they were away from home some catastrophe might befall their parents and therefore they did not want to leave. Following Anna Freud, psychoanalysts explained this fear as an unconscious expression of the child's hostility toward an overprotective parent. Presumably, the child concealed his unconscious death wishes from himself and others by manifestations of overconcern. His anxiety, the theory continued, stemmed from his unconscious guilt and his belief in the omnipotence of his unconscious. Unfortunately, the application of this theory, in the form of play analysis, often does not lead to a successful return to school.

Other psychiatrists, following Leon Eisenberg, found that about 75 percent of these children were relatively easy to treat with behavioral techniques that consisted of forcing the child to return to the school setting and keeping him there until his anxiety diminished. The mother, however, requires psychotherapy so that she does not sabotage these proceedings.

When Klein discovered that separation-anxious agoraphobics responded to antidepressant medication, he hypothesized that the younger versions of such patients—the severely homesick or school phobic—might likewise respond to treatment with that medication. Accordingly, he and his wife, Rachel Gittelman-Klein, organized a study of school-phobic children who had not responded to the usual treatment techniques. They investigated the psychological characteristics of such children and the effect of antidepressant medication in relieving their symptomatology and facilitating their return to school. The investigation confirmed the earlier observation about the children's anxieties with regard to their parents, but the effects of the experimental treatment cast doubt on the psychodynamic explanations.

When such children were treated with behavioral techniques alone, approximately half returned to school, but the children often continued to be distressed. When the behavioral techniques were combined with the medication, the children's anxiety and occasional depressive complaints diminished or disappeared, and they not only returned to school but returned to school happily. Behavioral techniques had accomplished some behavioral ends, but the antidepressant medication had benefited the children's subjective state, allowing a pain-free separation (see Gittelman-Klein and Klein, 1971). To us, the implication of these and related observations is that the psychodynamic reasoning advanced to explain separation anxiety has little to do with its basic cause.

Since separation anxiety is sometimes seen in depression and since depression is sometimes precipitated by separation from an important person, these observations are of theoretical as well as practical importance. We conjecture that one common component of a potential depressive's biology is an increased susceptibility to distress when separated from loved ones. Treatment of depression with antidepressants is accompanied not only by a decrease in depressive symptomatology but also by an increased toleration for separation from others who matter. We would like to attempt to make sense of this chemical and clinical observation in biopsychological and evolutionary terms.

Freud had proposed a learning theory of separation anxiety, explaining it on the basis of the infant's experience. Presumably, the infant notices that he is subject to discomfort (being wet, hungry, and thirsty) when his mother is absent, and that his needs are met when she is present. Separation anxiety is accounted for by the anticipation of increasing discomfort when Mom is not around. Pavlov would have been proud of this simple conditioning model.

Observations of animals, however, indicate that they are distressed when they are separated from their nest or mother before they could have learned that separation means absence of relief from discomfort. Puppies, kittens, and chicks will produce a wail of protest *the first time* they are separated from their mothers. If they have wandered away, they emit retrieval signals that have the predictable effect of causing the mothers to search actively and attempt to bring them back home. Similarly, infant monkeys raised in groups without mothers will cry pitifully when they are separated from each other. Mothering as such does not exist in these groups, yet distress on separation is extreme when the infant is removed from his peer group.

The fact that separation anxiety may occur before the animal or child has experience with separation does not mean that separation anxiety is totally unlearned. Rather, it seems that learning may be engrafted upon the bedrock of an innate biological mechanism. Detailed studies of monkeys and the behavior of infants in institutions shed further light on separation anxiety, especially when we conceive of such behavior in an evolutionary context. What adaptive sense does it make for individuals to become anxious when separated from loved ones?

First, let us look at the interesting predictable sequence of events that occurs when young children (say, ages two to four) or monkeys are separated from their mothers. Initially, the infant monkey or child goes through a period of protest, crying disconsolately and moving around actively. After a while, the protest diminishes and a second stage occurs, called despair, in which the monkey or child stops moving and crying and looks despondent or depressed. After another variable period of time, a third stage ensues in children but not in monkeys, a stage called detachment. The depressive symptoms disappear and the child seems normal. However, if he is reunited with his mother, he acts strangely apathetic and indifferent, turning away from her and toward his new caretakers.

In speculating on the possible evolutionary utility of this behavior, we note that when an infant is at first separated from his mother or caretaker, he is at increased risk. He has no protection against predators, hunger, or thirst. It is evolutionarily useful, therefore, if he raises a ruckus and searches actively, before suffering the actual pain of starvation. Such behavior is likely to attract the attention of his caretaker and restore him to his protected position before any damage has occurred.

If, however, help is not forthcoming after some time, it probably pays now for the child to keep quiet. Further noise and expenditure of effort would exhaust his metabolic resources and might notify predators that there is a meal available. From an evolutionary perspective, his chances of survival would be increased if his environmental interactions were acutely decreased, even though he remains conscious and able to signal possible rescuers. One way in which this might occur is through evolutionary selection of those with inhibition of the brain's pleasure centers under certain circumstances. By throwing the child into a state of despair, such inhibition would adaptively prevent him from continuing to appeal for help and to explore his surroundings.

The despair that accompanies the cessation of activity, the reaction to acute loss, also seems to be a technique for dissolving the bonds of affection. It apparently functions as grief does in adults, weakening ties and eventually freeing the individual to form new interpersonal bonds. The manifestations of grief—including physiological changes—are virtually identical to those seen in depression. Many aspects of vital depression seemingly resemble a spontaneous grief reaction.

The evolutionary utility of the detachment phase can be seen as building on the despair, further freeing the child by actively inhibiting his old attachments and enabling him to form bonds with new caretakers. In other words, the detachment phase allows successful adoption by other adults. Chimps may try to adopt orphans, but they fail. The detachment phase has yet to evolve in our primitive primate cousins. The infant who has reached the detached phase may eventually—after a period of intense clinging—develop a new relationship.

Thus, pathological separation anxiety, as in school phobia, seems to represent an exaggeration of a normal reaction often triggered by a trivial event or family loss. The individual's threshold is very low; he is vulnerable. Similarly, vital depression—at times precipitated by events—seems to represent an unusually low threshold for sustaining prolonged grief or despair reactions, together with an inability to experience pleasure.

Protest and despair reactions may be co-evolved control mechanisms related to similar protection processes seen in the lost toddler. Complex mechanisms may have developed that lower a threshold and fire off separation anxiety, or despair, or both. That the antidepressant medications work on both vital depressions and separation anxiety may indicate that their effect is simply to raise threshold levels in the inadequate central-control mechanisms, thus blocking either or both symptom patterns.

Separation anxiety is frequently unrecognized except when it appears as school phobia or agoraphobia or panic attacks. This is unfortunate, because people who are cursed with vulnerability to separation suffer frequently from anxiety and depression, and their sustained efforts to cling to the loved one can themselves have unfortunate psychological effects. They may become relentlessly intrusive and demanding, driving the loved one off by these self-defeating tactics. The therapeutic implication is that if separation anxiety—in its less obvious forms—were more frequently recognized, much anguish might be avoided. A trial of antidepressant medication with patients who are separation-anxious may bring surprisingly quick relief in situations where prolonged psychotherapy has not been helpful.

The dilemma of someone with a chronic undetected depression of probable biological origin—whose major manifestation is an insatiable need for the love and support of others—sometimes leads to other psychological strategies to allay the unquenchable needs, usually without the person's awareness. In order not to drive others off, such an individual may try to anticipate their expressed and unexpressed wishes, keeping his own wishes in abeyance. Thus, he may be predisposed to become passive and compliant. Being assertive, giving vent to his own wishes, is seen as a risky business because of the possibility of antagonizing others or provoking their withdrawal. Furthermore, since it is painful to want something and not act on it, the individual is likely to suppress or repress his self-assertive and selfish desires, unconsciously pushing them out of awareness.

This coping mechanism, typically regarded as neurotic, may be the kind of compromise that is the best of a bad bargain for someone with extremely strong needs for others and an extremely strong fear of separation or rejection. At the expense of being passive and self-effacing, the dependent person avoids the greatest catastrophe of all: losing the love, care, and esteem of valued people. This, too, has implications for therapy. If such dependency is decreased by medication, one cannot expect the ex-depressive instantly to give up well-learned interpersonal maneuvers. Not just medication but a relearning psychotherapy may be necessary.

Is *aggression* related to depression? Depression is often assumed to stem from the person's failure to express anger appropriately. Presumably, he or she holds the anger in, turns it inward, and therefore—through the mysterious workings of the mind—becomes depressed. It is commonly believed that depressives do not express anger outward, but this belief has not been subjected to empirical confirmation. In describing a recent detailed longitudinal study, Myrna Weissman and Eugene Paykel state: "Not only has hostility increased during the acute depression, but there was no evidence of any inhibition of hostility after recovery. Interpersonal friction remains substantially increased rather than decreased. Once again those simple formulations which relate depression in a direct way to the internalization of hostility and the inability to externalize it receive no support" (1974, p. 169).

Psychiatrists in the past may have theorized about depression on the basis of patients who did not manifest overt hostility during the therapy session. Any generalizations formulated on such a basis—which assumes that the patient's reactions to the therapist encapsulate her problems and represent her behavior in the real world—overlook the critical role that may be played by the patient's reluctance to antagonize someone who represents her only hope.

Aside from such unvalidated theory, however, the idea that increased anger may be present in biological depression makes some neurochemical sense, and it is supported by animal research. Animals will attack if pain is induced in them; they will attack if their nest or young are threatened; they will defend their territory if intruders trespass; and they will compete for mates. Chemicals that increase or decrease certain biogenic amines differentially increase or decrease these different forms of aggressive behavior, supporting the idea that the various forms of aggression are regulated separately and are different from each other. It does not take a wide leap of the imagination to infer that variations in such amines play a role in human irritability, anger, and sexual jealousy. And, indeed, some biological depressives exhibit not only the former behaviors but also a pathological, sometimes paranoid, form of sexual jealousy.

Depressed patients who respond positively to antidepressants become less irritable and angry, contrary to the common psychodynamic explanation, which would suppose that the relief of depression and the outward expression of anger would go together. Similarly, pathological jealousy often disappears. These observations strongly suggest that biogenic amine function is related not only to mood but to assertiveness, hostility, and sexual drive.

We are tantalizingly close to and frustratingly distant from an understanding of the ways in which chemicals and aberrant physiology affect mood. We know that the apparent biological factors in the disorders of mood are closely interwoven with such psychological factors as low self-esteem, extreme dependency, and high irritability. The depressive becomes withdrawn, the manic becomes impulsive, the masked depression can malfunction in any of a number of ways. These attributes in turn produce further psychological and social complications—for example, marital and employment difficulties, escape to alcoholism, and the threat of suicide. Moreover, basic biological abnormalities have predictable secondary psychological consequences—i.e., attempting to cope with unsolvable problems, people use psychological techniques that are only partially successful. These may reduce some symptoms but may in turn cause others.

Biopsychology in Personality Disorders

Several of the personality disorders lend themselves to an analysis of possible interactions of physical and psychological causal factors—hysteroid dysphoria, hyperactivity, antisocial personality, and alcoholism and drug abuse. Similar analyses could be done with other personality disorders, particularly those that seem to be close to the schizophrenias, but the data are fuller for some of those on which we are focusing and these are good illustrations of our point of view.

Hysteroid dysphoria. When everything is going well for patients with hysteroid dysphoria—when they are in their "normal" state—they are often very active, with enormous energy and flair. But they are extremely sensitive to rejection from others, changing mood abruptly and becoming profoundly depressed. The depression is frequently accompanied by an overwhelming feeling of lethargy and a need to go to bed and to overeat sweets. Traditional psychoanalytic thinking has described such behavior in terms of pathological defenses and unrealistic, self-aggrandizing fantasy goals; more recently, some psychoanalysts have labeled these patients borderline, suggesting a relationship to schizophrenia. We think there is no relationship whatsoever to schizophrenia and that we can make some biological sense of the hysteroid dysphoric's behavior.

We see the hysteroid dysphoric's primary problem as maintaining a tolerable mood despite inordinate sensitivity to rejection. These women's seductive attempts to elicit approval and avoid rejection are directly related to this goal. Our alternate explanation is not accidental but is the consequence of the development of new medication and treatments. When such patients are treated with psychotherapy, as is still usually the case, the focus is on aspects of behavior that seem modifiable—the patient's relations to others and her interpersonal tactics. Mood instability and the dependence on external sources of applause for self-esteem are considered secondary to internal conflicts that must be resolved if these emotions and behaviors are to change. The discovery that specific medication can directly change the mood instability of these patients now suggests that their interpersonal tactics and conflicts are not primary but rather secondary reverberations of their basic instability of mood.

We hypothesize that in everyone there is a biological mechanism that responds positively to the experience of social approval, applause, and admiration. In the earlier discussion of shame, guilt, and rejection, we spoke of the influence of these factors in the development of an internalized conscience. It seems to us that processes of these kinds make evolutionary sense, for the individuals who obtain the social approval of their parents and peers by abandoning disapproved behaviors and adopting desirable ones—by incorporating their ego-ideal—have a survival advantage.

Clearly, the particular ego-ideal the child develops will depend on the circumstances under which she is raised and will vary widely from culture to culture, class to class, and family to family. The mechanisms that produce the ego-ideals, however—a love of applause and a striving toward making ourselves applause-worthy—seem built in. This proclivity to think, feel, and behave in accordance with the wishes of loved ones does not seem confined to humans. Higher apes likewise imitate and adopt social models.

Some early psychoanalytic thinkers and many learning theorists have ignored these evolutionary realities, arguing that the wish to imitate the parent was only a secondary phenomenon related to the parent's response to the child's physiological needs. Although other theorists, such as Harry Stack Sullivan and also the psychoanalysts who focus on narcissistic disorders, have emphasized the motivating force of the need for approval, they have failed to move from that position to what seems to us to be the obvious next step. We believe that the need to receive applause is a primary, biological, innate source of gratification that can serve as a direct molder of behavior.

In hysteroid dysphorics, we believe that the mood-control mechanism is faulty in that it produces an excessive need for approval. Such people swing wildly in both directions, overresponding to both approval and disapproval. Some may also have been exposed to peculiar standards for obtaining such approval. We have observed clinically that many appear to have been treated with great indulgence by their fathers and to have had narcissistic mothers (who, indeed, may have a similar genetic predisposition) as a female model.

One can understand the clinical characteristics of the hysteroid dysphoric as derived from her basic mood vulnerability—overreaction to both applause and rejection—combined with psychological techniques developed to compensate for this vulnerability. For example, the fickleness and giddiness may be seen as a direct expression of mood instability. Hysteroid dysphorics become euphoric at anyone's applause. Their shortsightedness and emotional reasoning can be seen as a domination of judgment by intense mood. Their theatricality and seductiveness are exaggerated devices for eliciting admiring masculine attention—often in the pattern of their mothers and with the goal of undiluted approval by the fathers. The hysteroid dysphoric sees others merely as sources of admiration and cannot develop a discriminating appreciation of their real complexities and subtleties. When the other person is no longer a source of continual admiration, there seems to be no reason to continue the relationship. The tearfulness, abusiveness, and vindictiveness are hypersensitive responses to disapproval, compounded by an aggressive response to frustration.

Although these patients speak frequently of loneliness, they are distinguished from those with other forms of depression in not being dominated by separation anxiety. If they are in the company of a man who is dull and unadmiring, they will remove themselves as quickly as possible. The patient dominated by separation anxiety, however, will accept—and indeed cling to—any type of companionship.

We believe that our hypothesis is supported by our observation that hysteroid dysphorics do not respond to the most frequently used antidepressants, the tricyclics, but do respond to the other major group, the MAO inhibitors. Klein is currently conducting a controlled clinical comparative trial of these two different classes of antidepressants.

As mentioned, with treatment, the hysteroid dysphorics' mood lability is stabilized in both directions: they require less approval and admiration, and do not become as upset when rejected.

We can make only a tentative guess as to why these patients respond only to a particular kind of antidepressant. There may be a clue in the variation between their normal energy and flair and the lethargy accompanying the dramatic response to rejection. The swing resembles that of a person placed on a chronic stimulant drug, such as Dexedrine, in moderate doses for a long time, and then suddenly withdrawn. When drug administration ceases, the individual moves from high-flying ebullience into a short-lived, paralytic lethargy accompanied by —as with the hysteroid—abrupt increase of appetite, especially for sweets.

We hypothesize that everyone's brain normally produces mood-elevating agents to serve as stimulants and internal sources of reward. We conjecture that these rewarding agents are released by social approval and appetitive activity when the individual is engaged in the chase. We likewise hypothesize that social disapproval and disappointment may trigger the sudden cut-off of such internal stimulating agents by biologically built-in regulatory controls. The evolutionary utility of the sudden cessation of such built-in mood-elevating agents is that it would help us to learn through immediately painful experience to avoid activities that are disappointing, socially disapproved, and therefore ultimately dangerous. In behaviorist terms, the brain chemical would serve as a rewarding agent for activities that produced social approval and its withdrawal would act as a punishment when we engaged in activities that produced social disapproval. We hypothesize that the hysteroid dysphoric seems to have an overactive approval-disapproval mechanism, so that when she is approved of she is chronically high, but when disapproved of is thrown into an abrupt withdrawal. Monoamine oxidase inhibitors might prevent the rapid destruction of the hypothesized intracerebral stimulants, so that when the patient is rejected, mood only dips normally instead of dropping disastrously.

It is possible, of course, that there are also phenocopy versions of the hysteroid dysphoric. Hypersensitivity to criticism and rejection has traditionally been explained on psychological grounds—for example, one may have been raised in an extremely rejecting and disapproving family; or familial experience may have given one unconscious, extremely critical attitudes, making him unduly sensitive to criticism from others because he unconsciously assumes that their criticism is as severe as his own; or the person may have unconscious wishes to dominate others and can best do it by acting in a martyr-like fashion. All these explanations and many others seem reasonable. The effectiveness of medication in altering this complex pattern of reaction suggests, however, that the biological explanation may be preferable.

Further clinical observation and study are required to document our explanation.

Hyperactivity. In exploring biological mechanisms that may be implicated in the personality disorders, we find the response of the hyperactive child to medication particularly relevant. Hyperactive children, afflicted with restlessness, inability to concentrate, inability to attend in a focused way, decreased response to reward and punishment, mood fluctuation, and often learning difficulties, react to treatment with stimulant drugs such as the amphetamines with a dramatic 60 to 80 percent positive response. In psychiatry, we are lucky if we can get the seriously ill patient back to his previous level of functioning. With hyperactive children, we are very frequently able to do what we can rarely do with adults: enable the patient to function better than he has ever functioned in the past. The stimulant medications not only slow such children down but also increase their ability to attend, increase their responsiveness to instruction, and mute their impulsivity. The medication frequently expands their ability to act in ways that are gratifying to others and to themselves as well.

In adults who were hyperactive as children and continue to be restless, inattentive, forgetful, disorganized, irritable, impulsive, and moody, stimulant medication often decreases restlessness and impulsivity, increases attentiveness and mood stability, and helps them to tolerate stress better and to initiate and sustain better relationships.

In general, patients—both children and adults—who respond to the medication do not become tolerant to it and do not require larger and larger doses. The failure to develop tolerance differentiates these people from "speed" abusers, who must rapidly escalate their dose to obtain the desired effect.

Animal studies can help us to make neurobiological sense of these drug reactions. In a number of studies, stimulant drugs have been shown to increase an animal's sensitivity to reinforcement. That is, stimulant drugs increase the effects of reward and possibly even of punishment so that animals learn habits more quickly and with greater degrees of success. This finding is provocative, because stimulant drugs make hyperactive children more responsive to reward and punishment.

A much more suggestive finding comes from a study of hybrid dogs that were being used by psychologist Samuel Corson in Pavlovian experiments. Corson found that a fraction of the dogs were restless in the training school and refractory to reward and punishment. He administered a variety of drugs to the animals with no beneficial effect until, aware of the syndrome of hyperactivity in children, he tried amphetamine. He was delighted to find that the stimulant medication quieted the dogs, and, like hyperactive children, they were better able to learn. This reaction to amphetamine was not typical of the other dogs he studied, however. Many of the fox terriers behaved in a stereotyped manner, with repetitious, purposeless movements, and showed increased activity. Eventually, researchers examined the brains of the dogs neurochemically; we will return to their findings shortly.

At about the same time, one of us (Wender) was entertaining the hypothesis that hyperactive children and adults both suffer from depletion of dopamine in the brain. In the Spanish-influenza epidemic at the end of World War I, adults in whom the virus produced an inflammation of the brain sometimes developed Parkinson's disease; autopsies on those who died indicated that parts of the brain concerned with the regulation of movement, and now known to contain large amounts of dopamine, had been destroyed. In children who recovered from such brain infections, the post-encephalitic behavior disorder was indistinguishable from naturally occurring hyperactivity. The obvious inference is that the virus had attacked dopamine cells in the children and had produced the alteration in behavior.

Another clue came from our knowledge of drug action. Currently, special research is being done on three of the biogenic amines—norepinephrine, dopamine, and serotonin. The antidepressants, so useful in vital depressions, primarily affect serotonin and norepinephrine, and dopamine to a much lesser degree. Amphetamines, which are effective in the treatment of hyperactive children—as antidepressants are not—affect all three biogenic amines and dopamine to a much greater degree than do the antidepressants. Since amphetamine stimulates dopamine more than the tricyclic antidepressants, one might expect to find less dopamine in the brains or in the fluids surrounding the brains of hyperactive children. One would also expect to find less of the breakdown products of dopamine in the brain and in the surrounding fluids.

To return now to the hyperactive hybrid dogs who responded to amphetamine, an examination of their brains did show decreased amounts of dopamine and its principal metabolites. Studying the fluid that surrounds the brain, the so-called cerebrospinal fluid, a researcher at Yale, Bennett Shaywitz, also found that a small group of hyperactive children showed less of the dopamine's breakdown products in the fluid. An obvious inference is that their brains were manufacturing less dopamine. Because the number of children was small and because of problems with the technique, these results are suggestive, not conclusive.

In other words, hyperactivity may be a dopamine-deficiency disease. This might make it the polar opposite of schizophrenia, which some have postulated is a dopamine-excess disease. In behavior, hyperactive children and adults are in some respects the opposites of schizophrenics. The average hyperactive person, for example, is extraverted, the average schizophrenic introverted. Many preschizophrenic children are unusually good and unusually easy to condition, in contrast with their hyperactive brothers, who are refractory to ordinary methods of discipline.

We do not want to carry this parallel too far, for the data do not make a perfectly neat picture. Some children have both borderline schizophrenic and hyperactive attributes, for example, and reactions to stimulants in such children are atypical. Further, hyperactive children often benefit from such drugs as Mellaril, whose effects would be to decrease the effectiveness of dopamine stimulation.

Antisocial personality. Because the disorder is of great social importance, it is worth speculating how the new biology might conceptualize antisocial personality. Antisocial individuals, formerly called psychopaths, are, as we have said, characterized by the inability to form emotional attachments to others, to identify with them, or to care for them. As with hyperactives and alcoholics, their siblings in the family of the Unnamed Quartet, they are unresponsive to the stimuli that usually create good citizens.

This psychological state has also been reported as a characteristic of children who were reared in sterile, badly staffed orphan asylums. Such children have been described as superficially sociable but without any ability to form deep, lasting, close relationships. As we said in the discussion of separation anxiety, these children seem indistinguishable from children in the detachment phase. It is as if the orphan children had been permanently locked into that detachment phase by overuse of the mechanism.

Before we explore this concept further, let us digress for a moment. A common belief among psychiatrists is that the personality development of antisocial persons has been faulty in the area of conscience (superego). Without the monitoring of conscience, the theory continues, the antisocial personality can express sexual and aggressive drives without repression and without the neurotic symptoms that might indicate internal conflict. When antisocial persons have been given systematic structured interviews, however, it turns out that they do have a high level of appetite loss, sad feelings, insomnia, breathing difficulties, and palpitations—neurotic symptoms that are very similar to those seen in panic disorder and vital depressions.

To us, the appearance of these symptoms in antisocial individuals provides more evidence for the hypothesis that an evolutionarily derived "lost-toddler retrieval mechanism," involving protest, despair, and detachment, plays a role in several disorders. For some people the threshold for activation of parts of this built-in biological mechanism may be set too low and easily triggered, on the basis either of particularly bad early experiences or of some biological, perhaps genetically transmitted, malfunction.

Looking at all three phases, one might speculate as follows. Those whose thresholds are too low for the protest phase would develop panic disorder upon separation from important people. Similarly, those whose thresholds are too low for the despair phase would tend to develop severe vital depressions. And those whose thresholds are too low for the detachment phase would develop antisocial personality. Since neurophysiological regulators are not neatly compartmentalized, one would expect to find many people who manifest combinations of the symptoms—for example, people with derangements of both the protest and the despair levels and therefore likely to develop panic disorders and vital depression. A recognizable category, identified as depressed antisocial personality, conceivably reflects derangements of both the despair and the detachment levels.

The theory makes a testable prediction. We know that the antidepressant drugs appear to raise the threshold for the release of the built-in primitive reactions that produce panic disorder and depression. We can hypothesize, although there are no data, that antidepressant medication might be of value to the very young antisocial child whose detachment mechanisms are overactive. Antidepressants seem to be of little or no value in the treatment of the adult antisocial personality, perhaps because such people have lived a detached existence for so long that the possibility of forming caring bonds has passed the critical stage and the psychologically learned overlay of detachment is now autonomous. But if there were some way to identify the uncaring child early in life, treatment with antidepressant medication might raise the threshold of his detachment mechanism and thereby allow him to develop normal bonding to others and to become socialized. This is entirely speculative, of course, but considering the propensity of antisocial personalities for fragmented lives and social disturbance, systematic research of this kind is warranted.

Alcoholism and drug abuse. A common psychodynamic formulation attributes the behavioral effects of alcohol or barbiturates (goofballs or downers) to the relief of repression. Evidence is adduced from the frequency of sexual or aggressive behavior under the influence of alcohol, and is supported by the uninhibited behavior (cathartic abreactions) of patients treated with intravenous barbiturates. This formulation is oversimplified, however, because the behavior of the intoxicated person largely depends on the social setting and expectations within which the drinking occurs. For instance, the solitary drinker or the patient who is sedated with barbiturates and left in a quiet room does not suddenly release repressed drives by, for example, smashing the furniture or masturbating. If anything, such a person, under unstimulating circumstances, will simply lapse into drowsiness.

Nonetheless, in a stimulating social setting the intoxicated person does behave in a disinhibited fashion. Rather than viewing this process as a release of repression with a consequent outpouring of unconscious drives, one can explain it as resulting from the dulling of those neurophysiological systems that produce tension, anxiety, and inhibition of impulse in anticipation of social discomfort. As they mature, people learn to check emotional impulses toward immediate gratification during normal social interaction. In such a context, one is in a sense on constant alert, continually concerned about the positive or negative impression he is making. Such concern produces a vigilant state accompanied by muscular tension and sometimes by fear and anger. It is no accident, therefore, that most civilizations use intoxicating substances, particularly alcohol, as an aid to social conviviality. This phenomenon has been succinctly expressed by the psychoanalytic maxim that the superego is soluble in alcohol. Here again we postulate constitutional differences in social anxiety and thus in the need for alcohol.

Drugs other than alcohol and barbiturates have quite different effects. Cocaine and amphetamine, which are strong stimulants and have been shown to be related to increased amounts of biogenic amines in the brain, seem artificially to increase the kind of intense excitement associated with pursuit and appetite, producing concomitant states of elation and excitation. For this reason, people with decreased zest for appetitive pleasures—that is, whose appetitive center is depressed—might turn to the use of such agents to try to return to a relatively normal state. It is also possible, however, that people with quite normal reactions to pleasurable stimuli might turn to these agents in the search for a supernormal experience—a high.

Similarly, the use of opium and its derivatives, such as heroin and morphine, may well be related to the experience of consummatory pleasure. The use of these drugs is associated with a lack of interest in drive satisfaction, such as food and sex, and with a feeling of somnolence, as if the opiates had artificially reduced (satisfied) the biological drives. One might expect people with defects in their consummatory apparatus to turn to opiates, and, in fact, opiates were the standard treatment for severe depression during the nineteenth century. However, people with a normal interest in consummatory objects might also turn to these agents in search for a supernormal experience.

Biopsychology in the Schizophrenic Illnesses

That many forms of the schizophrenias are hereditary is certain. To quote W. S. Gilbert: "Of that there is no possible doubt, no possible probable shadow of doubt, no possible doubt whatever." But what is being transmitted? Unfortunately, our knowledge of chemical and psychological processes is at an elementary stage with regard to our understanding of delusions and hallucinations, thought disorder, social withdrawal, and a host of other bizarre manifestations of schizophrenia.

Two hints concerning chemical processes come from three sources: observations of amphetamine psychosis; theories as to how antipsychotic drugs work; and increasing knowledge about psychedelic drugs. Because the symptoms of amphetamine psychosis—the hypervigilance, the paranoid ideas, the delusions, and the auditory hallucinations—can be blocked by antipsychotic drugs whose action we know, we have a clue concerning which brain chemicals may be involved. Among other actions, amphetamines increase the activity of nerve cells that use the biogenic amine dopamine as a neurotransmitter. The antipsychotic drugs interfere with the action of dopamine. In a rough model, when dopamine is released from the first cell, it inserts itself, like a key in a lock, into the receptor in the second cell. Antipsychotic drugs may jam the locks, preventing the dopamine from stimulating the second cell. Why dopamine should produce psychosis, we do not know.

We do know that dopamine is involved in arousal, and that some schizophrenics and amphetamine psychotics are hyperaroused. We observe the same actions of amphetamine in monkeys and cats. They become excessively vigilant and appear to be frightened. How such excessive activity of the portions of the brain that use dopamine might produce hallucinations is unclear. How it may relate to delusions we will attempt to explain shortly. A dopamine theory of schizophrenia does not demand that too much dopamine be produced. Available data suggest that the cells that respond to dopamine may be too sensitive; they may overreact to normal amounts of dopamine.

The relevant knowledge about psychedelic drugs concerns two phenomena mentioned earlier: there appear to be some psychedelics to which the brain does not develop tolerance; and the normal brain itself possesses the chemical mechanisms for synthesizing some psychedelic substances. The presence of these drugs in the normal brain can be demonstrated. One hypothesis is that everyone's brain manufactures psychedelics—as it makes its own stimulants—but that the brain of the schizophrenic, for reasons that are entirely obscure, fails to go through the normal process of breaking them down. As a result, they accumulate and produce psychotic symptoms.

One tantalizing piece of evidence comes from the functioning of particular cells in a lower portion of the brain that are inactive only during dreaming sleep (an hour and a half to two hours a night, but most of the dreams are not remembered). LSD has the property of turning off these cells. However, LSD hallucinations are primarily visual, while schizophrenic hallucinations are primarily auditory.

Why schizophrenics become withdrawn is also not known, although biogenic amine systems seem to be related to the withdrawal experienced in depression. Another piece of evidence is that when amphetamine is administered to hyperactive children an adverse effect is sometimes seen, apparently related to too large a dosage, in which the children become excessively focused on trivial matters and appear socially withdrawn. Since amphetamine does the same thing in hyperactive children that it does in adults—release dopamine—there is some evidence that excessive dopamine activity can lead to preoccupation and apparent introversion as well as hyperarousal. In speculating about evolutionary sources of these behaviors, we are reminded that hyperarousal is ordinarily generated by dangerous situations, and that at such times an alert freezing—that is, withdrawal—while scanning the environment for signs of peril, may be an appropriate response. In the schizophrenic, such an evolutionarily derived mechanism may be exaggerated.

Since antipsychotic drugs do not cure schizophrenia but ameliorate the symptoms, sometimes only turning a severe schizophrenic into a borderline schizophrenic, it is clear that the dopamine theory is highly incomplete. One refinement is the assumption that antipsychotic drugs do not block the activities of dopamine entirely, and there is some recent confirmation of this. Although the list of "ifs," "buts," and "maybes" is in fact longer, there has been at least some progress in making neurochemical sense of the schizophrenic psychoses.

With the aid of psychological theorizing, we may now apply the biological and chemical data to try to construct a hypothesis to explain delusions. We begin by postulating that there is a built-in neurophysiological match-mismatch mechanism that continuously compares the data of life with the inferences we sustain about ourselves and the world. If the data support our inferences, the mechanism says "You're right" and we develop feelings of certainty that we have substantiated our hypotheses about life. If the data do not fit our inferences, we feel doubtful and perplexed and may have to change our minds. When this mechanism is used sensibly, we pay attention to all the evidence, for and against. If I believe that I am a fine machinist, pianist, or poet, I should be weighing all the evidence pertinent to that belief, internal and external, counting both successes and failures.

This process of hypothesis testing is complicated by several obvious problems. First, all data we receive are not equal. Some facts are clear, and others are uncertain. In general, we give more credence to straightforward data than we do to muddled or ambiguous information. But the process is also influenced by our desire to come up with hypotheses we like. We may put more effort into clarifying supportive data than contrary fact. For example, we have a natural desire to think well of ourselves, so data supporting this opinion are pursued, seen clearly, and remembered easily. Contradictory data, which would make us think poorly of ourselves, are ignored and forgotten. This is the underlying mechanism of the well-known maladaptive system of wishful thinking.

Another problem is that the bases for most of our beliefs—our attitudes and values—are not scientifically reasoned from direct data. They come from conclusions taught to us when we are young, when we are in a poor position to check what we are taught. There is some evidence from developmental psychology that that which is taught early in life is more permanent and more deeply rooted than that which is learned later. This is voiced in the perhaps apocryphal saying of the Jesuits: "Give me the child until five, and you may have him thereafter." Beliefs engendered early in life may persist in the face of much contradictory evidence, because the new evidence is weighed as less reliable than that provided during the period of social enculturation. Clearly, early sexual and religious indoctrination may have lifelong effects that fly in the face of adult experience. Once strong convictions exist, especially when they are supported by the culture or subculture in which the individual functions, disconfirming evidence is ignored or disbelieved.

With a childhood in which beliefs and attitudes are diligently inculcated and an adult life in which these attitudes are promulgated by the community, anyone can believe anything devoutly, no matter how absurd, and defend it to the death. In times of social change, people with beliefs that are being superseded, as well as those with new beliefs, huddle with their like-minded brethren, thus splinting their doctrines against the forces of both social contradiction and new data. The threat to long-standing beliefs brings with it the threat of personal disorganization.

Does social indoctrination provide an explanation for delusions, then? Some psychiatrists have asserted that delusions develop because of very peculiar upbringings, but the weight of evidence is against this assertion. The schizophrenic sticks out like a sore thumb against his or her cultural and familial background, regardless of how unusual that background is. The Haitian schizophrenic who believes that he is possessed by a voodoo god is perceived as ill by other Haitians even though the culture believes in possession by devils. The difference is that the psychotic gets it all wrong. He is not participating in a socially defined drama. He is writing his own script, and doing it badly.

Many primitive tribes believe that an enemy can work fatal magic on a person should a wizard or shaman obtain hair or nail clippings from that person. Such beliefs are similar to the beliefs of paranoid patients that malevolent forces are persecuting them through subtle poisoning, telepathy, or radio waves. Nonetheless, the primitive cultures alluded to are not psychotic and their "paranoid" cultures do not indicate that paranoid delusions are simply a cultural phenomenon. Culturally accepted beliefs do not constitute delusions, since cultural solidarity provides adequate proof of their truth for most members of that society—in other words, there is safety from psychiatric categorization in numbers. Societies do have difficulty, however, categorizing *subcultural* beliefs that go against the majority viewpoint of the culture. A small sect is more suspect than a large one with an established historical tradition. The former is often thought of as part of the lunatic fringe, while the latter's members may be regarded as pillars of the community. In general, people regard their own beliefs as facts and those of others—in proportion to distance—as fallacy; but here, too, difference and distance cannot be equated with delusion.

Thus, we need some further explanation for delusional conviction. One important lead is the sense of overwhelming certainty that can be produced by a wide variety of drugs—marijuana, hashish, LSD, peyote, nitrous oxide, ether—and that may occur in brain disorders such as epilepsy. In one classic example, a psychologist—it may have been William James—decided to sniff ether for scientific reasons. While on his ether trip, he experienced an overwhelming supernal insight into the ineffable nature of the universe. Realizing that this profound truth was destined to be ephemeral, he had the foresight to write down these eternal verities. The following morning he found that he had written: "The entire universe is pervaded by the smell of turpentine." Not bad as eternal truths go.

James also observed that laughing gas could produce contentless certitude: "The nitrous oxide intoxication in which a man's very soul will sweat with conviction and he is all the while unable to tell what he is convinced of at all" (1890, Vol. 2, p. 284). James's description of the feelings accompanying this kind of experience vividly conveys its difference from ordinary consciousness:

> With me, as with every other person of whom I have heard, the keynote of the experience is the tremendously exciting sense of an intense metaphysical illumination. Truth lies open to the view in depth beneath depth of almost blinding evidence. The mind sees all the logical relations of being with apparent subtlety and instantaneity to which its normal consciousness offers no parallel; only as sobriety returns, the feeling of insight fades, and one is left staring vacantly at a few disjointed words and phrases, as one stares at a cadaverous-looking snow-peak from which the sunset glow has just fled, or at the black cinder left by an extinguished brand.
>
> The immense emotional sense of reconciliation which characterizes the "maudlin" stage of alcoholic drunkenness—a stage which seems silly to lookers-on, but the subjective rapture of which probably constitutes a chief part of the temptation to the vice—is well known. The centre and periphery of things seem to come together. The ego and its objects, the meum and the tuum, are one. Now this, only a thousandfold enhanced, was the effect upon me of the gas: and its first result was to make peal through me with unutterable power the conviction that Hegelism was true after all, and that the deepest convictions of my intellect hitherto were wrong. [James, 1979 reprint, p. 218]

Thus, drugs may generate beliefs and convictions that cannot be swayed by the paltry forces of logic or contradictory evidence. These drugs seem to be firing off some internal brain mechanism that releases a poignant certainty.

We believe that in schizophrenia this occurs as a pathologically induced, super "Ah-ha!" experience. Everyone has had the experience of being profoundly puzzled. Things just don't fit together. We go over our problem repeatedly, looking for a pattern. Suddenly the light dawns and—"Ah-ha!"—we are transfixed: "Push the lever *in,* not down!" "You don't *have* to get married!" or, profoundly, "$E = MC^2$."

A new proposition has been generated and everything falls into place. There is a close, perhaps a perfect fit between the data and the belief. The "Ah-ha!" experience might also have evolutionary value, because the feeling of relief and exaltation more often than not probably does reflect a better solution to the problem and in that way enhances the probability of survival.

In the acidhead's trip, an intoxicant seems to be producing the "Ah-ha!" feeling of "It's all clear to me now." Some trivial part-truth ("You've got to do your thing, man") is seen as the Answer. Once out of the trip, the individual frequently has only the memory of transcendental certainty. When feelings of doubt begin to emerge, supported by evidence from the world of reality, acid-trippers are faced with battling their own skepticism. It is probably no accident that both the acid-tripper and the religious mystic frequently arrive at a conviction of unity, that all is One, and that drawing careful distinctions among things (I am not you) is simply a sign of being deceived by the Veil of Illusion and not piercing to the underlying Reality. By wiping out contradictory distinctions, vague all-embracing doctrines retain the "Ah-ha!" sense of beatification.

Of course, there is some scientific sense in postulating that an underlying unity is a basic attribute of the universe. However, the point is that the feeling of certainty need not rely on any match with reality.

In connecting the development of schizophrenic delusions to effects common in drug intoxication and spontaneous mystical enlightenment, we also note that the subjective psychological experience of the deteriorating schizophrenic is analogous to the psychological context in which religious conversion experiences frequently occur. The potential convert is in the midst of torturing self-doubt, physical deprivation, exhaustion, and prestigious attacks upon his ability to reason clearly (Werner Erhard's *est*, a recent panacea, is a clear example of an environment manufactured for conversion).

In the stages of schizophrenic delusion formation, the kind of schizophrenic who prior to illness has a good intellectual development and no strange personality characteristics (a good premorbid schizophrenic) begins to develop worries and apprehensions as he becomes ill. He begins to feel put upon and to see mysterious significance in prosaic matters. "What did Joe mean by tugging on his ear as he talked about Bill?" "What did my boss mean by saying 'Goodbye' instead of 'Good night'?" There is a growing sense of confusion and bewilderment. We view this as an early stage in the malfunctioning of the match-mismatch mechanism that monitors the similarities and discrepancies between our life experience and our hypotheses about the world. As the mechanism continues to fail, sizable discrepancies begin to be ignored. Fleeting ideas that would usually be criticized and rejected begin to gain conviction—a state often referred to as delusional mood.

Finally, the mechanism misfires altogether in a state of psychotic illumination—"Ah-ha!" cries the psychotic. "It's all clear now, I'm meant to save the world." Once this conviction is reached, a whole train of secondary conclusions follows. One has to preach and convert as the beliefs develop into an entire system explaining away all contradictions, if contradictions are noted at all.

The natural history of the acute schizophrenic break in the good premorbid schizophrenic is important because it resembles an extended version of a single LSD trip. Both the recovered schizophrenic and the ex-LSD user who has had a mystical experience begin after several months to lose confidence in their beliefs. The patient or the acidhead may start to notice the unlikeliness of her statements. As she recovers, more doubts are expressed, and finally she may say, "Did I really believe that?" Often, on recovery, the ex-schizophrenic will say that her experience was just like a dream that she can barely remember.

The acute schizophrenic, the acute LSD user, and the religious convert all have an attribute in common: they typically backslide from their illuminated state. Antipsychotic medication will speed up this process for the acute schizophrenic and will interrupt the LSD delusion, perhaps by accelerating the healing of the faulty match-mismatch mechanism.

A further parallel can be drawn between chronic delusional states and chronic LSD intoxication. Some schizophrenics experience repeated psychotic episodes with accompanying delusions. With each recovery, a residual deficit remains, with progressively muddier thinking and loss of self-criticism. A similar development may occur with some chronic LSD users, although some students of the acid culture report that former heavy users—if they have avoided drugs that in large doses are known to cause brain damage, such as amphetamines—cannot, after a while, be distinguished from non-users. Before recovery is completed, however, some acidheads are indistinguishable from persons who have suffered repeated schizophrenic episodes. One possibility is that the match-mismatch system has permanently stripped its gears, so that clear propositions can no longer be formed and fuzzy ideas are greeted as lucid, illuminating, and convincing.

We have presented this lengthy digression not as a convincing proof but as an example of our own thought processes, spelling out our notions about the genesis of delusions in order to exemplify how reasonably sophisticated biological psychologizing can metaphorically borrow known mechanisms (in this case from computer technology) and use them to explain the operations of the mind. Inventing mechanisms is not new. Freud repeatedly postulated mechanisms to explain observed mental operations. In some instances, his disciples have reified these concepts, turning metaphor into reality, talking as if somewhere in the mind the clever Id is devising ways to outwit the stern and unbending Superego. Reification may be misleading, but postulating mechanisms, Freudian or cybernetic, is not.

Before leaving the schizophrenias, we wish to emphasize several points: it is a devastating disease, and if two million people in the United States have it, four or five times as many—those close to the schizophrenics—also suffer from its consequences. When an autonomous, loving, functioning person is transformed into a parasitic, egocentric, incompetent one, the effects on the other family members can be worse than those produced by death. Even its milder forms, often viewed as idiosyncrasies, can be profound sources of suffering. Thus, we regard an awareness of the possible biological components of this disorder as of major importance.

We hope it is clear that despite our heavy emphasis on biology and chemistry in this chapter, we are well aware of the possible psychological contributions to mental illness. It is well known that psychological experience—for example, battle stress—can profoundly affect the chemical, hormonal, and physiological functioning of the body. In psychiatric illnesses, a psychological experience can frequently be identified as the precipitating factor in a vulnerable person. Vital depressions are sometimes produced by losses, grief, or financial misfortune. The mood of the hysteroid dysphoric plummets when the current object of her affection departs.

Our overall view is that genetic factors may make an individual vulnerable to certain forms of psychological experience; in this vulnerable person, those psychological experiences may in turn alter brain functioning and thus alter later psychological experience; medication can, in some instances, restore the disturbed chemical functioning of the brain.

The notion of vulnerability, as useful in psychology as it is in physiology, refers to a difference in susceptibility (a quantitative difference) rather than a difference in kind (a qualitative difference). For example, in the condition called agammaglobulinema, the individual has a decreased ability to form protective antibodies to infection. He will become infected when exposed to an amount of bacteria that a normal person can fight off. The normal person might be infected only if exposed to a much larger amount of bacteria. The difference is in degree of resistance.

The same concept may apply psychologically. Biological differences among people may make them more or less resistant to disturbing events. Some people may become mentally ill with very little exposure to disturbing experience, in the form either of inadequate child-rearing or of adult stress. Some people may withstand most childhood or adult stress but succumb if the pathological circumstances are extreme. Still others may endure great psychological hardship and yet retain their mental health.

A related factor is the important variations in personality that accompany the diseases. Dependency is increased by depression; insensitivity to others is seen in mania; frightened clinging and lack of autonomy are seen in separation anxiety. Just as the illnesses occur along a spectrum, we assume that there are variations in the accompanying personality difficulties—for example, we expect to find persons with mild chronic separation anxiety or rejection sensitivity. Attributes of this kind not only manifest themselves symptomatically but may also play a role in molding other aspects of personality. As mentioned, an increased tendency to separation anxiety probably facilitates development of a severe conscience. Rejection sensitivity probably fosters an increased desire to obtain such an exalted status that others would never be rejecting. Such people may therefore have an inflated ego ideal.

The implications of psychological vulnerability are at least two. (1) Biologically mediated psychological illness can sometimes be prevented by organizing the susceptible person's life differently. For example, the separation-anxious child should not be sent to camp if she is currently undergoing a period of separation anxiety. (2) Some medications may be used prophylactically. We have treated vital depressives who respond well to antidepressants and may be taken off them without redeveloping depressive symptoms but are so susceptible to minor stresses that in only two or three months they again experience intense depression. For such persons, continuing treatment with antidepressants should be considered. Obviously, we would prefer to diminish vulnerability, chemically or otherwise. At present, we cannot. We can only help our patients to avoid those experiences most likely to trigger episodes of illness, treat them with appropriate medication if they become ill, and maintain them on appropriate medication as long as the likelihood of relapse is major.

It should be stressed that many normal personality attributes as well as diseases and disease spectrums probably occur on a biological basis, with variations as environmentally produced phenocopies. Many psychological theorists attribute variation in personality attributes almost wholly to early life experience. We agree that personality characteristics can shape early life experience and thus affect subsequent personality, but these fundamental attributes may themselves in part be biologically determined.

In addition, there are other kinds of biological bases to personality. Consider the phenocopies of low self-esteem that are the psychological consequences of obvious biological deficiencies. Biological abnormalities often cause painful psychological experiences. In coping with such experiences, the individual uses compensatory devices; these may themselves cause problems, or they may miscarry and become rigidified into personality characteristics. Everyone is acquainted with the little-Napoleon syndrome, in which men of short stature act pompous, overbearing, condescending. Some people attempt to compensate for various physical or mental deficiencies by acquiring possessions, by display in their clothing, or by body-building. Others seek power or prestige or sexual conquests. All these compensatory devices may backfire, however, because of the negative reactions of others to vanity, boasting, and attempts at manipulation and control.

On the other hand, compensatory devices sometimes can achieve the success that bolsters self-esteem. This was first observed by Alfred Adler, who coined the now outmoded term "inferiority complex." Adler observed that many people focused their energies on attempts to compensate for a real or perceived deficit and that in so doing they often became successful. Biological factors, then, generate comprehensible psychological reactions that can either strengthen the personality or cause difficulties.

CHAPTER 7

The Threefold Nature of Unhappiness: Some Examples and Some Difficulties

We have presented two main sets of reasons for believing that there are biological bases for much disordered feeling and behavior: first, the relatively clear evidence for the inheritance of many of the conditions; second, the distinct effects of medications on many of the illnesses. Because these effects differ sharply from the effects of medication on normal people, we think the drugs may be repairing the malfunctioning control systems that seem to underlie mental illness.

A respectable minority of psychiatric opinion has always held that the major psychoses, such as schizophrenia and manic-depressive illness, have a biological component, and this idea has begun to compete seriously with Freudian theory in the popular mind. For instance, a recent book, *The Psychological Society,* by journalist Martin Gross, convincingly reviews the evidence for the biological bases of schizophrenia and manic-depressive disease. Gross, however, has fallen prey to the common misconception that psychiatrists identify only two kinds of mental disorders—the psychoses and the neuroses. After arguing for a biological basis to the psychoses, he attacks the idea of neurosis, stating that it is simply fancy medical terminology for anxiety, that anxiety is a part of everyone's idiosyncratic natural temperament, and that it is precipitated if the individual comes in conflict with society. He believes that society holds up a demanding conformist model that does not allow for individual constitutional variations, and thereby induces needless anxieties in all those whose makeup does not allow them to accept social demands. "Most of mankind is therefore left with two basic conditions to contemplate. One is insanity, which will strike a small percentage of us with its onslaught of tragedy.... Or, faced with the dilemma of sanity, we must find a way to a better existence" (p. 325).

Gross's argument is an interesting but narrow one since it asserts that only major illnesses have clear-cut biological roots. We have endeavored to show that this is simply not true. Many mental illnesses that do not fall within the categories of schizophrenia or manic-depressive disease have clear biological roots. Moreover, the major psychotic illnesses may have a host of genetic minor relatives, referred to as spectrum disorders. Although there are congenial elements in various of his formulations, his belief that all other expressions of guilt, anxiety, fear, and so forth are due to the clash of each person's special constitution with society is much oversimplified.

The idea that the psychoses are largely biological but the neuroses largely psychological is held by psychiatrists as well as lay persons. Solomon Snyder, an outstanding psychiatrist and biochemist, has made fundamental advances in the understanding of brain function. In his stimulating book *The Troubled Mind,* he quotes Thomas Szasz as follows: " 'It is customary to define psychiatry as a medical specialty concerned with the study, diagnosis and treatment of mental illness. This is a worthless and misleading definition. Mental illness is a myth. Psychiatrists are not concerned with mental illnesses and their treatments. In actual practice they deal with personal, social, and ethical problems in living.' " Snyder then continues: "Szasz's concepts are especially appropriate for the neuroses. The gradation between normal and neurotic behavior is continuous and subtle. No specific brain dysfunction has been linked to any neuroses. Thus, why bother with elaborate classifications which mislead the public into believing that the clusters of different neurotic symptoms are as well defined as the bacterial species causing different forms of pneumonia?" (p. 18).

Snyder goes on to disagree with Szasz with regard to manic-depressive disease and schizophrenia, where there is "fairly strong proof that these are true biological diseases, every bit as real as diabetes or rheumatoid arthritis." However, he clearly agrees that the neuroses— that is, the milder emotional disorders—may consist only of problems in living. Further, when Snyder describes such disorders as phobia and antisocial personality—for which we have cited evidence of biological components—he does so exclusively in terms of psychological causes and mechanisms.

Thus, although Gross and Snyder represent an advance over an exclusively psychogenic viewpoint, their stance is still too simple. We suggest instead that human misery and unhappiness can be understood in terms of a threefold framework: reality factors, mislearning or maladaptation, and mental illness, with mental illness including a broader range of disorders than just the psychoses.* The details of this schema are not eternal revelations and are open to scientific experimentation and analysis. The factors overlap and influence one another; there are subtle variations that are difficult to categorize; and conceivably one could group them differently. However, an overall distinction of this kind seems clearly supported by current knowledge, as we will elaborate below. An understanding of the probable sources that contribute to an individual's unhappiness can give the psychiatrist, psychotherapist, or counselor—and the individual—a better idea of the possibilities for ameliorating the suffering.

Realistic unhappiness consists of unpleasant, distressing sensations and feelings that are justified by circumstances in that they are characteristic responses of people in interaction with any of a variety of misfit environments to which they cannot adapt or from which they cannot escape. One possible grouping of kinds of reality is: catastrophic reality, interpersonal and preferential reality, developmental reality, social reality, and the reality of inborn limitations.

Some realistic unhappiness is easily recognized, such as that due to death, natural cataclysm, accident, desertion, and major physical illness. Religion, cathartic cultural rituals, friendship, stoic endurance, and organized private or governmental assistance are the chief supports in response to catastrophes of this kind. People who are overwhelmed by such sorrow—for whatever reason—can also sometimes be helped by therapy, in the form of either support or exploration of any mixed feelings in the reactions to the event.

Personal unhappiness of a situational nature—for example that related

---

*Philosophers and theologians posit existential sources of unhappiness. Philosopher Ben Mijuskovic, for example, maintains that the nature of consciousness inevitably condemns man to loneliness; and Søren Kierkegaard held that man's despair and dread are related to his sinfulness and can be relieved only by religious faith. It seems to us that such viewpoints are open to question on several bases. Observationally, not everyone is subject to overwhelming loneliness or unhappiness; such reactions, in fact, might well be explained in terms of the other factors we describe.

to an unsatisfying marriage or job—is often inadequately recognized, and if recognized is often regarded as of purely psychogenic origin. Several of our case histories deal with unhappiness of this kind, emphasizing the therapist's function in helping the patient to recognize his or her attitudes toward the situational stresses, to analyze the realistic possibilities for change within the situation, to compare the relative strengths of the patient's own competing wishes, and to consider the likely consequences of, for example, ending the marriage or changing jobs.

Manipulation of the environment in this way can make a profound difference in satisfactions, although of course a repetitive pattern of abandoning mates or jobs would lead one to suspect that the answer lies elsewhere. Some therapists automatically assume that attempts to change aspects of one's life are simply ways of avoiding basic inner problems. This can be unfortunate. In fact, the traditional psychoanalytic therapeutic contract demanded that patients make no major life changes. Since such therapy often went on for several years, even opportunities that knocked several times must have been missed.

Situational unhappiness can also arise from inevitable developmental changes associated with the life cycle, and from the failure to recognize stresses arising from the new demands—temporary or otherwise—that are being made on the individual. Adolescence is a major and familiar example, but an important and less widely recognized instance is that of the mother who must care for three or four young children close in age to each other. Until the children are somewhat independent, she cannot, without help, maintain her usual wifely, domestic, and outside interests; something has to give, and too often it is the mother's emotional equanimity.

A related source of stress has become more prominent with the rise of the feminist movement—the attempts of women to cope simultaneously with professional and household demands. The assumption of the responsibilities of a family can function similarly in men. Recently, other normal developmental stages—such as the rise up the career ladder and then the increasing awareness of the finitude of growth and life—have been recognized by Daniel Levinson and others as precipitating depression and other emotional reactions.

Developmental stress can be seen in three-year-olds not allowed to climb jungle gyms, in innately shy people, in underprivileged youths unable to find employment, in college-educated people in clerical jobs, and above all in schizophrenics who are aware of their inability to meet social demands. It is also a major source of the unhappiness that comes with the changes of advancing age.

All these developmental stresses require recognition of their inevitability and coming to real terms with real boundaries.

Some sociologists and social philosophers attribute much of contemporary malaise to the changes wrought by modern technology. Arguments of this sort are superficially appealing, impossible to document, and reminiscent of the Noble Savage myth, but nonetheless, they should not be dismissed. Man evolved slowly over a million years to fit a number of expectable social and physical environments. Despite the popularity of the view that man is of infinite flexibility, he probably shares some characteristics with his animal relatives, among them finite adaptability. Apparently, he evolved in small foraging tribes in which he was a member of a group of familiar persons, his extended family and the tribe itself. One of the major peculiarities of modern urban Western culture—especially in the United States—is that man has largely dissociated himself from intimate life with the extended family and the tribe. After having been raised within his limited neo-local family, which often consists only of his parents and siblings, with relatively infrequent contact with other biological relatives, he or she picks a spouse and together they go out to face the cold, cruel world by themselves.

This mode of existence developed in Western countries only since the industrial revolution, and has spread only with the increased movement and freedom accompanying motorized transportation (especially the automobile), the dislocations of two world wars, and the creation of mass housing. The popularity of Alvin Toffler's lucid book *Future Shock* testifies to the widespread recognition that everything seems to be moving too fast. Insofar as a sense of comfort and participatory emotion stems from membership in a familiar group, one would expect that ways of living that mandate against participation in close groups of this kind would deprive many persons of a warm sense of belonging. It is easy to speculate that such modes of existence predispose to feelings of isolation and loneliness.

If such are the life circumstances of the young couple, the situation has been far worse for the female half of it. The man goes out into the world, where he is able to form relationships with job and business associates, other adults with whom he may share some commonality of interests. Such is not the lot of the housewife and mother. Despite the fact that our culture has—at least in the past—placed great value on the virtues of being a wife and mother, her life has become singularly peculiar. A hundred years ago, the young wife and mother may have worked on the farm, surrounded by other female relatives, so that she had adult companions during the day and participated in an adult social life. Similarly, in the large cities, members of ethnic groups often participated daily in an extended family group, and various social castes lived in relatively compact neighborhoods that permitted elaborate social rituals, whether on the front stoop or via the calling card.

But in the modern kingdom of heaven, the suburb, the young housewife spends most of her day in the company of her small children. She has few adult social contacts and little feeling of belonging to an adult community. Telephone bills skyrocket and television soap operas and game shows draw huge audiences. Under such circumstances, it is very common for young women to become dissatisfied and depressed.

Until recently, our culture told such women that this was a proper, satisfying way of life, and certainly material want has not been the issue. It has often been very difficult for women in this position to acknowledge to themselves that theirs was not the fairy-tale existence they had expected when they grew up. At the same time, the function of the middle-class church as a purveyor of generalized solace has been diminishing. As a result, in affluent circles, a disproportionately large number of patients seeing psychiatrists has consisted of such women.

Because the presumed glories of suburbia long hid the lurking emptiness, young women who became depressed or dissatisfied under such circumstances were often considered neurotic. Considerable effort was directed toward exploring their early experiences and their personality structures in an attempt to determine what was causing their mysterious dissatisfaction. Although individuals and their reactions vary, we believe that many of these women have been reacting appropriately to a situation historically and culturally so bizarre that it is likely to produce dissatisfaction even in those who are psychologically well put together. This observation was made pointedly by Betty Friedan in *The Feminine Mystique* but at times seems forgotten by some of our colleagues; it bears reemphasis.

An analogous reaction occurs in both men and women as a response to the stultification of corporate and bureaucratic life, to the competitiveness and ethical shortcuts of the marketplace, to the impersonality of urban living, and, paradoxically, to the boredom of surfeit that comes with constant stimulation without mastery. The resultant apathy, vague discontent, and restlessness—again, varying with the individual—sometimes send the unhappy man or woman to the psychiatrist. And the psychiatrist, unfortunately, does not always adequately weigh the reality behind the complaints.

Another realistic factor affecting people's feelings about themselves is what Robert W. White has called "one of our most fundamental and biologically important affects," the "feeling of efficacy" (1965, p. 203). If an individual feels that he cannot constructively manage the environment—because of personal limitations, family restrictions, or economic, social, or political circumstances—low feelings of efficacy develop, accompanied by a decreased sense of competence and a lowered self-esteem. In contemporary urban society, a large proportion of the available jobs—blue-collar, white-collar, or no-collar—provide no feelings of efficacy or the inner satisfaction and sense of self-fulfillment that can accompany such feelings.

Remedies for the depressions and dissatisfactions that stem from modern life and our rather unusual social organization cannot be expected from the psychiatrist. In the past, psychiatrists have bravely, and perhaps arrogantly and naïvely, assumed the role of the priesthood and taken on all problems. It is most likely, however, that solutions to such problems of living will come only from long-term changes in social organization. New formats for social existence such as communes are attempts to remedy or ameliorate contemporary loneliness and isolation, but they bring their own problems—such as clashing goals and temperaments—and have provided durable solutions for only a minute percentage of the population. A more widespread response to current forms of anomie has been the growth of alternate psychological treatments—humanist therapies, various forms of encounter groups, techniques for achieving alternate states of consciousness. In their focus on growth, on intimacy, on actualization of potential, on sensuality, or on achieving distance from the mundane world, they recognize that many of the unhappy people who come to them are not suffering from illness but from various effects of modern life.

In relating our social structure to common dissatisfaction, we must of course look at the hopeless unhappiness of underprivilege as well as the subtle unhappiness of privilege. Psychiatrists, particularly those who work in urban public clinics or in association with social welfare agencies, daily see a vast panorama of human misery—a seemingly endless parade of unfortunate souls in tragic life circumstances. Along with the usual psychiatric illnesses, one sees a compound of the effects of gross poverty; the consequences of ignorance (limited occupational attainment, superstition, misinterpretation and fearfulness of ordinary life events); addiction—to narcotics, to psychedelics, and most common and by far the most severe, to alcohol; legal entanglements such as petty thievery to maintain a drug habit, resulting in multiple arrests; sexual deviations not tolerated by a disapproving society, resulting in disgrace and legal penalty; deprivation-associated illnesses such as tuberculosis and untreated life-threatening ones such as hypertension; and the sad results of making a mistake in one's choice of life that leads to self-constructed traps and blind alleys. Some personal ineffectuality may be the result of a limited heredity, but an overwhelming conglomeration of misfortune is the product of the accident of birth in a subculture with built-in limitations resulting from racial and ethnic prejudice and cumulative patterns of coping with constricted circumstances.

Those on whom such misfortunes have fallen are often anxious, depressed, demoralized, and confused. It is their disorganized behavior and psychological symptoms and the absence of any social mechanism for effectively dealing with such problems that lands them in the psychiatrist's or the mental health clinic's office. Although some churches do their best to succor the poor and to prop up the demoralized—sometimes succeeding remarkably well—psychiatrists inherit the residue of human problems. But psychiatry has no special explanation for the misery of these people, nor is any arcane system of theories required. People have been constructed over millions of years of evolution to be anxious, depressed, and confused when they are starving, unable to meet the most basic physiological or psychological needs, possessed of self-destructive habits they cannot break, or pursued and rejected by the society of which they are nominally members. Not only does the psychiatrist not have (or need) any special theories to account for such distresses; he has no remedies for them. Society has used psychiatry as a repository for its manifold residual ills, and unfortunately many psychiatrists have assumed that they have the wherewithal to deal with them.

In this area of psychiatry, first called social and then community psychiatry, the profession has directed increasing attention to the role of these common problems in the origins of human misery. One can understand the compassion and guilt that turn a psychiatrist's attention in this direction, but there is no evidence that he possesses any special expertise to deal with the relevant social forces. Whether social or economic reform, social engineering, or community reorganization can mitigate or eliminate such problems remains to be seen, but the economist, sociologist, and political reformer are closer to the root issues than is the psychiatrist. Objectively caused distress requires actual changes in circumstances. Freud believed that the "evils" we have described, ordinary human adversity, were the expectable residues when neuroses were successfully treated. He did not expect that these residues would become redefined as illnesses that his ideological descendants would claim to cure.

The issue of realistic unhappiness is perhaps easiest to define in extreme situations. When we talk about poverty as a universal source of unhappiness, what we mean is that the fit between the human organism and the environment is so bad that anyone but a saint would be unhappy and there is no way out. It doesn't matter that there are considerable individual differences and constitutional fluctuations, given this grim inescapable reality.

With even a moderate standard of living, however, the question of what constitutes realistic unhappiness becomes far more difficult to answer. For some people certain environments are good fits, and for others the same environments provoke chronic unhappiness. The question of reactions to quasi-permanent caste status also enters here —the unhappiness that may accompany the lesser social roles assigned to women and minorities such as blacks and homosexuals. Not only is it difficult, moreover, to determine which personalities can be expected to react poorly to which environments; it is also difficult to decide whether the ingredients in those personalities are inborn or develop through experience. This brings us to a final major aspect of reality we wish to consider—the misfit with the environment that occurs as a result of inborn limitations.

Accepting the idea of inborn but normal limitations is difficult, and, indeed, social progress and personal growth often depend on the refusal to accept it. Further, many of the theories in this area are largely speculative. Yet we all incorporate some recognition of the idea into our thinking. We assume that in order to become a concert pianist or a sculptor one must begin with a considerable innate endowment. For the musician or artist with supreme goals but insufficient ability, inborn limitations are a realistic source of unhappiness. (An inability to recognize the misfit of goals and talent may require a different explanation.) The short man who wants to be a basketball player must similarly face his own limitations, and the girl with disproportionately heavy thighs and hips will have difficulty exercising herself into the ballet.

These examples are relatively easy to grasp, though even they may yield to extremes of perseverance and persistence. What we want to focus on, however, are even more tenuous examples, such as inborn variations within normal limits of cognitive skills, personality, and character, which cannot be regarded as illness or impairment but may produce unhappiness because they affect the individual's fit with the environment or his or her expectations concerning that fit.

Hard evidence relating early life experience to attitude and character is largely unavailable, since there have been few longitudinal studies observing development from birth to adulthood. Even good longitudinal studies cannot give precise answers to these questions, because such studies are not experimental but naturalistic, in the sense that the family and child were simply observed and not systematically changed. For instance, parents who talk a great deal to their children tend to have bright children. Does this prove that the talking *made* them brighter? Of course not, since parents who talk more to their children may be brighter than other parents, and the children's higher intelligence may thus merely be hereditary.

In order to test scientifically whether the amount that a mother talked to a child had an effect on the child's intelligence, we would have to design an experiment of this kind: two groups of mothers of equally normal or low-normal intelligence would be identified and their usual speech patterns observed. If all the mothers had similar speech patterns, some would be instructed to continue as usual, while the others would be encouraged to talk more to their children. Observers would check the interactions at regular intervals, and the child's intellectual development would be measured later. The Head Start enrichment programs for young children have been experiments of this kind, but the results are equivocal.

Ordinary naturalistic (as opposed to experimental) follow-up studies have given us some information on such matters, but it has largely been negative (Block, 1971). Longitudinal studies have to date clarified little about the consistency of personality over time or the effects of different modes of child-rearing on personality. The field of lifespan developmental psychology is only now becoming formalized, and we can look forward perhaps to more definitive work in the coming years. For example, a recent study (Scarr and Weinberg, 1978) examined the longitudinal effects of family background on intellectual performance during the first eighteen years of life. Using data on biological and adoptive parents and children, the researchers concluded that genetic differences among families account for the major part of explained differences in IQ among older adolescents.

Additional support comes from Alexander Thomas and Stella Chess, who since 1956 have conducted several longitudinal studies of children from birth to young adulthood. After investigating several hundred children from diverse socioeconomic and cultural backgrounds and of varying physical and mental endowments, Thomas and Chess have concluded that a child's natural temperament plays a major role in determining his behavior.

Even if it should be true that what one learns as a child is greatly affected by one's constitution, it is clear that adult unlearning may still be a useful process. For instance, let us assume that certain children are born with a great ability to anticipate the future and also to feel humiliated, whereas others simply do not anticipate clearly and also are able to shrug off social rejection. If two children, one of each type, were raised in extremely future-oriented, demanding families who require perfection in school work and shame their children when they fail to achieve it, the first sort of child might develop into an anxious perfectionist, continually striving for greater achievements; the second child might end up feeling disgruntled with his family and himself because he never met their expectations. If he could never satisfy his parents, no matter how well he did, he might give up trying and turn his attention toward aspects of life that were more immediately rewarding, such as peer relationships, sports, procrastinating, and even the escape and rebellion represented by alcohol and drugs. If, as adults, both enter psychotherapy, in each case the therapy might well focus on getting them to unlearn attitudes that reflect the interaction of the parents' needs and the child's nature—one therapist in effect saying, "Don't try so hard," and the other saying, "Try a little harder." Such therapy would encourage diminished identification with the parents and the realization that a life in a pattern different from that expected by the parents is justifiable.

As we pointed out in Chapter 5, when discussing nature and nurture, a famous passage from Freud deals with the problem of separating the influence of constitution and learning in the development of particular traits. In attempting to account for a young woman's homosexuality, he traced it to the birth of her brother, but was faced with explaining the fact that most women with younger brothers do not become homosexuals. He then commented on the ease of making a connection by working backward from a final stage as against the difficulty of looking forward and trying to predict a result. He went on to say that, in this particular patient, "consideration of the material impels us to conclude that it is rather a case of congenital homosexuality which, as usual, became fixed and unmistakably manifest only in the period following puberty" (1920, pp. 169–70). This is an example of Freud's frequent invocation of constitutional differences as an explanation for a personality development that seemed inadequately explained by life circumstances.

Despite the little data available to enable us to affirm clearly what aspects of personality either are directly constitutional or are largely determined by constitutional variations, we do suspect, along with Freud, that a wide range of attitudes, abilities, mood states, and activation levels depend on one's constitution. Perhaps, again like Freud, we are influenced by our professional exposure to pathological personalities, who seem more rigid and enduring, less flexible, than normal, less predictable people.

Physicians and philosophers for at least several thousand years have come to the same conclusion. In the second century A.D., the Greek physician Galen postulated four constitutional temperaments: melancholic, choleric, sanguine, and phlegmatic. In the seventeenth century, La Rochefoucauld stated: "Our happiness or unhappiness depends as much on our temperaments as on our luck." Speculations of this kind are bolstered by the evolutionary advantages that many of these traits conceivably provide: activity, curiosity, and adventurousness can be associated with a better provision of basic survival needs; interest in consummatory pleasures can contribute to the survival of both the individual and the species; caution, submission, and aggressiveness can represent alternate responses to competition and danger, each effective in particular circumstances. When these traits are manifested in extreme versions, we recognize pathology—manic states, antisocial behavior, anxiety, and depression—but their variations within normal limits may contribute to nonpathological personality differences that nevertheless affect the fit with the social environment.

The adoption research strategy that has been so successful in the study of psychopathology may prove illuminating here, as in the Scarr and Weinberg study mentioned earlier. It would be highly desirable to sort out more clearly the influences of constitutional traits, life experience, and the severe malfunction that can be identified as illness.

Does the low-activity, passive, distant, self-isolating child have the beginnings of schizophrenia, or is he simply manifesting a normal personality variation? Is the dependent, clingy four-year-old who refuses to go to nursery school manifesting a normal pattern of somewhat slow development, or is he showing signs of pathological separation anxiety that may develop into panic disorder? Does the hot-tempered, uncaring, self-aggrandizing child who is a source of puzzled concern to his well-meaning parents suffer only from a normal temperamental deviation?

Here we are already making progress. Such children can be tested through age-standardized measurements of their ability to attend to and to remain focused on problem situations. If an overactive, self-willed child also cannot attend in a focused way to standardized tasks, then he may have the pathological disorder of hyperactivity (often referred to as minimal brain dysfunction). If so, the parents and therapists will have a clearer idea of how to approach the child's malfunctions. It is this kind of improved diagnostic ability that should be sought in the entire area of personality.

We suspect that many emotional personality traits are inborn—but we cannot prove it. Included might be: need for people vs. indifference to them; easy acceptance of passive role vs. strivings for mastery; ease with others vs. anxiety about strangers, and shyness; ease of separation from attachments vs. separation anxiety; dominance vs. submissiveness and compliance; easy satisfiability vs. insatiability; proclivity to develop anticipatory anxiety and guilt; interpersonal perceptiveness vs. social imperceptiveness; empathy vs. self-centeredness.

The list could be extended indefinitely, and a fair case could be made that various kinds of upbringing are likely to produce, enhance, or inhibit the appearance of every one of these supposedly constitutional traits. Ignorance is ignorance. We are stating our guesses, not confirmed facts. However, a closer look at one personality dimension that has been popularly accepted and has been subject to considerable experimental investigation will give a better understanding of the difficulties entailed in studying such issues. The dimension is extraversion-introversion, and much of the material that follows derives from a useful review by Glenn Wilson (1977).

Although the terms "extraversion" and "introversion" have been in the language for at least several hundred years, their initial psychological use is attributed to Jung, who attempted to relate psychopathology to personality (he considered hysteria the characteristic neurosis of the extravert, psychasthenia [phobias, compulsions] the neurosis of the introvert, and schizophrenia a psychotic extreme of introversion). In common usage, however, extraversion refers to an orientation toward the external world, and introversion to a preference for introspection. An extended discussion of this supposed pair of personality traits comes from Hans Eysenck, who gives the following character description:

> The typical extravert is sociable, likes parties, has many friends, needs to have people to talk to, and does not like reading or studying by himself. He craves excitement, takes chances, often sticks his neck out, acts on the spur of the moment, and is generally an impulsive individual. . . . [H]e is carefree, easygoing, optimistic, and likes to "laugh and be merry." He prefers to keep moving and doing things, tends to be aggressive and lose his temper quickly . . . and he is not always a reliable person.
>
> The typical introvert is a quiet, retiring sort of person, introspective, fond of books rather than people; he is reserved and distant

except to intimate friends. He tends to plan ahead . . . and distrusts the impulse of the moment. He does not like excitement, takes matters of everyday life with proper seriousness, and likes a well-ordered mode of life. He keeps his feelings under close control, seldom behaves in an aggressive manner, and does not lose his temper easily. He is reliable, somewhat pessimistic and places great value on ethical standards. [Eysenck and Eysenck, 1964, p. 8]

Obviously, these verbal portraits represent complex extremes; most people are mixtures. We all know people who like parties and have many friends but also enjoy studying by themselves. Eysenck's answer to this would be that these traits simply tend to hang together and that it is only speaking statistically to say that someone with several extraverted traits probably also has several others and probably will not have many introverted traits.

Eysenck has also developed an extravert-introvert questionnaire (the Eysenck Personality Inventory), which includes items such as: "Are you usually carefree?" and "Do you like the kind of work that you need to pay close attention to?" By totaling their scores on the questionnaire, one can rate people as extraverts or introverts or somewhere in the middle (where most people fall).

With such a questionnaire, it is possible to analyze behavior microscopically and study how closely the various items are associated with each other. Within the group of extravert items, there are subclusters for sociability, for impulsiveness, and for liveliness, excitability, and activity level. In a situation of this kind, if we find that A tends to go with B, there are basically only three possible explanations: A causes B; B causes A; or a third factor, C, causes both A and B. In the extreme extravert, then, it is possible that sociability causes impulsiveness or that impulsiveness causes sociability, or that both are caused by some third factor, such as, say, excitability.

Whether the extraversion-introversion contrast might be inherited has been studied by examining the similarity between identical and fraternal twins on questionnaire measures of extraversion. Identical twins are indeed much more similar to each other than fraternal twins are. Further, fraternal twins are about as similar to each other as parents and children, or as ordinary siblings are to each other. Again, since the identical twins stand out as being unusually similar, there is a strong suspicion that hereditary components are at work, although differences between the twins point as well to nongenetic factors. Only an adoption study or a study of identical twins reared apart might resolve this question.

With regard to other personality characteristics, at least as measured by questionnaires, S. G. Vandenberg carried out a remarkably complete tabulation comprising 185 pairs of monozygotic twins and 908 of dizygotic twins. Eleven tests measured personality traits, needs, and attitudes in factors of many kinds; for example, those labeled energetic, conformity, masculinity, femininity, dependency needs, punitive attitude, responsibility, and so forth. In all but eight of the 101 variables, the monozygotic pairs were more alike than dizygotic pairs. Interestingly, the kinds of variables that most often emerged in both members of identical-twin pairs seemed to measure the degree of sociability and energy, a concept very close to that of degree of extraversion or introversion. In another investigation of twins—79 pairs of monozygotic twins and 68 of dizygotic twins—Irving Gottesman demonstrated a strong genetic component for social introversion.

Theories concerning biological factors that might underlie extraversion and introversion are controversial. For instance, Eysenck presents a complex theory that implies that introverts are good conditioners—that is, learners—as compared to extraverts, and that therefore introverts learn to be afraid much more easily than extraverts, which leads to a more civilized socialization among introverts than extraverts. Unfortunately, the theory implies that in general someone who conditions well on one task will also condition well on another. To be concrete, let's say that someone has learned to withdraw her finger when she hears a bell signal prior to getting a shock, and quite similarly has learned to wink her eye when she hears a buzzer signal to avoid getting an air blast on the eyeball. Eysenck's theory postulates that people who learn to withdraw their fingers quickly will also learn to wink their eyes quickly, but such a correlation is practically nonexistent.

Eysenck's theory can be modified, however, if one does not see the learning of social fears as simply a general case of conditioning ability. J. A. Gray has postulated that introverts are more sensitive to threats of punishment and extraverts more oriented toward the pursuit of rewards. An extension of the theory holds that this should be reflected in risk-taking, with the extraverts seeing only the optimistic side and the introverts only the pessimistic.

For experimental confirmation, one would have to show that extraverts and introverts did indeed systematically show differences in behavior under different circumstances of reward and punishment. That would not necessarily be the basic source of all the other traits, however, but might simply be one more associated trait. Unless there were some way to affect experimentally the postulated reward and punishment centers—for example, by drugs—we could not come to unequivocal conclusions.

A more naturalistic test would be to show that some measurement of response to the anticipation of pain was more closely correlated to all the other introverted traits than those traits were to each other. If one could measure the reaction to anticipated pain very accurately, however, and the other personality traits only fairly accurately, then the resultant pattern of correlations would not identify the primary cause.

Despite the forbidding complexities that keep certainty out of our grasp, it does not seem unreasonable to conclude that some personality traits are real; that these traits are at least partly hereditary; that there may be understandable physiological bases for these hereditary personality traits; and that the actual behavior that occurs during development will often represent the interaction of the developing child's constitution and the type of circumstances under which he or she is raised. To explain behavior exclusively on the basis of heredity is clearly foolish, but so are estimations that depend entirely on life experience. In part, the relevance of these conclusions here is that a person's unhappiness may be the result of attempts to conform to expectations that are not realistic in terms of certain constitutional but nonpathological limitations.

Still another implication of constitutional differences is that people with problems stemming from their conflict with the environment will react differently—in terms of their own propensities—to possible remedial approaches. The combination of restless temperament and boring circumstances, for example, might lead to change, hobbies, travel, religion, psychotherapy, jogging, or alcohol, depending on personal proclivities—plus training and culture.

Some recent research on personality traits has added revealing refinements. A longitudinal twin study by Robert Dworkin and his colleagues (1976) shows that different traits manifest evidence of heritability at different ages. To give specific illustrations, on one of the measures used in the study, depression is among the traits that show significant heritability in adolescence but not in adulthood, ego strength is among those that show significant heritability in adulthood but not in adolescence, and anxiety and dependency show heritability at both ages. Dworkin's finding might conceivably reflect differential gene regulation at different ages or differing nature/nurture interactions as environment changes with age. The finding helps to explain why personality tests of normal people have been disappointing as long-term predictors. It also means that age is a variable that must be considered in future research on the genetics of personality.

An area of probable constitutional differences that we have neglected is that of innate differences between men and women. Although we have bravely jumped into the sea of controversy regarding organic and psychological factors in general, we are not courageous enough at the moment to swim in these particularly chilly waters. We think it is impossible to ignore the obvious sexual personality differences, but they have undoubtedly been socially and culturally influenced. Stereotypes cannot be applied in individual cases. Other than saying that, we are standing back and watching the current debate with interest.

Some people who do not appear biologically ill, do not have a pronounced constitutional variation, and do not live in an unduly oppressive environment nevertheless seem continually to mishandle their lives so that they end up recurrently disappointed and miserable. Most of the books on popular psychology are written about this group, although, unfortunately, these books usually confuse such people with those afflicted with genuine illness or those trapped by realistic limitations.

One point about which such books are in general agreement is that people produce their own misery on the basis of learned patterns of behavior that continually misfire. We agree that mislearning and lack of learning are the roots of many personality limitations, which then result in inadequate management of one's world. Such learned maladaptive patterns can be reasonably attributed to experience, especially experience when young. Some mislearning can arise from family expectations and training, producing intrapsychic conflicts, self-defeating attitudes, and an inaccurate world view. Other mislearning can come from the surrounding culture, either reinforcing or contradicting the family subculture.

It should be clear, however, that we believe that many of these learned maladaptive patterns occur secondarily to constitutional variations and to illness. The developing human being does not simply receive passively the imprint of the environment, but because of peculiarities of makeup will far more easily develop certain skills, believe certain facts, and adopt certain opinions and attitudes rather than others. Further, there seem to be marked differences in flexibility and the ability to unlearn, so that much early learned foolishness persists and may itself prevent the learning of useful new information and new ways of responding. As psychiatrists help people review their histories, the learning of maladaptive patterns seems generally understandable. Talking to nonpatients, however, one finds that many people unlearn similar maladaptive patterns. Despite behaviorist and psychoanalytic theory, we know little about the constitutional makeup or peculiarity of experience that allows some people to change while others are stuck with old, nonadaptive behavioral, emotional, and cognitive patterns.

In at least one respect, we agree completely with Freudian theory: mislearning in the area of sexual attitudes is at the root of much unhappiness. Sexually repressive social attitudes may cause severe personal limitations by miseducating the young child. Many kinds of adult sexual unhappiness are the secondary result of teaching the young child that the sexual organs are dirty or shameful or untouchable or vulnerable or even hateful.

The idea that such childhood enculturation is a common cause of adult maladaptation seems so well established that it would be almost heresy to doubt any aspect of this received truth. Supportive evidence does, indeed, come from William Masters and Virginia Johnson, who in their programs for dealing with sexual inadequacy have found that a notable proportion of their complete failures (1970, p. 213) are with people raised in orthodox religious communities who cannot seem to overcome prohibitions, instilled at an early age, against sexual activity. Yet many people raised under the most stringent and punitive sexual circumstances develop healthy sexual attitudes and the ability to respond to sexual partners with pleasure, love, and appropriate behavior. Here again, it may be that predispositions toward sexual inhibition or fixation are a prerequisite if puritanical family attitudes are to produce enduring sexual conflict, guilt, or malfunction.

Sexually repressive social and family attitudes can also damage a youngster by denying him or her useful elementary knowledge. The widespread illegitimate pregnancy among teenagers, in an age when safe and convenient contraception is readily available, is a clear example of the role of ignorance in getting into trouble. Not only do certain family attitudes mean that youngsters receive inadequate information at home, but in addition such attitudes have an impact on other possible sources of information. The introduction of meaningful sex education into school systems, including explicit discussion of the likelihood of conception and the mechanics of contraception and abortion, has been prevented in many communities by organized activist groups. Surveys concerning the degree of knowledge among teenagers about the elements of sexual reproduction have clearly shown that many have only the very limited, often erroneous, knowledge they have picked up in the streets from their equally ignorant friends. Obviously, society is still in considerable confusion regarding sexual attitudes. Television, the movies, and literature indicate that we have come a long way since Victorian times. Yet restraints on sex education and the contents of school libraries indicate that many segments of society are still ambivalent and uncertain about what healthy sexual expression is and how best to achieve it.

Because sexual repression has been an obvious source of unhappiness, little attention has been given to the reverse phenomenon, which is an increasing problem in our permissive society—the anxiety and the real consequences resulting from the expectation that sexual behavior is the natural outcome of all dating and is a reflection of maximum masculinity or femininity. Aside from its effect on the illegitimate birth rate among teenagers and on venereal disease, this expectation can produce extreme tension among those who are unsure of their own sexuality or who dislike being pressured into acceptance of all partners.

Popular models of personality limitation deal as well with the excessive repression by a punitive family of such urges as anger or dependency. Others emphasize parental deprivation rather than parental restriction—the failure to provide love, attention, or good modeling of rational self-control. As mentioned earlier, it is widely believed that the young child is directly affected by the esteem in which he is held by his parents. Harry Stack Sullivan, in particular, believed that if the parents are unloving toward the child, he will not learn to love himself. This is at some variance with Freud's view that the child from birth is deeply self-absorbed, in the phase that Freud called infantile narcissism and omnipotence, and that later feelings of lowered self-esteem are the inevitable accompaniment of the child's discovery that he is not all-powerful. Adler considered early infantile feelings of inferiority to be major determinants of later psychopathology, and in his famous concept of the inferiority complex he directly relates the child's necessary recognition of how inferior he is to the mighty adults by whom he is surrounded. Freud's and Adler's theories seem to make feelings of inferiority and low self-esteem a universal necessity, since every child must experience his own lack of omnipotence and his own weakness compared to adults; Sullivan's formulation is at least consistent with the wide variation in feelings of self-esteem from person to person.

Still other theories emphasize that parents, in their role as models, may actually teach maladaptive ways of behaving with other people by being constricted, aggressive, submissive, inattentive, or uncaring. In particular, it is often asserted that parents serve as the nuclei for attitudes toward other people in later life (transference), so that, for example, a woman's attitude toward her boss may reflect her attitude toward her father, or a man's attitude toward his lover or wife may reflect (directly or rebelliously) his feelings about his mother. More elaborate theories conjecture that parents may evoke mixed feelings of hatred and love, or fear and desire (ambivalence), and that these feelings then serve as the basis for later intractable internal conflicts in which one continually oscillates between one state and another, unable to arrive at a stable equilibrium.

Other theories postulate that the important issue is that early experiences can affect one's evaluation of the world and oneself—one's world view. The term "world view" refers to the idea that we react to the real world not only as it may be but as we are taught and learn to perceive it. The world is too rich to deal with in all its complexity. In language and in our minds we simplify by paying attention only to certain aspects of experience and, as Harry Stack Sullivan said, by "selectively inattending" to others. To give some obvious examples, the Eskimos have several dozen different words for snow, distinguishing among crusty snow, wet snow, dry snow, lump snow, and so forth. There is no Eskimo word for "parrot," however. South American Indians of the tropical forests have many words for parrots and no words for snow. Societies pay attention to the important aspects of their environment and communicate subtleties of these distinctions to their children.

To cite illustrations from more familiar cultures, most people in the United States speak the same language but do not have identical conceptual frameworks. The important point made by many interpersonal theorists is that individuals coming from the same overall culture still may nevertheless move around with different models of the world. Models of this kind have been referred to as "cognitive maps," "assumptive worlds," or systems of "personal constructs." For example, the sexually repressed mother who comes from a Victorian or puritanical religious tradition may teach her daughter that men are sexual animals, ever eager to take advantage of unwary prey. She thus conveys two lessons to the little girl: first, she must be wary of the sexual attentions of the men she meets; second, sex is bad. Or the ambitious, upwardly mobile sales executive may preach to his son that life is a competitive, dog-eat-dog struggle. If the boy absorbs his father's message, he may later look at all experiences with other men in terms of competitive advantage. He will not ask himself if such-and-such is a nice or an interesting guy, someone who might be pleasant to go fishing with, but, rather: Can he get the better of me? Such people have begun in childhood the construction of a possibly lifelong distorted model of the world. Similar misleading cognitive maps can be formed in cultural subgroups. Groups that preach Christian love, and teach their children not what is but what ought to be, are often singularly blind about interpersonal aggression. These people are reluctant to recognize hostilities in others and themselves, and are subject to great guilt if they do find themselves reacting with such feelings.

All of us use distorted cognitive maps, but some are worse than others. The nature of the distortion has been described as having three components: first, inaccuracy or bias—for example, the young woman who sees all men as lechers; second, deletion—for example, someone who fails to perceive that aggression and hostility exist in the world; third, stereotypy, which is linked to generalization—for example, a child who is taught that all blacks have rhythm or that all Jews engage in sharp business practices.

Generalizations can be useful when they are correct. We teach our children to be wary of angry dogs whether they are chihuahuas or wolfhounds, and not to touch things that are too hot whether they are stoves, matches, or boiling liquids. But the generalizations that interfere with selective, discriminating, appropriate responses to individual people can be both socially and personally harmful. The cognitive maps that are necessary for living interfere with our functioning when they are inaccurate or idiosyncratic. Such experiences and attitudes might develop in the family, or within a social setting, or in both.

Some family indoctrination or training may be adaptive under some circumstances but not others—as, for example, when a family emigrates from one culture to another and the children find that the attitudes of their parents clash with those of their new peers. Regardless of the relative merits of the two cultures, the friction is potentially maladaptive and a possible source of unhappiness.

Elements of the surrounding culture itself can produce mislearning, with consequent profound disappointment and unhappiness. Among the candidates for current cultural myths are the expectations that life can be constantly exciting, that jobs can be consistently fulfilling, that immediate satisfaction of sexual drives is of high priority, that a college degree should guarantee one a good job, that education should be fun, and that material possessions will bring happiness.

Finally, as Jerome Kagan points out in *The Growth of the Child*, the whole idea that early experience is indelible has not been documented. After all, blood cells are continually replaced and neurotransmitters continually replenished; it is reasonable to assume that parts of the memory for emotional events can also be changed over time. As Kagan summarizes:

> The total corpus of information implies that the young mammal
> [human or infrahuman] retains an enormous capacity for change
> and, therefore, for resilience in the growth of psychological compe-
> tences *if environments change;* if an initial environment that does not
> support psychological development becomes more beneficial.
> [1978, p. 43, Kagan's italics]

Kagan's statements have several implications. First, the influence of early childhood experience on adult behavior may be greatly overrated. Second, the influence of early experience may depend on susceptibility. Third, where early childhood experience has been enduringly influential, psychotherapy might conceivably be one of the later beneficial environmental changes that could help to reverse its effects.

Having taken a look at the possible contributions of reality and mislearning to unhappiness, we return to our primary concern—mental illness. In our view, as we have said, mental illnesses consist of poorly functioning brain regulatory mechanisms that produce distressing symptoms, upsetting, ineffective actions, and some degree of involuntary impairment (for a technical elaboration of this definition, see Klein, 1978).

We believe that adoption studies, responses to medication, and studies of brain chemistry point to a biological component in mental illnesses and to heredity as a large contributing factor. In some illnesses, such as some of the schizophrenias and hyperactivity, the biological component seems to produce the illness by itself; in others—such as acute schizophrenia and some forms of depression—psychological stresses may combine with biological vulnerability to trigger the illness. Here again, Freud is in substantial agreement with this position. In one of his last papers, "Analysis Terminable and Interminable," he states:

> The aetiology of every neurotic disturbance is, after all, a mixed one.
> It is a question either of the instincts being excessively strong—that
> is to say, recalcitrant to taming by the ego—or of the effects of early
> (i.e., premature) traumas which the immature ego was unable to
> master. As a rule there is a combination of both factors, the constitu-
> tional and the accidental. The stronger the constitutional factor, the
> more readily will a trauma lead to a fixation and leave behind a
> developmental disturbance; the stronger the trauma, the more cer-
> tainly will its injurious effects become manifest even when the in-
> stinctual situation is normal. [1937, p. 220]

In keeping with his conflict theory of psychopathology, Freud's view of biological vulnerability was largely restricted to an excessive strength of instinct. Our view includes this as only one possibility. We are more prone to emphasize biological vulnerabilities that interfere with the built-in socialization patterns of our species.

As we have seen, some disorders previously explained on strictly psychological grounds respond to medication in a way that strongly suggests biological components. The outstanding example, to which we have referred repeatedly, is the panic disorder, which may in turn lead to panic phobia and generalized anxiety state. Controlled studies of the effects of medication leave no doubt that this illness responds dramatically to antidepressant medication. Some hysteroid dysphorics, who seem plainly to be suffering from psychological difficulties related to low self-esteem and overreactive, manipulative styles of life, also respond remarkably well to one specific subgroup of the antidepressants, suggesting that they have a vulnerability understandable on physiological rather than psychological grounds. Many hyperactive children who have failed to respond to psychotherapy respond to stimulant medication by functioning better than ever before.

Further, the spectrum concept of mental illness is now becoming more appealing. Among the relatives of the patients with the major psychoses, for example, one finds a range of people with apparently minor disorders who seem to share the genetic loading of the sicker patients. Among the biological relatives of adopted schizophrenics, one finds a high proportion of the so-called borderline schizophrenic or schizotypal personality. And among the relatives of severe depressives are a host of persons whose lives are compromised by moderate shifts in mood that are given psychological and sociological explanations but that respond well to antidepressant medications. Adolescents identified as suffering from emotionally unstable character disorders, whose lives are plagued by constant shifts between giddy hedonism and a hostile, sullen despair, can sometimes be stabilized by lithium, though in the past there has been a tendency to slough off their symptoms as typical adolescent turmoil. These adolescents have families that tend to manifest a variety of mood disorders, thus again raising the issue of genetic predisposition.

In addition, conditions that as yet we are unable to treat effectively, such as antisocial personality, alcoholism, and even some proportion of criminality, all of which have been explained by a variety of psychological and social causes, give evidence in adoption studies of having biological components. Psychological and social causes obviously enter into these illnesses but seem insufficient to explain some of their characteristics.

Other evidence of biological factors where none were heretofore suspected includes that of the subgroups of children with severe separation anxiety that prevents them from going to school or camp or staying overnight with friends or relatives; the specific response of such children to antidepressant medication has been impressive.

Conceivably, extreme psychological stress can by itself produce mental illness in someone with normal brain chemistry, but nothing definitive is known. Similarly, we do not know why some people can withstand horrendous psychological pressure without developing mental illness.

The mentally ill person often also fails to make the best of his or her situation and may develop a host of realistic secondary complications. The alcoholic who develops cirrhosis of the liver, the manic who exhausts all his financial resources, and the agoraphobic who exhausts her family all have realistic reasons for unhappiness that are basically secondary to a primary diseased state.

The interweaving of mental illness and other sources of unhappiness makes it difficult to isolate the influential sources and also complicates the ultimate symptom picture. For example, the biologically handicapped schizophrenic may be raised by a biologically handicapped mother in such an eccentric way as to produce learned personality distortions in addition to the schizophrenic malfunctions. Further, schizophrenics occur disproportionately in the lower economic classes (cause and effect have never been adequately sorted out here), and realistic deprivations and a lack of elementary resources aggravate the schizophrenic's difficulties. Poverty alone may disrupt family lives sufficiently to compound any tendency toward disorder or to influence individuals to seek modes of escape that resemble symptoms of mental illness.

Basically, however, we return to our belief in the biological underpinnings of mental illness. This belief has the invaluable property of being disprovable; it is not simply the result of aesthetic ruminations —whether armchair or couchside—to which no convincing refutation can ever be given.

The moral, as we see it, is plain. Both the mental-health professional and the informed lay person must shift gears. The exclusively psychogenic approach is clearly outdated. We must not, however, revert to the stereotype of the exclusively organic approach, because this, too, does less than justice to the complexities of human life. A biopsychiatric approach can provide the framework that integrates current knowledge and allows for progressive scientific advance.

It should be clear that the biopsychiatric approach does not hold that psychotherapy is always a waste of time but that *by itself* it is useless for disorders in which constitutional deviations and physiological abnormalities are the basis of the malfunction. Ignoring these realities can only lead to unrealistic hopes and therapeutic disappointments. Taking them into account can for many people result in a rational pharmacotherapy augmented by an appropriate form of psychotherapy.

For some illnesses, the current roster of treatments is still grossly insufficient. Only research will help develop the proper treatment for these unfortunate sick people. Mindless repetition of wishful shibboleths obfuscates the situation, substituting unfounded certainty for the necessary research. It can also worsen the lives of the sick, since they must add to the illness itself guilt over their failure to overcome resistances and defenses. Of course, they can—and do—blame their illness on their parents' cruel and irrational behavior, but this small comfort does nothing for the symptoms and dissipates the family solidarity that patients need to support them through their illness and its secondary consequences, such as unemployment and social isolation. Too often, the final result is utter demoralization.

The task of distinguishing among sources of unhappiness is often made more difficult because all of them can lead to demoralization. Demoralization, as we use the term, is the belief in one's helplessness, engendered by any one of a number of serious defeats, such as dissolution of a marriage, loss of a job, inability to get a promotion, failure to reach an academic goal, or especially affliction with chronic physical or mental illness. Sometimes life deals a blow that cannot be swept under the rug, that thoroughly shakes a person's self-confidence and makes him feel ineffective against uncontrollable events. He may be brutally shown how far his achievements, aspirations, or character are from his goal. This may lead to a reevaluation by a downward shift in self-image—the group of attitudes and evaluations one holds toward oneself. Rather than seeing himself as capable and effective, he changes his self-image in the direction of helplessness and incompetence. As Robert White points out, experiences of efficacy—mastery—and non-efficacy mold one's self-esteem, and for the adult the most realistic stable form of self-esteem depends on an objective estimate of his strengths and weaknesses. Because most lives lack dramatic content, demoralization as a result of major defeats is probably less common, however, than demoralization from illness, particularly chronic illness. But, regardless of the cause, the demoralized person sees himself as a loser surrounded by winners.

The bad effects are not likely to stop there. Demoralization frequently arouses a whole set of secondary unpleasant emotional states, including shame, guilt, anxiety, and depression. A demoralized person is ashamed that he is not living up to community standards or is failing in his job. He may feel guilty if he believes that the demoralizing experience is a punishment for actual or fantasied deeds. She may be anxious because she feels unable to deal with the responsibilities she has accumulated. He may be depressed because his helplessness will prevent him from achieving his goals. Because the future seems stripped of positive potential, she is completely pessimistic: life is going to continue to be unrewarding, and constructive effort will be useless.

An important distinction between demoralization and vital depression must be emphasized. The demoralized person is pessimistic about the results of his own efforts, while the person with vital depression is pessimistic about everything. The demoralized person can relish a gift and experience consummatory drive-reducing pleasure such as food and sex if it does not require a high level of attention and if no demands are placed on him to get going in an appetitive, hunting, seeking way. He can enjoy a vacation, a lively party, or a good meal, but probably will not want to plan them himself. But the person with vital depression cannot enjoy even those pleasures that are given to him directly without any effort on his part; all is weary, stale, flat, and unprofitable.

Nevertheless, of the chronic illnesses likely to produce demoralization, depression is probably the most common because a major feature of depressive mood is the profound conviction of one's massive incapabilities. The demoralization produced by biological depression may persist after the depression disappears. In many instances, this seems the result of the process of learning—or mislearning. Because of the depression, one has indeed been nonfunctional, incapable of attaining goals in life. When the depression is relieved, the sense of incapability, formerly justified, may persist on its own momentum.

One of the unfortunate aspects of demoralization is that it produces a vicious circle. With low self-esteem, the expectation of failure, and the lack of anticipatory hope, demoralized people naturally tend to fail to experience success. In one of the popular phrases of behavioral science, their expectations become a self-fulfilling prophecy. Pessimism breeds defeat, which breeds pessimism. That this can sometimes be countered by the assumption of a positive optimistic outlook has lent credence to the belief that hope engenders success, which engenders hope, and so forth. Demoralization can slowly respond to the instillation of optimism, encouragement, and benevolent pats on the back. This is the well-known power of positive thinking, or what has also been called a virtuous circle (Wender, 1968).

The fact that demoralization frequently does respond to hope probably lies behind the misnamed nonspecific effectiveness of a wide variety of psychological interventions, including not only psychotherapy but mind-healing of all types, especially those associated with religious belief and conversion. The effectiveness of these interventions stems from the fact that they can often produce a hopeful faith. If the demoralized person's belief in his own effectiveness can be stimulated, if he somehow can be roused into action, successful experiences may then negate his feelings of defeat and permit him to further muster his energies and dig out of the hole in which he found himself.

In this respect, too, he is different from the vitally depressed patient. Telling vitally depressed people to buck up is a useless enterprise and also convinces the biologically depressed person that the encourager is a damned fool or at least has no appreciation of the depressed person's state of mind.

The power of positive thinking usually requires external assistance, however, for only the rare individual can be truly self-reliant, given the complexities of modern living. The demoralized person needs to try again, but under conditions of social solidarity and group support, both emotional and practical. People will fail, make mistakes, and experience rejection. The power of positive thinking is a weak reed unless the demoralized person can turn to others. This probably explains the wide popularity of self-help groups.

The condition of demoralization—a shift toward feelings of pessimism and hopelessness—has been produced as an animal analogue by psychologist Martin Seligman, who has subjected animals to unavoidable, irregular stresses—to "no-win" situations. After a while, these animals give up. Seligman considers this a model for pathological depression. We think it more clearly resembles human demoralization. It would be interesting to learn whether the animals respond better to antidepressants or to amphetamines, which, as we shall shortly elaborate, further distinguish depression and demoralization.

Turning to an evolutionary framework, is there any biological utility to the experience of demoralization? It is possible that severe disappointment acts to inhibit the brain regulatory mechanism that we have postulated as underlying appetitive hunt and search activity; that is, the mechanism that produces feelings of energy and optimism. This may make evolutionary sense. If one has been severely and repeatedly disappointed, it may pay to cut down on environmental interactions for a while, since one may be in a developmental stage in which current capacities do not match current goals. Keep a low profile, let it blow over, and await a brighter day.

Thus, although we have defined demoralization as a learned mood, here, too, we suspect that learning builds on unlearned predispositions. People probably do learn to be helpless, given sufficiently massive, uncontrollable disappointments, but the ground has been prepared evolutionarily, endowing them with a low threshold in the hypothesized mechanism that inhibits appetitive search behavior under conditions of chronic disappointment. This hypothesis is borne out by drug responses. Demoralization often does respond to adjunctive stimulant medications—amphetamines—along with psychological uplift treatment; it helps the patient to mobilize his resources. Antidepressant medication usually does not stimulate the demoralized patient into action. After the biologically depressed patient has responded to antidepressant medication, he is frequently left with a residual demoralization. At this point, stimulant medication often proves very helpful in instigating rewarding activity, whereas it would have been useless during the early phase of the biological depression. These differences indirectly indicate that something besides learned changes in attitude is central to disappointment-induced inactivity. Our earlier distinction may hold here, with the amphetamines helping demoralization through their effect on appetitive drives, and the antidepressants being less useful because they have more influence on consummatory pleasure regulation.

A phenomenon related to personal demoralization, massive socioeconomic demoralization, is a social situation of great importance and disastrous potential. It may seem simplistic to postulate the same mechanism for such widespread behavior, but one sees attempts at self-treatment by the underprivileged by means of drug addiction and alcoholism—the plagues of the inner city—which temporarily relieve the demoralization blues. The potential dangers of drugs are of no consequence to the down-and-out. The implications for what might be required to reverse the situation are discouraging, for reality here is a mélange of accumulated barriers: prejudice, inadequate and inappropriate education, poverty, high unemployment rates and dead-end jobs, historical role, social pressure, and cultural norms. All this is added to the individual's own physiological predispositions and particular learning experiences.

Demoralization, then, is a good example of the interplay of the kinds of factors that the psychiatrist may be asked to sort out and miraculously change. With supportive psychotherapy and stimulant drugs, the psychiatrist may be able to jog the patient into sufficient movement to bring reinforcing rewards from life. But for the patient demoralized by his own limitations, by intransigent personal circumstances, or by overwhelming environmental disadvantages, there may be nothing the psychiatrist can do.

CHAPTER **8**

The Psychotherapies

The number of psychological procedures that have been used in efforts to ameliorate human mental misery is immense. The latest count—computed, appropriately enough, by an IBM systems analyst—is up to 250, and includes such exotica as Bioplasmic Therapy, Burn-Out Prevention, Neurotone Therapy, Photo Counseling, Rebirthing, Soap Opera Therapy, Vita-Erg Therapy, and Zaraleya Psychoenergetic Technique (Herink, 1980). An attempt to review and evaluate even all the mainstream psychological therapies that have been used would be valiant but fruitless. Compounding the difficulty of sheer numbers is the problem of deciding where to draw the line between psychotherapies and other helping agencies. What about therapies that have a religious component or may be based firmly on religious belief? Or those based on social activism or communal living? Some of the most striking reports of psychological cures may be found in William James's *The Varieties of Religious Experience,* a book that provides ample anecdotal confirmation of the therapeutic potency of religious conversion. Here we can only draw attention to the overlap and decide arbitrarily to restrict ourselves to nominally nonreligious therapies and those that do not involve permanent attachment to a particular community.

Another factor that complicates the life of the would-be objective investigator of the psychotherapies is the fragmentary and variable data concerning the effectiveness of the various techniques. There are hundreds of anecdotal clinical studies attesting to effectiveness and additional hundreds of studies that attempt to evaluate psychotherapy scientifically. But because they study small numbers of often undiagnosed patients, frequently do not use credible controls, and do not adequately define symptoms, techniques, and goals, the results often are not understandable or open to generalization. Many show that patients improve with psychotherapy, but it is not clear whether the improvement can be attributed to the psychotherapy, to suggestion, to maturation, to circumstances, or to the natural course of the illness. In addition, in any group of patients studied, some improve, some do not improve, and some worsen. Because improvement totals usually do not specify how different kinds of patients reacted, it is difficult to determine which subgroups might do better in psychotherapy, which show little change, and which might be harmed.

Through gradual improvement of research standards, a sufficient number of adequately designed studies now support overall agreement that psychotherapy at least alleviates discomfort and increases the sense of well-being in some kinds of patients (Smith, Glass, and Miller, 1981)—in line with the common-sense observation that talking to someone about one's troubles is usually better than keeping them bottled up. But, beyond that simple statement, agreement disappears. Researchers are particularly divided concerning the usefulness of psychotherapy with the major biological disorders, such as schizophrenia and vital depression. We ourselves, for example, do not believe that the evidence indicates that psychotherapies have any appreciable effect on schizophrenia, though other investigators have come to different conclusions (see Klein, 1980). Similarly, we strongly doubt that they have any effect on vital depressions. (Interestingly, the latest data analysis from the Boston–New Haven collaborative study of the relative merits of interpersonal psychotherapy and pharmacotherapy in depression indicates that psychotherapy is useless in endogenous [vital] depressions.) They might have some stabilizing effect in some of the other biological illnesses.

In a study prepared for the National Academy of Sciences in 1978, Morris Parloff and his colleagues at the National Institute of Mental Health summarized the scientific data on the effectiveness of psychotherapy. Parloff's group included such traditional therapies as psychotherapy, psychoanalysis, family and group therapy, and behavior therapy, but did not study the newer and more flamboyant techniques, such as primal scream, transactional analysis, gestalt therapy, encounter groups, and the various sensory and body therapies. The Parloff summary included the following: patients treated by psychotherapy "show significantly more improvement in thought, mood, personality, and behavior than do comparable samples of untreated patients" (p. 1). However, in a small percentage of cases, as yet unidentified, combinations of therapists, techniques, and patients can produce negative effects. Patients with symptoms of anxiety and mild depression tend to show greater improvement in psychotherapy than patients with somatic complaints. Patients with "high motivation, acute discomfort, a high degree of personality integration, previous social success and recognition and a capacity to be reflective and to express emotion are particularly suited for most forms of psychotherapy," although requirements for success in some forms of behavior therapy may be less rigorous. "Above all, the decision to enter therapy itself indicates a commitment to change" (p. 2).

With regard to the effectiveness of psychotherapy in specific disorders, Parloff reports the following:

Schizophrenia. For institutionalized patients, the effectiveness of individual or group psychotherapy as the major treatment remains ambiguous. (We believe that no appreciable effect has been demonstrated. See Klein, 1980.)

Patients discharged to the community often do not have the social skills required for adequate adjustment, but as yet there is no clear role for psychotherapy in improving this situation. Since family response to the discharged patient seems an important factor in his ability to function, work with the relatives may have as high a priority as work with the patient himself (Parloff et al., pp. 4–5; Kanter and Lin, 1980).

Depressive disorders. Several approaches—a structured interpersonal therapy, various behavioral methods, and cognitive behavior therapy —may all be effective, alone or in conjunction with drugs, for many depressed patients.

(Unfortunately, most psychotherapy studies of depression have not bothered systematically to describe the patients' difficulties. As ordinarily investigated, vital depressions are confused with demoralization, hysteroid dysphoria, the affective disorders of hyperactivity, and the demoralization that is frequently a reaction to easily identified events—and that is short-lived with or without therapy. For a group of demoralized patients, warm friendly support may be more effective than drugs, which work only for vital depressions and do nothing for others except to give them dry mouths and constipation. On the other hand, antidepressant medication has repeatedly been demonstrated to be effective—to an important degree—in 70 to 80 percent of individuals with vital depressions. Without specifying exactly the sorts of depressed people being studied, assertions about psychotherapy—like assertions about drugs—are meaningless.)

Neuroses and personality disorders. Inadequate studies suggest that about two-thirds of patients treated for anxiety benefited from psychotherapy. It has been effective with about half of the patients treated for various phobias, but agoraphobia appears extremely resistant to treatment. (Our experience is that simple phobias respond positively in as high as 90 percent of the cases to either psychotherapy or behavior therapy; we agree with the comment on agoraphobia, as indicated in our recommendation of drug therapy.) Obsessive-compulsive disorders in their extreme form have been difficult to treat (p. 6).

Sexual dysfunctions. Although success with such symptoms as premature ejaculation, vaginismus, and anorgasmia has been reported by psychoanalysts, psychotherapists, hypnotists, and behavior therapists (and, we might add, practitioners using the Masters and Johnson techniques), the nature of the studies does not permit comparison of their effectiveness (p. 7).

Marital discord. Here individual therapy seems less effective than conjoint, couple therapy, or group therapy. Behavior therapy may be useful in specific aspects of marital interaction (p. 8).

In response to meager data of this kind, the National Institute of Mental Health is only now beginning large-scale research on the effectiveness of psychotherapy. Such research will attempt to discern differences in effectiveness in terms of different kinds of therapists, patients, disorders, and therapeutic techniques.

The contrast between the apparently flourishing field of psychotherapy and the little that is known definitively about it may seem difficult to understand, but we think it can be explained in terms of the following factors: belief in the self-evident effectiveness of psychotherapy, inappropriate early conclusions from improvement, the need and desire to help and be helped, failure to distinguish among possible sources of problems, failure to specify goals, and new standards of evaluation.

A question that is often asked is whether the effectiveness of psychotherapy *requires* scientific proof. Most accurate human knowledge was discovered long before the era of the scientific experiment. Most of man's technology until the eighteenth century was entirely empirical. Good clay pots were not constructed on the basis of theories of sols and gels or solid-state physics. The useful treatments that were discovered before the scientific age were the product of generations of trial and error.

Our oldest rule-of-thumb technology is probably applied psychology. People have parented, taught, and governed others for ages. Virtually none of the explicit and implicit bases for such behavior have been demonstrated in the laboratory, and when demonstrated they have been in such an abstract form as to be almost unusable. Most ideas about human behavior are tacit, used without formulation into rules. Every child knows that if you kick someone in the shins he is likely to get angry. As the child grows older, he learns how to control his own behavior, sometimes in very subtle ways, and learns to get other people to do what he wants. Such knowledge is recapitulated in the development of every (well, almost every) individual, and it is taken for granted that some people are more talented than others in the art of human relationships. That being so, why should it be difficult to believe that experienced and sensitive psychological workers can produce appreciable psychological changes in their subjects, especially with the benefit of accumulated, subtle, applied psychological wisdom? Further, controlled evaluations of treatment have been introduced only in the last twenty or thirty years, and many scientific medical advances were made before that time.

We are not talking about intuitive psychological art, however, but about whether people can affect psychiatric illness, ingrained learned maladjustment, and realistic unhappiness. Because only a handful of researchers have attempted to clarify whom they were treating, exactly how they were being treated, and precisely how the consequences were measured, the research provides vague conclusions about a heterogeneous group of patients whose problems represent an unknown mix of illness, maladjustment, and demoralization. The scientific results are chaotic, and it seems obvious that relying on clinical sensitivity means continuing to provide inadequate treatment in many instances.

Since the scientific research is unsatisfactory, another question that arises is why early studies on psychoanalysis and psychotherapy were persuasive. In part, the answer comes from the nature of the patients treated. Freud and his followers initially derived their theories of causation and treatment while working with symptomatic, sexually inhibited Viennese. Adler presumably derived his techniques from dealing with ambitious middle-class patients. Jung, in turn, formulated his theories working with middle-aged, successful, religiously troubled persons whose problems were not sexual but involved questions of purpose and philosophical meaningfulness. The influential American psychologist Carl Rogers began his work with relatively healthy college students. It is possible the therapies used were relatively effective and easily accepted by these kinds of patients, and that confusion and ineffectiveness have resulted from their application to other kinds of patients.

Another reason why initially convincing therapy no longer convinces may be related to confusion of the therapist with the therapy. Therapists' reports on their work tend to describe those specific behaviors of their own that they remember. They are often quite blind, however, to the specific characteristics of their own personality and their own incidental behavior during work with patients, although both of these could conceivably be the most important psychological ingredients.

In contrast, the followers of Carl Rogers, for example, claim that much of the effectiveness of therapists stems from their nonspecific, human characteristics, such as genuineness, empathy, and unconditional positive regard for the patient; specific therapeutic techniques, such as free association, the interpretation of dreams, role-playing, and so forth, are seen as irrelevant. But the naïve observer, reading only the therapist's report of the therapist's behavior, would attribute the reported success to the specific techniques employed. The therapist may in fact have succeeded in relieving the patient's symptoms, but for reasons other than those he postulated. Another therapist using the same specific methods might find them ineffective and might attribute the lack of effectiveness to the originator's bias, exaggeration, or deceit. But if genuineness, empathy, and positive regard—or other as yet unidentified and unconfirmed therapist qualities—are the major effective ingredients of therapy, and the follower lacked these qualities, then using the prescribed technique would be insufficient.

Finally, the patient's expectations of new modes of therapy and new healers of great reputation, plus simple cathartic relief, have undoubtedly been responsible for many of the initial clinical-case reports of effectiveness. But as the novelty has diminished and as dynamic leaders have been succeeded by pedestrian imitators, effectiveness may have dwindled.

If, then, scientific evidence for psychotherapeutic effectiveness is lacking, and even informal evidence at times palls, we are faced with the question of why psychotherapists continue to develop such intense loyalties to the particular schools they espouse.

The question is not difficult to answer, especially when one looks at the history of medicine, which is dominated by the prolonged use of ineffectual or even harmful treatments. For years, physicians bled patients (tapped pints or quarts of blood from their veins), applied suction cups, burned and blistered the skin, and administered a wide variety of mysterious potions, including bat wings and newt eyes. Oliver Wendell Holmes remarked at the end of the nineteenth century that if most of the pharmacopoeia were dropped into the sea, it would be so much the better for mankind and so much the worse for fish.

Until the era of experimental medicine, proponents of conflicting, inadequate treatments quarreled vociferously and interminably. Physicians—like shamans, witch doctors, and magicians—were passionately attached to worthless treatments. Although fraudulence—a conscious, cynical desire to maintain a source of income and prestige—probably explained some of it, and an understandable and possibly unconscious desire not to look a gift horse in the mouth probably was also involved (as Confucius reputedly said, "The wise man does not examine the source of his well-being"), most of the enthusiastic support for treatments of unknown effectiveness can be attributed to less venal and even to commendable factors.

There are at least three possible explanations. The first is the physician's and the patient's desperate need to do something. Passive observation is intolerable. For both parties, action of any sort is anxiety-reducing, and in the absence of other evidence this alone can reinforce belief. A patient does not want to consider himself lost to hope. The physician will not willingly perceive himself as impotent. To quote Oliver Wendell Holmes again:

> There is nothing men will not do, there is nothing they have not done, to recover their health and save their lives. They have submitted to be half-drowned in water, and half-choked with gases, to be buried up to their chins in earth, to be seared with hot irons like galley-slaves, to be crimped with knives, like cod-fish, to have needles thrust into their flesh, and bonfires kindled on their skin, to swallow all sorts of abominations, and to pay for all of this, as if to be singed and scalded were a costly privilege, as if blisters were a blessing, and leeches were a luxury. [1889, p. 378]

A second factor contributing to the perpetuation of unhealthful practices is the high spontaneous recovery rates for many medical and psychiatric disorders. Most patients with most illnesses get better by themselves even in the face of detrimental therapies. Spontaneous recovery affects not only the patient but also the physician. The physician treating his neurotic patient with the newest form of therapy is like the rain dancer stomping around on the hot, dusty plateaus of the Southwest. Many neurotics do improve willy-nilly, and it does rain a few days a year even in the deserts of Arizona. Neither the physician nor the rain dancer/witch doctor is going to abandon his powerful role and stop his ministrations in order to see what happens without intervention (even if the community considers such cessation ethical). Both get occasional and striking payoffs: cure and rain, respectively.

The animal literature tells us that rats who have been trained to pull a bar for an occasional and unpredictable reward will optimistically continue to press the bar long after the food has been withdrawn—like habitués of one-armed bandits in Las Vegas and Atlantic City. Similarly, witch doctors and psychiatrists whose efforts pay off periodically and unpredictably are likely to become addicted to their own behavior.

The way in which a patient can make the therapist believe in his own efforts is strikingly illustrated in an anecdote recounted by Jerome Frank. The therapist in question was a Kwakiutl Indian who, after observing the grossly fraudulent techniques of some practitioners, entered shamanistic training skeptically, but after his own therapeutic successes came substantially to believe in himself: "He pursues his calling with conscience . . . is proud of his successes and . . . defends heatedly against all rival schools [a particular fraudulent technique] whose deceptive nature he seems completely to have lost sight of, and which he had scoffed at so much in the beginning" (quoted in Frank, 1974, p. 58).

Of course, witch doctors and psychiatrists will attempt to mitigate the disappointment of failure by an effort to determine why intervention worked in some instances and not in others. The witch doctor/rain dancer is never at a loss to explain his failures. The lack of a downpour—or, say, the failure of Little Deer's sore arm to heal—resulted from chanting the complex sacred formulae with subtly ruinous mistakes, or slightly violating miscellaneous rules of protocol or formal behavior. His psychotherapeutic counterpart is likewise never at a loss for explanations: the patient's resistances were too great, his ego strength was not substantial enough, his secondary rewards from illness were excessive, and so on. Or the doctor may even discover faults within himself—the negative countertransference (negative feelings toward the patient) had not been worked through, the sessions were too infrequent, therapeutic attention had been directed to maladaptive behavior that was only a smoke screen for the real underlying pathology, interpretations had been poorly timed, *ad infinitum.*

There is an irony even in the apparently self-critical statements made by therapists (or by shamans). It is much easier for the therapist to attribute his lack of progress to a mistake in the application of a potent treatment than to admit that the treatment—the mastery of which has involved immense effort and time, and on which he prides himself—is itself impotent. It is analogous to an eighteenth-century physician blaming himself for the death of his pneumonia patient by claiming that he used his mustard plasters, leeches, and cupping too unaggressively. Then as now, the physician would rather claim ineptitude (or a slip of the scalpel) than ignorance.

A third reason why faith in various psychotherapies persists despite lack of convincing evidence is that the hope and expectation of cure that the doctor generates in the patient is one of the doctor's strongest therapeutic tools, since it mobilizes the demoralized patient's resources. The combination of hope and high expectation is a real, effective, common ingredient that cuts across all therapies, just as demoralization—which it treats—is a common complication that cuts across illnesses. Enthusiastic proponents of a therapy more effectively arouse the patient than do skeptics, doubters, and impartial evaluators. Thus, the healer who moves from being a cool agnostic to being an impassioned and devout member of any psychiatric school will almost certainly discover that his therapeutic effectiveness has increased *if* his patient's limitations are largely the product of demoralization and despair. If the patient is sick, passion is less than curative. Warmth, empathy, and involvement are better for hopelessness than they are for cancer. Believable support helps demoralization. It is worthless for biological depression.

The true believer *is* very likely to be more effective, but he is unlikely to recognize that his effectiveness is related to style and not to content. His fervor, professional aura, self-assurance, and therapeutic enthusiasm are his potent tools, not his doctrine. Consider your response as a patient with an ulcer, confronting the two following doctors. The eclectic: "Your ulcer is a rather uncommon sort . . . a number of studies have been published with very conflicting results . . . there are several general treatments and it is difficult to determine which, if any, would be helpful to you . . . let's just try them one after another and see which, if any, would be helpful." Or the enthusiastic believer: "Although your sort of ulcer is uncommon and much nonsense has been written about it . . . I have been extremely successful with the following therapeutic plan, which is a bit complicated but almost always works." To the extent that anxiety aggravates a peptic ulcer and peace of mind facilitates healing, it is not difficult to anticipate which patient is likely to experience the better therapeutic result—or at least to give the more enthusiastic testimonial.

A primary reason for the floundering in psychotherapy, we think, is that most psychotherapists—and schools of psychotherapy—have failed to distinguish among mental illness, mislearning, and reality as sources of unhappiness, and thus have stacked the cards against themselves. Each source of unhappiness, we believe, responds differently to psychological intervention.

The uses of psychotherapy, as we see them, are related to our basic threefold view of human unhappiness:

Unhappiness from mental illness—the bad feelings, faulty thinking, disadvantageous attitudes, or ineffectual or self-defeating actions that come from impaired brain regulatory mechanisms. These are such illnesses as the schizophrenias, some disorders of mood, hyperactivity, panic disorder, and hysteroid dysphoria, which seem to have a basic biological component. Because of their biological basis, we believe that psychotherapy alone is unlikely to be effective and that drug therapy is indicated. Psychotherapy *may* help patients to live with, adapt to, or compensate for biologically produced disabilities, but systematic evidence to this effect is lacking.

For some, this viewpoint will be less than heartening. We would all like to believe that we are O.K. and "born to win." If our life has been something less than totally rewarding, it would be wonderful to believe that a glorious future lies within us and that by transactional analysis, or rational emotive therapy, or Rolfing, or gestalt therapy, or primal screaming we will be able to cast aside the constricting folds of our self-inflicted cocoon and metamorphose into the beautiful, admirable, lovable butterfly that we know lies within—our true self. Potential assets may well lie within those afflicted with mental illness, imprisoned by the constraints of faulty brain chemistry. With proper medication, some will indeed emerge, but we believe that psychotherapy can only be an adjunct therapy for most of these conditions. In the present stage of our knowledge, even medication can sometimes produce only a drab moth in some illnesses—such as chronic schizophrenia; in such cases the butterfly fantasy is best recognized for what it is—a fantasy.

Unhappiness from mislearning or maladaptation—the learning of inappropriate or inadequate responses. Clear examples are sexual ignorance and constriction. Other possible examples are low self-esteem; fear of or rebellion against authority; and the inability to tolerate delayed gratification. Such forms of maladaptation may be amenable to psychotherapy. However, no one yet knows which psychotherapies, if any, are best for which maladaptations. Further, an area that remains to be explored is differences in people with respect to capacity to unlearn maladaptive behavior, to learn substitutive adaptive behavior, and to retain adaptive behavior during periods of stress.

The primacy of early learning is a factor of unknown strength here. A familiar instance of this primacy is the learning of language. Most children acquire language by exposure to it, mastering grammar, vocabulary, and pronunciation without effort until about age six or seven. After eight or nine, however, a new language is learned with more difficulty, and some people may never fully master it, even with study and practice. Much of this early learning occurs outside the family, from peers rather than parents; children of immigrant parents grow up largely with local accents, not parental accents. To what extent similar rules apply to other characteristics of human behavior is not known.

What seems to be true is that some people are flexible while others are not, but in everyone both flexibility and the ability to learn certain skills diminishes with age. Even a dull child learns his native tongue easily, while a high-IQ adult foreigner may have a difficult time with the same language. Just as there are rare adults who can fully master a difficult foreign language within a few weeks, there are other talented people who can unlearn and undo the effects of early psychological experience. Others can change early learned attitudes, values, and patterns of behavior only partially and with great effort. Obviously, such variations may account for different responses to psychotherapies.

Realistic unhappiness. Examples can range from the bored housewife in suburbia to the victim of a bad marriage to the homosexual in a small town (in contrast to the homosexual in San Francisco) to the poorly educated person dissatisfied with a dead-end job to the trapped welfare mother with young children and an absent father. The belief that therapists can help people with such difficulties is overly optimistic and on occasion misguided. Some psychotherapists try to persuade individuals to construe their difficulties as an internal problem rather than a rational response to a troublesome situation. More objective psychotherapists can help people to recognize the realistic nature of their problems and reaffirm the desirability of change, but often can do no more than that.

The demoralization that can result from any of these three sources of unhappiness reflects an acute or chronic state of having given up—a situation in which one is unable to muster the energies to overcome stresses that ordinarily could be handled. Demoralization sometimes does respond to supportive psychotherapy of any kind. Both individual and group psychotherapy can diminish anticipatory anxiety and demoralization by providing settings that enhance self-esteem and allow some sense of accomplishment. The avoidant person, for example, may learn that some social assertiveness is not disastrous; in therapy, a dependent person can recognize her capacity for greater independence. The resultant relief of anxiety and demoralization facilitates the patient's ability to employ new—and possibly successful—adaptive techniques.

The confusion of illness, maladaptation, and reality is not surprising, and involves the idea of phenocopies. In many instances, it is not easy to tell if a problem is learned, biological, or both. For example, feelings of low self-esteem are an almost inevitable accompaniment of biological depression, but there is little doubt that low self-esteem can arise purely on the basis of childhood experience. Similarly, low self-esteem, justified or unjustified, can accompany realistic experiences of failure. Thus, low self-esteem requires different treatment approaches depending on its probable origin. Biological sources may require biological remedies; psychological sources may indicate that psychotherapy can help; realistic sources may require a social remedy beyond the competence of the psychiatrist.

Most schools of psychotherapy do not recognize the possibility of phenocopies, and assert that all but the most severe, gross instances of malfunctioning are psychologically produced. In the real world, however, problems usually occur together. Illness or maladaptation frequently lead to demoralization and to such realistic sources of unhappiness as inability to handle one's job. The mentally ill person who responds positively to medication may have to unlearn maladaptive behavior patterns that accompanied the illness, and he may need vocational rehabilitation as well.

Many of the studies that show the effectiveness of psychotherapy do not discuss the magnitude or the quality of the changes produced. This point is well illustrated by a large-scale study of the effects of drugs and psychotherapy in depressed women who had been successfully treated with antidepressant medication. Following recovery, they were then put by lot (random assignment) into four groups. One group had medication plus weekly psychotherapy; a second group had medication and relatively infrequent checkups; a third group had a placebo and weekly psychotherapy; while the fourth group had a placebo and checkups. The investigators were interested in two questions: Would psychotherapy prevent relapse as well as medication, and would psychotherapy improve familial relations better than medication? The answer was no to the first question and a partial yes to the second. Psychotherapy did not prevent relapse, while medication did. Psychotherapy, but not minimal-contact checkups, improved the patient's interpersonal relations in those patients who had not relapsed. Drugs and psychotherapy had different effects on different aspects of the patients' symptoms.

The summary point to be made here is that psychotherapists are handicapping themselves if they do not recognize their own limitations. Only by working in cooperation with appropriate other remedial approaches can they not only maximally benefit the patient but also give psychotherapy its best chance of succeeding.

In addition to problems presented by failure to recognize the sources of the patient's distress, psychotherapy evidences difficulties deriving from failure to specify goals. The use of a single word, such as "treatment" or "cure," implies that there is one goal toward which psychiatrists should strive. But "treatment" and "cure" are ambiguous terms. An examination of the ways in which these words are used by physicians who treat physical illness may be helpful in developing an understanding of the different kinds of goals that can be sought.

Traditionally, physicians in public health talk of three types of prevention, including conventional ideas of treatment as one of the types. The first type, primary prevention, is protection of the individual from developing a disorder. Immunizations against smallpox or education of parents concerning the role of sex instruction in child-rearing would be examples of this. The second form, secondary prevention, corresponds to treatment or cure in the ordinary sense—such as surgery for appendicitis, antibiotics for pneumonia, insulin for diabetes, and psychotherapy for a neurotic depression.

Here, it is extremely important to emphasize that all physicians take it for granted that there are two differing forms of treatment: short-term and prolonged. In the first, the treatment is given for a short time and the illness disappears—out comes the diseased appendix, or with the administration of the antibiotic the pneumonia disappears. This curative form of treatment seems to be the type that most psychotherapists have in mind, although not necessarily in a short-term version.

The other common form of physical treatment—suppressive treatment—is underrecognized by most psychotherapists. This is treatment that must be continued if the chronic or current disease is to be kept in check. Insulin does control diabetes but does not cure it. Antiepileptic medication may control seizures but does so only as long as it is administered.

Psychotherapists do employ both forms of treatment, but they tend to emphasize their successful cured patients and to downplay the others. Sometimes psychotherapists see patients at infrequent but regular intervals, implicitly recognizing that intermittent contact is necessary if the disorder is to be kept under control. Such treatment is sometimes called supportive, symptomatic, or superficial, as opposed to deep or reconstructive. This is a valuable kind of therapy, we feel, which can benefit many demoralized patients over extended periods of time, providing an indispensable crutch or splint. Of course, if psychotherapy is being inappropriately given to patients whose psychological distress stems from chronic biological problems, it is no great surprise that such therapy may continue indefinitely.

Two additional aspects of treatment are shortening rather than curing illnesses, and making the patient more comfortable while the illness runs its course. Many patients with tuberculosis would recover without treatment. New antibiotics do cure the illness in some patients who might have died, but usually they accomplish the more modest but useful goal of shortening the course of the illness in patients who would have recovered spontaneously. Neither the physician nor the patient regards this as a trivial result.

That psychiatry may at times accomplish this was demonstrated by Jerome Frank (1974, p. 154) with a small study of psychoneurotics. Frank found that psychotherapy accelerated the rate of growth (social effectiveness) that apparently would have taken place without it. He found that over a five-year period the patient who received psychotherapy did no better than a comparable person who did not, but that for the first several months the patient having psychotherapy achieved a more rapid resolution of his difficulties.

This is not a negligible result; much of medicine is concerned with expediting natural healing processes. Similarly, much of medicine focuses on controlling discomfort while the body heals itself—as when we take aspirin and nose drops for a cold. Psychotherapy can function analogously, especially in disorders related to development and temporary conditions, such as adolescent stresses, reactions of grief, and responses to the demands of young children.

The third type of prevention, tertiary prevention, occurs in rehabilitation medicine and refers to treatment directed at minimizing the limitations caused by an incurable disorder. In days past, the physician could neither prevent nor treat polio, but with braces and exercises could minimize the debility of the recovered polio patient. Similarly, the psychiatrist may help to design social milieus that permit the partially recovered ex-hospital patient to live a more normal existence.

Traditionally, the glamour of some psychiatric therapies has resulted from their claims that they can cure underlying illness. However, even therapies that claim cure sometimes make use of indefinite treatment that looks more like tertiary prevention. In more conservative psychoanalytic training, for example, the duration of the trainee's analysis can range up to seven to ten years, with periodic reanalyses recommended to deal with recurrent problems. Other therapies more realistically recognize what they are doing—for example, Alcoholics Anonymous and Synanon bluntly state the need for lifelong treatment.

In medicine, the nature of the illness dictates which goals are available. One might attempt to terminate an ongoing process with restoration of complete health, to cure with future immunity, to ease pain in a deteriorating process, and so forth. Similar recognition of available options is essential if psychotherapy is to be used most effectively.

An additional aspect of all forms of treatment accepted in medicine is the frequent necessity of trade-offs. Therapy often produces new symptoms, which are accepted if they are not as bad as those they are replacing or if the original symptoms are severe enough to warrant some risk in treatment. Some people die from immunizations. Operations may prove fatal. On rare occasions, certain antibiotics may totally impair the body's ability to fight infection. The physician always lives with calculated risks whenever he treats, and his aim can only be to recognize them and to try to diminish them. In the treatment of mental illness, such risks are more obvious with medication, but they do exist with psychotherapy—primarily in the use of intensive therapy with people of fragile personality structure. Still another risk is that an exclusive focus on psychotherapy may delay the administration of effective biological therapy. The various cautions we are recommending can help to reduce such risks.

Further confusion in the field of psychotherapy has occurred when a fourth, perfectly legitimate personal goal has been mixed with the other three. This goal, which has gained much popularity and interest recently, is in a sense a kind of supernormal health—an enhanced personal growth. Traditional medicine has evaluated its success in terms of eliminating or preventing the negative—for example, preventing polio, repairing broken bones, or helping the paralyzed with crutches, but not training Olympic athletes. The goals of those who seek to actualize potential in some ways more closely parallel those of educators—whether intellectual or physical—than those of physicians. Education and training can range from helping the retarded to learn basic skills or teaching the cerebral-palsy victim to use a motorized wheelchair to advanced seminars in astrophysics and classes in karate. There is no reason why therapists should not attempt to reach analogous high-performance psychological goals with healthy individuals (who are sometimes those afflicted with realistic social or developmental unhappiness). The confusion has arisen because in some instances the nominally growth-promoting techniques have been used with persons who are not healthy and for whom other techniques of treatment, pharmacological or psychological, would be far more beneficial.

Another problem with the growth-promoting therapies is that values here play a much larger role than in more traditional psychotherapeutic techniques, although no psychotherapy is value-free. It is easier to agree that anxiety and depression are undesirable states than, say, to agree that greater self-assertion, sensuousness, and freedom from responsibility will lead to greater happiness. What constitutes the good life is not blindingly obvious.

Although it is easy to understand why inadequately tested therapies have attracted followers, an opposite kind of reaction is equally familiar. For centuries, intelligent lay persons not only have questioned the helpfulness of medical treatment but have wondered if the best treatment was no treatment at all. The harmfulness of pills and physicians has been the butt of jokes and jibes for millennia. In *Bartlett's Familiar Quotations* we find, to cite just a few:

> Like the diet prescribed by doctors, which neither restores the strength of the patient nor allows him to succumb... [Demosthenes, fourth century B.C.]

> There are some remedies worse than the disease. [Publilius Syrus, 42 B.C.]

> Better to hunt in fields for health unbought,/Than fee the doctor for a nauseous draught. [John Dryden, 1700]

> Man may escape from rope and gun;/Nay, some have outliv'd the doctor's pill. [John Gay, 1728]

With a tradition of this kind about physical medicine—which cannot even agree about the most effective treatment for the different forms of cancer, despite stark measures of outcome—it is not surprising that there has long been a reservoir of mistrust among both scientists and the public about psychiatry's more baroque treatments.

Thus, as science has developed more sophisticated methods of measuring medical effectiveness, at least part of psychiatry has attempted to follow the leaders. As mentioned earlier, large-scale public-health, controlled drug studies were first initiated in 1946 when streptomycin was developed in England. With the discovery of the tranquilizers in the 1950s, psychiatry, too, began to learn more stringent testing procedures, and more recently such procedures have been used with psychological techniques.

Sophisticated testing of drugs now involves preliminary animal tests for safety; preliminary clinical trials, without controls, to assay possible usefulness; and finally, controlled trials. The controlled trial defines the condition and the treatment as clearly as possible in order to facilitate the necessary replication of the study by others.

Here psychotherapy is immediately in trouble. Diagnoses of patients are by no means easy to specify, and psychotherapeutic techniques are rarely easy to describe. One-way screens for observation and audio and video recorders have made it possible to check on what the therapist has done, but specifying in advance what she should do remains an enormous problem in psychiatric research. Very few kinds of therapy have produced manuals that give the therapist specific instructions on how to proceed in order to conduct that particular therapy.

After such initial specification, the patients are divided into comparable groups, one group having the active treatment and the other group (the control) having every aspect of the treatment except the active ingredient. To deal with the problem of comparable groups, it is important that the patients be divided on the basis of random assignment and not on the basis of the experimenter's selection (random assignment is like tossing a coin to determine whether a patient is placed in the active or in the control group). The experimenter might be picking up subtle differences that would make the groups not comparable to each other. For instance, he or she may want to believe that the treatment works and therefore may unconsciously put the healthier patients in the active treatment group and the sicker patients in the control group.

The group that does not get the active treatment receives a placebo treatment—one that looks identical to the first but lacks the supposed therapeutic ingredient. If an X-ray treatment is being tested, for example, both groups would be taken into the radiology room and both would have the radiation apparatus aimed at them, but only the active treatment group would actually receive radiation. The placebo or control group allows for the effects that hope and expectation produce in the patient and also allows for spontaneous improvement.

Even in cancer, hope and benefit may play some therapeutic role. For many other physical illnesses, the placebo effect is striking. The expectation of deriving benefit from pills, lotions, and potions produces real, appreciable benefit in a sizable fraction of the subjects having placebos. Individuals told that injected saline is morphine frequently experience substantial relief from severe pain. Anxious or depressed persons given inactive pills often feel better than those with similar problems who are given no pills. Whatever accounts for this effect, it must always be taken into account, particularly in situations where one is measuring subjective changes. In breast cancer, the physician can measure the size of the cancer and whether the benefit is permanent or only temporary, regardless of what the patient reports; in a test of a pain killer, the physician must depend entirely on what the patient says. Whether its power comes from expectation, trust, belief, or suggestibility, the placebo effect must always be reckoned with. Failure to acknowledge its importance or to use control groups has resulted in the adoption of scores of ineffective treatments.

In addition to responding to the placebo effect, many illnesses—even cancer—get better by themselves. In many illnesses—such as the acute schizophrenias, the major mood disorders, and panic disorder—there is a recurrent pattern of relapse and recovery, even without treatment. If there is no control group, it is easy to assume that the treatment preceding spontaneous recovery has been the effective force.

As should be apparent, psychiatric research presents some special problems. In cancer research, it is not too difficult to find comparable patients to divide into two groups. But, in psychotherapy research, how is one to attempt to produce matched (adequately similar) samples if, as some therapists maintain, no two persons are exactly alike? The experimentalists may twist and turn, devising rating scales that measure anxiety, depression, values, existential doubt, and interpersonal relations, but the adamant non-experimental psychotherapist may claim that all such efforts are futile because the two groups are not really equal.

However, the hard-nosed statistician never claims that two groups of patients are exactly equal; they are matched only within the limits of chance. The statistician further tells us that random assignment assures that the two groups of people do not differ—except by chance—even in important respects that we are ignorant of and hence cannot measure. This is not trivial. Random assignment saves us from our own ignorance.

The "uniqueness of the individual" viewpoint is an interesting philosophical position and of course a valid one. Recognition of uniqueness is essential in many educational and therapeutic contexts; but in some areas we may be able to function only by attending to our common human features, not our distinct ones. As the philosopher Ludwig Wittgenstein observed, the believer in the absolute uniqueness of all human beings—that is, the believer in universal solipsism—cannot meaningfully state his position without self-contradiction, because it implies that his unique readers would not understand his unique language. The extension of the "everyone is unique" argument to psychotherapy leads logically to inaction, for if the patient is completely unique, there is no way of knowing what might be effective. Hence, the psychotherapy researcher continues the search for the common factors in patients, ailments, and treatments.

Once the experimental and control groups have been designated, the next stage in experimental evaluation is the determination of how any changes are to be measured. In medical examples, the effects of treatment can be stated in a relatively straightforward manner: After a specified period of time, how many of the patients are alive or dead? Of those who are still living, in how many has the disease recurred and in how many has it apparently vanished? Or, less dramatically, in how many has acne or migraine subsided? In psychiatry, it is more difficult to describe change, but nevertheless it is usually possible to specify and measure objective target characteristics one wishes to change. In general, psychiatric treatment is concerned with symptomatic distress and social effectiveness and thus might focus on such symptoms and behaviors as hallucinations, suicide attempts, apathy, panic attacks, lack of assertiveness, compulsive rituals, or promiscuity.

Another problem here is who is to make the judgments concerning the patient's improvement. The people who presumably know the patient best are the therapist and the patient. However, therapists' ratings are likely to be unconsciously biased in favor of improvement. Physicians disagree about the effectiveness of their particular varieties of treatment for almost all disorders—from lumbago to hernia repair; it is highly likely that in an area such as psychotherapy, where criteria of improvement are so much more elusive, similar or greater biases will be a problem.

In drug studies, the therapist can be permitted to make observations and judgments if he does not know whether the patient is receiving an active medication or a placebo. If he is biased in favor of medicine, he may judge both groups as more improved than they actually are; if biased against medicine, he may underestimate the results of both treatments, but the difference between the groups will stay the same. But it is impossible to use this procedure with the psychotherapist who is treating the patient. Similarly, the patient theoretically can judge his comfort best, but he may be influenced by expectations, hope, and desire to please the therapist.

The judgments of others can be applied by having them rate before-and-after psychological tests or interviews. In that case, impartiality is achieved at the expense of sensitivity, since such independent evaluators cannot appreciate the subtle aspects of the patient's functioning. Various functional criteria provided by family members or others are also useful—such as whether formerly hospitalized patients have returned to work, are participating in family activities, are paying the bills, and so forth—but this material does not help in judging more subtle changes. The most demanding researchers these days try to use all these sources of information—therapists, patients, objective observers, and the family.

This, in general, sets forth the requirements for adequate research in psychotherapy, but it has not touched on one of the major problems—determining what treatment the control group is to receive that looks like psychotherapy but does not have the specific elements of psychotherapy. Talking to a friendly person might be considered a placebo, for example, in contrast to such specific techniques as the couch-bound analysis of free associations and dreams, the examination of particular patterns of interpersonal responsiveness, the inspection of repetitive patterns of behavior within a group, or the encouragement of primal screaming, but it might be difficult to be sure that the friendly person didn't inadvertently enter into one of the specific areas of treatment being investigated. Researchers have often resorted to patients kept on a waiting list (without treatment) as a comparison standard. This presents ethical problems in instances of severe illness. Investigators are still wrestling with such difficulties, and are especially eager to sort out possible specific and nonspecific effects of psychotherapy.

This is a crucial question in psychotherapy research because it is possible that all psychotherapy modalities, despite their apparent wide differences, may derive their effectiveness from the same nonspecific elements. These nonspecific aspects may include the following (Frank, 1974, pp. 325–30): (1) Expectation of benefit—improvement accruing from the expectation that by following certain rules and procedures recommended in a relationship with a trusted authority in an identified place of healing, one will obtain the desired goals. This probably includes an unconscious and irrational hope of a magical cure—the kind of hope that first generated the occupations of shaman, priest, and doctor. There is some evidence, however, that maximum expectation of benefit requires congruence between expectations and what actually occurs in therapy (Frank, 1974, p. 164). The patient must have at least some idea of what to expect. The expectations are also enhanced by a cohesive explanation (not necessarily true) of why the therapy works; through such an explanation, the terror of the unknown is somehow diminished. (2) New opportunities for learning, both experientially and cognitively. Examples of such learning might be therapist behavior and values that seem worthy of adopting, positive responses from the therapist that counteract early negative reactions from family members, or specific ways of changing sexual or phobic behavior. New learning in therapy includes relief at finding that the therapist (and in group therapy, other patients) is not overwhelmed by whatever bizarre fears and behaviors one confesses (a relief similar to that produced by confession in the Catholic Church). (3) Success experiences, such as new insights, behavioral changes, or acknowledgment of responsibility. (4) Decrease in sense of alienation through the relationship itself; acceptance by the therapist counters feelings of unworthiness and contributes to the need for social experience. (5) Emotional arousal.

Support for the idea that the effectiveness of psychotherapy is based on nonspecific factors recently emerged in a study by Antonette Zeiss and her colleagues (1979). The investigators randomly assigned sixty-six depressed outpatients (moderate to severe unipolar depression) to one of three different types of treatment: interpersonal-skills training (e.g., training to increase assertiveness and social interactions); cognitive training (e.g., training to decrease irrational beliefs and negative thoughts); or training to increase mood-related pleasant activities. All treatments significantly alleviated depression, and no treatment had specifically greater impact on the special behaviors on which that particular treatment had focused. The authors speculate that improvement was related to the patients' increased sense of mastery and personal efficacy, regardless of treatment technique.

Similarly, Klein and his colleagues (in press) in a study of approximately two hundred phobics have shown that, in a high-prestige phobia clinic, behavior therapy and supportive therapy did equivalently well. The supposedly specific desensitizing and relaxing behavioral treatments were of no additional value. Klein suggests that the common feature of these therapies was their ability to persuade the patients to confront their phobic situations in real life. Through this exposure, the patients' fears become extinguished. The therapies, then, have essentially a priming or instigational role. The real therapy went on after the session.

The extent to which psychotherapeutic effects depend on nonspecific factors is unknown, but such factors are of therapeutic benefit only if the patient's belief system matches the therapeutic modality. An Australian aborigine will not benefit from a trip to Lourdes, and a devout Catholic's hopes for a cure will not be raised by the bone-pointing ministrations of a shaman. A psychoanalytic patient may regard primal-scream therapy as ridiculous, and a follower of gestalt therapy may believe that psychoanalytic intellectualization ignores crucial aspects of human functioning. Fortunately for innovators, patients vary enough in their enthusiasms to provide willing novitiates for all new forms of treatment. The potent nonspecific benefit of novelty is captured in the medical adage: "Hurry to use a new medicine before it loses its effectiveness."

Since placebo treatment as a requirement for research is relatively recent, what can we make of the decades' worth of uncontrolled, naturalistic data that have been presented as evidence for the effectiveness of various psychotherapies? In theory, such data have compared the natural history of psychiatric disorders without treatment with the histories of similar persons who have been given psychotherapy. Although certain psychiatric illnesses do have statistically predictable courses—that is, in people suffering from these illnesses we can predict what fraction of them will be in psychological state A now or in psychological state B at a later time—in general, we cannot predict what will happen to a particular patient. Thus, although naturalistic case histories can serve as a means of generating hypotheses, they are valueless for testing them.

Moreover, patients do not enter psychotherapy at random but because they wish to do so. They thus form a special subgroup of those who suffer from a particular illness. This is most evident in those who join Alcoholics Anonymous. Persons who enter AA have a good chance of becoming and staying dry. However, only alcoholics who are strongly motivated to dry out enter AA. Although accounts by members lead one to believe that participation in AA has per se played a major role in successful bouts with alcoholism, the doubter wants to know how much benefit has been due to motivation, how much to actual participation, and how much to the specific belief systems and practices of AA. Similarly, we cannot determine the relative importance of self-selection in causing beneficial effects from psychotherapy. Further, since past clinical reports on psychotherapy did not consistently describe the type of patients treated or the details of the therapy, interpretation of these reports is impossible.

Thus, although it may seem cavalier, we remain unimpressed by the accumulation of many years of devoted but uncontrolled case studies. Nevertheless, we believe that some forms of psychological treatment are effective in some patients treated by some therapists some of the time. We believe that not only can these therapies mitigate symptoms and hasten relief but they can also produce changes that would otherwise not have occurred in behavior and feelings. We also believe that some treatments are ineffective and others are injurious.

The field can best progress in testing these beliefs if: (1) patients are distinguished in terms of the probable sources of their problems—illness, mislearning, or reality factors; (2) goals of therapy are specified more clearly.

In 1980, the United States Senate considered, without any conclusion, whether the government should extend its current level of financial support for psychotherapy. Further, what should the therapist's professional qualifications be? Not surprisingly, representatives of various professions, including nurses (R.N.s), psychologists (Ph.D.s), and psychiatrists (M.D.s), testified that their professional status was quite sufficient for them to independently prescribe and conduct psychotherapy and to receive governmental reimbursement for their efforts, and that government support should increase.

What does our review of the facts concerning psychotherapy suggest in this regard? Although many different forms of psychotherapy, as compared to no therapy at all, appear to make patients with moderate illnesses feel better, there is distressingly little information as to whether this improvement in feeling is maintained after therapy or is associated with improvements in functioning. Further, critical review of the data, with reference to serious illnesses such as schizophrenia or vital depression, does not demonstrate even this degree of benefit (Klein, 1980).

When this unimpressive set of findings is linked with the almost uniform inability to show that one form of therapy produces better results than another, it should be clear why the claim that psychotherapy is a social good that requires increased financial support for highly trained, expensive personnel is greeted with skepticism.

If, as we think, Jerome Frank is right in saying that at the core of all forms of psychotherapy is the decrease in demoralization produced by the generation of hopeful expectancies in the context of a trusting relationship, then it really is not too surprising that controlled clinical trials of different forms of psychotherapy have been unable to demonstrate any particular superiorities. It follows from this that the personal qualities of the therapist and the prestige of the setting within which he practices may be of more significance than any specific training or techniques. In their extensive review of the psychotherapy literatures, M. L. Smith et al. (1981) were unable to find any relationship between the type of therapy or the qualifications of the therapist and the benefit produced.

Experimental studies contrasting the professional backgrounds of various kinds of therapists are almost nonexistent. A study by H. H. Strupp and S. W. Hadley (1979) of distressed college students found that college professors untrained in psychotherapy did just as well as a group of trained psychotherapists whose professional experience averaged twenty-three years. A program for training nurses as psychotherapists (Marks et al., 1978) has documented their very satisfactory performance. It is not clear, however, whether the same results could not be obtained if such a training program were applied to any group of intelligent, personable, well-motivated people. A number of articles document the psychotherapeutic effectiveness of relatively untrained volunteers.

We believe that therapies that can only be carried out by highly trained, expensive professionals should demonstrate, by experimental comparative trials, that they can produce specific benefits that are unobtainable by simpler therapies, or by personnel with lesser training, before they claim extended public support.

Requiring that the standards of systematic, experimental study be applied to psychotherapy has been said to be unfair since such standards are not required for other medical specialties. This is probably true, but two wrongs do not make a right. The other medical specialties have achieved their enviable position because of a series of dazzling objective successes that often obviously require a high degree of technical skill. Further, the degree of understanding of what has gone wrong with a person who is medically ill is clearly far more advanced than in the case of psychiatric disturbances. Psychiatry should be proud to apply such measures to its own professional procedures, thereby setting a model for medicine as a whole.

We advocate developing new methods of organizing care for those afflicted with mental disorders. The properly trained psychiatrist, we believe, is the best person to *evaluate* whether the troubled patient is suffering realistic unhappiness, personality limitations, or a psychiatric illness with a major organic component. Further, the psychiatrist is the only professional who can be sufficiently conversant with both the psychosocial and the physical methods of treatment, since he can both prescribe for and supervise the entire range of useful interventions. Still further, all patients considered for psychotherapy or any form of care for emotional disorder should have a general medical evaluation reviewed by a psychiatrist knowledgeable about how medical disease may mimic emotional disorder.

As we have emphasized, the essential feature of our recent remarkable successes has been an improved ability to diagnose illnesses that are treatable with medication. It is crucial, therefore, that all patients be given modern, informed, psychiatric evaluation and prescription of care. However, the use of an expensive, highly trained psychiatrist as a *treating* psychotherapist seems an extraordinary waste of training and ability, since it is quite likely that these procedures, when prescribed, can be carried out with equivalent benefit by personnel with only a moderate degree of training.

We can predict that these recommendations will be greeted with disapproval by the professional groups currently active in the system of mental-health care. Those psychiatrists or psychoanalysts who are primarily identified with carrying out individual psychotherapy will protest that their level of skill and training allows them to produce profound beneficial results that are unobtainable by other methods. We urge them to show the evidence that will allow the scientific evaluation of this claim.

Many psychologists, social workers, and nurses will resent our statement that they do not have the background that would enable them to conduct a sufficiently broad evaluation to allow a synthesis of both the psychosocial and the organic factors. Also, the fact that these groups are not legally allowed to prescribe medication will make many of them uneasy with our biopsychiatric approach, which emphasizes that for many patients medication is not only useful but is the best available treatment.

If psychologists, social workers, and nurses cannot perform the optimum diagnosis, and cannot prescribe medication, it then becomes clear that both evaluation and prescription absolutely require the services of a properly trained psychiatrist. (We repeat that many currently practicing psychiatrists have not received proper training.)

Such conclusions may well be attacked as a form of psychiatric imperialism rather than a reasoned judgment derived from available facts. We assert that the current organization of clinical care for those with emotional and mental disorders is out of date. Its reorganization will occur only if an informed citizenry demands it.

Listing and describing the range of psychotherapies would generate a chapter as coherent as the histories of the nineteenth-century Balkan states. One must attempt to group them in accordance with their common features, but unfortunately they lend themselves to grouping in a dismally vast number of ways. We might focus on what the therapist does, or what the patient is requested to do. Some therapies are didactic, some Socratic. Some focus on conscious processes, others on the unconscious mind. Therapies may be conducted with individuals, couples, families, groups, even crowds. Some explore the present, some the past. Some examine the contents of lives, some the forms. Some work primarily with reason, others with emotional expression. Any simple pigeonholing principle is bound to fail.

There is a second thing we cannot do. We cannot discuss all the therapies in the eminently sensible terms of which are best for what kinds of problems, because the data are conspicuously absent. Nor can we base such judgments on the experience of practitioners, since few have used more than one system and none have used very many.

Accordingly, no individuals have had enough experience with the variety of approaches to the same sorts of problems to be in a position to make educated clinical guesses concerning the relative value of many different therapies. We constitute no exception.

We will, then, present one approach to categorizing psychotherapy. Our presentation will at best be true; we shall have to abandon any hopes for its being beautiful. Although the various psychotherapies overlap, for descriptive purposes we divide them into the following groups: the intrapersonal therapies—those that focus primarily on experiences within the individual; the interpersonal and related therapies—those that focus on the person's relation to others; the multiple-person therapies (group, family, couple; these therapies are not unique types and use approaches and techniques from the other therapies, but their effects are special enough to warrant being categorized separately); the behavior therapies; the abreactive and cathartic therapies; and the state-altering therapies.

Intrapersonal Therapies

The intrapersonal theory of greatest venerability and the one that enjoys the honor of historical priority is psychoanalysis. Summing up its therapeutic techniques, beyond what was said in Chapter 2, is difficult not only because the theory is complex and the literature vast but also because consensus as to what is crucial has changed with time.

Major theoretical contributions of psychoanalysis are the conflict-based origin of symptoms, and the concepts of psychic determinism, the dynamic unconscious, psychological defense mechanisms, infantile sexuality, and transference. *Psychic determinism* refers to the hypothesis that no mental phenomena happen by chance—that seemingly meaningless thoughts, emotions, and actions are all meaningful products of the workings of the mind. As we said earlier, the *dynamic unconscious* refers to the belief that behavior and feelings are affected by the interplay of forces in the individual—such as drives, wishes, memories, and emotions—that may be outside his conscious awareness. Psychoanalysis holds that when drives and wishes produce ideas that are unacceptable to the individual's conscience (superego), *defense mechanisms* may act to repress the conflict-laden ideas to the dynamic unconscious, where they may still affect feelings and behavior in the form of symptoms. Of the unconscious forces, Freud felt that those generating the most difficulty arose out of *infantile sexuality* and expressed themselves during psychoanalysis in the form of *transference*.

Freud asserted that in the course of development the infant and child derived erogenous pleasure at a surprisingly early age and from hitherto unsuspected sources—for example, from the mouth during the first year, from the anus from about ages one to three, and from the genitals at ages three to five. Reaching the genital stage was associated with resolving the oedipal conflict—working out one's rivalry with the parent of the same sex over competition for the parent of the opposite sex. It was assumed that incorrect handling of the stages of infant sexuality would affect later personality. A child who experienced excessive oral gratification or suffered excessive oral frustration might fixate on the oral zone.

If fixated on an early stage of development, a person might never progress through the later stages to full adult sexuality. Further, the sexual fixation might have pervasive effects on the person's subsequent personality development. Someone whose personality had oral coloring would, of course, like eating, drinking, and smoking, but more important, might develop interpersonal oral traits, such as dependency (sucking) or sadism (biting). An anal character might be extremely obstinate, parsimonious, and orderly—or, conversely, extremely untidy. Most psychoanalysts have moved away from such concerns as oral and anal characters, but the oedipal conflict, and its hypothesized relationship to development of conscience (superego), still attracts considerable attention—especially in the broadened form of inevitable rivalries of many kinds between generations.

Treatment in psychoanalysis has focused on making the unconscious conscious by means of free association and interpretation, including dream interpretation. Presumably, free association allows the individual to become aware of his unconscious—with the assistance of the analyst's interpretations—by noting in the midst of conscious material indirect and symbolic allusions to other material. The use of symbolism to explain and understand behavior has always played an important role in psychoanalysis, and the extreme difficulty of validating symbolic interpretation has continued to plague scientific evaluations of psychoanalysis.

Early analysts thought that insight into the underlying sexual trauma or conflict would cure the patient, but as the field grew and patients did not conform to this pattern, psychoanalytic theory became increasingly complex. Symptoms are still seen as reactions to conflicting forces within the individual, but the nature of the possible conflicts has expanded from simple sexual trauma and conflict to more generalized unacceptable desires—such as hostile impulses against parents seen as inadequately supportive—and their possible consequences (shame, guilt, loss of love, personal injury). The major therapeutic goal, simply stated, has remained the bringing of the unconscious conflicts into awareness, and enabling the patient to come to terms with them. Coming to terms may be accomplished by consciously renouncing wishes that cannot be gratified, understanding the unrealistically childish nature of the origin of the wishes, more realistically assessing the consequences of carrying out the wishes, or relinquishing the fear of the consequences of the wishes.

As psychoanalysis developed, the relationship between the patient and the therapist—the transference—became of primary importance. Early in his therapeutic endeavors, Freud had noticed that his patients developed intense, often irrational feelings toward him. These feelings encompassed the entire range of feelings that can exist between people, but the two most obvious—and, Freud felt, important—were sexual and aggressive. Freud hypothesized that the nature of the psychoanalytic situation was such that patients were prompted to reexperience and to relive feelings they had had about important people in their past life—generally, but not always, their parents—and to direct these feelings toward the analyst. This phenomenon he called transference.

Freud's initial reaction was that transference was an impediment to treatment and must be removed. Positive transference, intense sexual feelings and a desire to please the analyst at all costs, resulted in the patient's excessive agreeableness and willingness to accept all psychoanalytic interpretations. Furthermore, the patient, usually of the opposite sex, became more interested in the pursuit of the analyst than in the pursuit of treatment. Similarly, negative transference, hostile feelings toward the analyst, also interfered with work toward therapeutic goals. Instances in which the patient exhibited his whole neurosis in his relationship with the analyst were designated as transference neuroses. Freud eventually came to believe that by working with these revivifications of past problems one could change the patient's attitudes and behaviors and thus free him from his neurosis.

For the analysis of the transference or the working through of the transference neurosis to be effective, the patient had to do two things. First, he had to recognize that his behavior toward the analyst was inappropriate, or neurotic. He had to accept the painful fact that the feelings and attitudes he experienced were not generated by what was happening in the real world. Next, he had to experience, in addition to recognize, the irrationality of his behavior and thus begin to develop the motor power for changing it. The theory, and the hope, was that the irrational behavior displayed in the psychoanalyst's office was only one instance of irrational behavior that the patient displayed in his relationships with other people. Presumably, by recognizing his neurotic attitudes and behaviors in the safety of the psychoanalyst's office, he might learn to change them there, and then be able to change them in the real world.

Freud focused on the irrational components of these emotions, but we should mention that recently psychotherapists have become aware of the rational components of both positive and negative feelings of this kind. How many women, either before or after marriage, have the experience of pouring out their hearts to a constantly sympathetic, sensitive, high-status individual who responds positively to their sexual preoccupations and who listens attentively to their expressions of feeling for a full hour at a time? On the other hand, what is an appropriate realistic reaction when someone states his most deeply held feelings and the listener does not condescend to reply to them? Or, in replying, interprets the speaker's ulterior motivations, generally in an implicitly critical and demeaning light?

The emphasis on transference constituted both a theoretical and a practical change. Initially, psychoanalysis had been directed at *intrapsychic* events. Now it was directed at *interpersonal* events. Initially, it had attributed psychological problems to repressed desires. Now it began to attribute them to maladaptive patterns of behavior, formed on the basis of relationships early in life and repeatedly lived out. This was a major change in focus and constitutes the bridge to the interpersonal therapies.

As analysis and its offshoots developed, countless variations on these major principles evolved, including, in non-Freudian descendants, a retreat from the idea of the centrality of sexual and aggressive drives. Among the early rebels, for example, Adler emphasized the inferiority complex in a therapy eventually called individual psychology; Jung's analytical psychology emphasized mystical and religious elements of personality; and Otto Rank wrote of birth trauma, brief therapy, and the role of the will. Later, the ego psychologists focused on stages of development, and other theorists looked to the intricacies of early object relationships (relationships with important persons). Existential analysts tried to weave notions of man's freedom in with concepts of his psychological bondage, and a recent radical development has been the proposal by the French psychoanalyst Jacques Lacan that the basis of psychoanalysis should shift from a focus on instinctual drives to a focus on language.

The development of psychoanalysis has been noted by many to parallel that of a religious cult. As in the history of Christianity, for example, a modest, easily comprehensible beginning leads to immense, intricate theories. Doctrinal differences cause breakaways by schismatic groups. Some of the heterodox survive, change their labels, and continue regarding themselves as the true spiritual descendants of the Master. Psychoanalytic circles have grudgingly accepted newer findings in the same way that the Catholic Church eventually permitted a belief in the heliocentric view of the solar system. Embarrassing assertions of the past are excused as metaphors, whereas the newer views are found to have been implicit in the beliefs of the Founder.

Among such changes in psychoanalysis is relaxation of the formal requirement of four or five therapeutic hours per week, with the patient supine and the analyst removed from the patient's field of vision. The modified forms of therapy based on psychoanalytic theory are generally referred to as either dynamic or analytic psychotherapy; dilute versions of them probably constitute a substantial portion of private and clinic practice today, among psychologists and social workers as well as among psychiatrists.

Psychoanalysts and psychoanalytic psychotherapists have participated in very little rigorous research, but we can speculate that psychoanalytic treatment would be most plausible for people who need to sort out their feelings, wishes, attitudes, and values, people who find the theoretical framework congenial and are willing to accept the duration and cost of treatment.

Increased awareness of possible contributions to who one is and what one really wants is undoubtedly interesting and might be useful. However, the relationship of self-knowledge to therapeutic benefit—especially in terms of specific problems—is unknown. It also has not been demonstrated whether this so-called self-knowledge is accurate or merely an acceptance of the analyst's views.

Even if self-knowledge is desirable, is psychoanalysis the best way of acquiring it? In focal areas, self-knowledge may perhaps be best achieved not by analysis but by talking with others facing similar problems. For example, homosexuals, battling spouses, and women depressed by the triviality of housewifery often seem to derive more benefit from talking to other homosexuals, acrimonious couples, or dissatisfied housewives than they do from individual psychotherapy. Furthermore, an accurate picture of one's interpersonal behavior is often best revealed in group therapy. Gestalt and other therapies maintain that their methods provide a faster and more complete means to insight. But perhaps there are different forms of insight about different areas of personal functioning, and different personal responses to possible ways of knowing oneself.

Interpersonal Therapies; the "Talking Cures"

Psychoanalysis at first focused on understanding striking and inexplicable mental illnesses. It attempted to explain the grotesque manifestations of hysteria, including deficits in memory, loss of bodily sensation, muscular paralysis, convulsions, and hallucinations. It attempted to explain the bizarre, ritualistic behavior of obsessional-compulsive neuroses and the intense, irrational fears of phobics. One of Freud's major works attempts to understand psychoanalytically the distorted meanderings of a paranoid appeals-court justice's diary (Freud, 1911), and one of Freud's classic case histories, that of the "Wolf Man," played a central role in speculations by psychoanalysis about the hard-to-understand obsessional neuroses (Freud, 1918).

As the practice of psychoanalysis continued, analysts began to see patients who were not as sick and who complained less about unusual symptoms and more about problems involving values, attitudes, and relationships—perhaps in part encouraged by the nonmedical aura of the treatment. Many of their complaints concerned their attitudes toward themselves, especially low self-esteem, their reactions to life experience, and the inability to love, to become close to others, to be assertive, to be compliant, to feel comfortable with others; or an inability to rid themselves of exaggerated self-demands, guilt, need for approval, and need for success.

Although the development of a variety of therapists and schools was in part the result of the rejection of substantial portions of Freudian theory, it was also related to the increase in patients who came to treatment with less dramatic but more common problems. Therapies originally deriving from analysis proper were those of such theorists as Harry Stack Sullivan, the formulator of interpersonal therapy; Karen Horney, who, like Sullivan, emphasized relationships and recognized the possible influences of culture and of experiences beyond childhood, but who, unlike Sullivan—and Freud—downplayed the possible role of biological factors; Erich Fromm, who included broader social concerns; and Eric Berne, whose transactional analysis devised catchy, easy-to-grasp ways of referring to the various defense mechanisms and forms of manipulative behavior identified by psychoanalysis.

Bridging medicine, psychology, and philosophy was Frederick ("Fritz") Perls, with gestalt therapy. This therapy's holistic approach, combining psychoanalytic concepts, reactions against psychoanalysis, gestalt psychology, mind-body integrations, the use of the imagination, and concerns with both pathology and growth, contributed greatly to the human-potential movement. From psychology came Carl Rogers with his influential nondirective therapy and the idea of the supreme importance of empathy; Abraham Maslow, also associated with the development of the humanistic, actualizing therapies; and Albert Ellis, whose rational-emotive therapy is one of several that concentrate on unrealistic attitudes. There are innumerable others, and considering them all together is a tremendous oversimplification. They do have features in common, however, perhaps the most important of which is their adherence to some version of the "talking cure" (the term devised by Anna O., the hysterical patient whom Breuer first described to Freud)—that is, therapist-patient exploration of the patient's problems.

Further, with some exceptions, they have tended to deal more with realistic unhappiness and maladaptive learning than with mental illness per se. Sullivan was known for his work with schizophrenics, and Rogers and his colleagues experimented inconclusively with treating schizophrenics on the basis of empathic relationships, but in the realm of illness interpersonal therapies have had most to say about depression and anxiety and problems in working and playing with others.

In focusing on aspects of human interactions that may shape personality and cause neurosis, many interpersonal therapists emphasize the formation of a world view. As we indicated in discussing mislearning, such a learned cognitive map may develop both within the family and within social and cultural subgroups, such as religious, class, and ethnic groups. Therapy is based on correcting distortions in such maps, enabling the individual to see more accurately the world in which he moves and to recognize how faulty perceptions may affect the comfort of his relations to that world.

Interpersonal therapists, like psychoanalysts, believe that early relationships—say, with the mother—are of critical importance; they do not emphasize the inhibiting or seductive effect on the infant's libidinal yearnings, however, but rather point out that the particular kind of relatedness will substantially influence the ability of the person to form subsequent relationships with others. If a mother is dependable, caring, and responsive to her infant's needs, for example, he will presumably grow up trusting others. But if the mother is erratic, negligent, or hostile, the infant may develop difficulties in establishing close relationships. Unconscious conflicts are not omitted from interpersonal theories but are not as salient as in intrapersonal theories.

For example, consider an adult man who reports feeling uncomfortable around women. In traditional psychoanalytic terms, this might be interpreted as a generalization of his unconscious incestuous yearning for his mother—with whom he confuses all other women—and his unconscious fear of castration should he act upon his oedipal wishes. The interpersonal theories might see his discomfort as the result of readily comprehensible interpersonal learning. He might feel uncomfortable not because of oedipal wishes but because his mother—or older sisters, or governess—had rejected him, belittled him, or pushed him around. He fears women as the bitten child fears dogs. Presumably, the discomfort can also produce unconscious conflicts. If he has normal heterosexual impulses, he will perhaps unconsciously feel anxious about women since he is pulled toward them and simultaneously fears the consequences of a close relationship with them.

Perhaps an even more important difference between interpersonal therapies and psychoanalysis is the emphasis on how the patient interacts with others in the here-and-now. Some of the therapies hold that, regardless of the origin of the behavior, it might be subject to change if the patient gets some idea of her effect on others. This idea is related to the assumptions underlying behavior therapy, in that the symptomatic behavior is seen as having some independence from basic character and as subject to environmental influences that do not depend on insight into the wellsprings of personality.

One of the conceptualizations used by interpersonal therapies in describing the maintenance of inadequate behavior is the self-fulfilling prophecy, the idea that expectations result in a kind of behavior that generates reactions in others that in turn reinforce the expectations. As a hypothetical example, if a woman has been brought up to distrust men and as a result is uncomfortable and rigid when with them, they are quite likely to withdraw quickly after initial interest, thus reinforcing the woman's distrust. The basic idea behind the term "self-fulfilling prophecy" is that one is at double jeopardy—one's feelings may be perpetuated by the learned behavior itself. The behavior may be intrinsically unhealthy or it may be an inappropriate remnant of a response that was once understandable. An example of the latter situation can sometimes be seen in children from broken and rejecting families: the children withdraw into themselves to avoid further disappointment. When adoptive parents or counselors reach out to them, the children's continued wariness may discourage the helpers, produce reduced efforts, and entrench the children's resistance.

In emphasizing not only the idiosyncratic experiences the infant has in her family but also cultural and social determinants of interpersonal relationships, the interpersonal schools have fostered examination of the possibility that different cultures may produce people with different personalities—that, for example, Jews, Italians, and Greeks are more expressive and less reserved than the English or Scandinavians. Some interpersonal therapies—for example, those associated with Erich Fromm—have also considered the contributions of social and political roles to subjective feelings of discomfort.

Although interpersonal therapies and psychoanalysis formulate their underlying theories differently, both relate curative efficacy to reliving one's behavior during a corrective therapeutic emotional experience, perceiving ingrained maladaptive responses as inappropriate to the therapeutic setting, recognizing unconscious contributions, and developing new, better response patterns. The interpersonal therapists, however, tend not to see development in terms of relatively fixed stages—such as the oedipal stage. Perhaps their reaction against this aspect of psychoanalysis has contributed to their relative neglect of the possibility of innate personality qualities—for example, an inborn sensitivity or aggressiveness that might affect both initial childhood indoctrination and reactions in treatment.

Interpersonal therapies may be best suited for learned maladaptive behavior, both of family and of cultural origin—for example, problems in achieving optimum distance from other people (getting too close or not getting close enough); difficulties with assertion and compliance—unassertiveness, bossiness, rebelliousness; difficulties in being able to express love for other people and receive love from them. Interpersonal therapy also seems well adapted for group treatment, where the patient can experiment with various behaviors with others in a close approximation to the real world.

One special aspect of illness in which interpersonal therapies may be particularly effective is invalidism. Mental illness, like any illness, may be used as a weapon in interpersonal relations. The syndrome of invalidism was well described at the beginning of the century by Alfred Adler, the early psychoanalyst who was the first of the Freud circle to be excommunicated. In physical invalidism, someone who is confined to a wheelchair because of genuine damage to his spinal cord may use his incapacity—consciously or unconsciously—to manipulate and control his family. Similarly, someone afflicted with psychological symptoms may secondarily employ these symptoms to manipulate others into greater concern and special ministrations. An anxious or depressed patient may also openly or covertly blame his problems on his family, inducing guilt coercively. In these ways, he may derive some compensations from a real problem. Even if the symptoms of anxiety or depression disappear, he may continue to exert the same controls on his family, especially since his enduring demoralization may heighten his need to be served.

Such interpersonal use of symptoms has been particularly well described by transactional analyst Eric Berne in *Games People Play*. In engaging in such maneuvers, the patient produces a self-perpetuating vicious circle that causes her more harm than benefit because it convinces her that there is no other way to cope. Pointing out the role of such behavior to the patient and the family may produce significant benefit both for the family and for the patient. However, focusing on, analyzing, and reducing such covert interpersonal power struggles, as helpful as it may be, should not be confused with treatment of the illness itself. By viewing alcoholism as a multiperson game, for instance, Berne confuses the consequences of the disorder with its causes.

Several of the other "talking" therapies that have diverged considerably from psychoanalysis are also worth special mention. We shall focus on gestalt therapy when we discuss group therapies and shall also say more about transactional analysis at that time. Another group consists of therapies that contain a large element of cognitive analysis of irrational attitudes, behavior, and anxieties—such as Aaron Beck's cognitive therapy, Albert Ellis's rational-emotive therapy, and William Glasser's reality therapy. These treatments assert that emotional upsets are entirely secondary to ineffective, irrational beliefs and attitudes. A depressed person feels depressed because he is constantly putting himself down as a result of unrealistic standards he cannot live up to. Modify the standards and the depression goes away, these theorists assert. All these therapies involve confronting the patient with his own irrational ideas, and Glasser's version adds the rejection of irresponsible behavior and the learning of other ways to behave. Beck and his group believe cognitive therapy to be especially well suited to the treatment of depression, and Ellis has frequently emphasized the treatment of sexual conflicts.

Facing in still another direction is Eugene Gendlin's "focusing," which seeks internal bodily awareness.

With the humanistic therapies that evolved from the work of Perls, Rogers, and Maslow, the emphasis dramatically shifted from specific complaints and pathology to the possibility that vague anxieties, depression, and dissatisfaction all derived from a failure to realize and express man's highest potential. As Maslow pointed out, human needs can be arranged in a hierarchy, and people attempt to gratify the higher ones only when the lower ones have been satisfied. Attention to growth and self-actualization seems to have accompanied the surfeit of means to gratify basic physical needs provided by modern technology for some segments of Western society. At the same time, it is possible that the dehumanization associated with technology has contributed to the desire for different kinds of experiences.

The paths to self-actualization have not been clearly marked, but among the goals espoused by humanistic therapists are sensitivity to one's own and others' feelings; genuine emotional experience rather than intellectual understanding; recognition and gratification of instinctual needs; greater awareness of the contributions of sensory experience to enriched living. Extension and elaboration of these ideas have resulted in additions to the interview form of therapy, such as groups involving various physical and emotional exercises and forms of physical contact designed to increase sensory awareness and to break down inhibitions against intimacy. The multitude of encounter groups that did not call themselves therapies ensued, many rushing to flout not only conventional boundaries for group behavior but also physical and emotional therapeutic taboos.

As experimentation increased, goals continued to change in the direction of an elusive spirituality, as in psychosynthesis and Arica training. Psychosynthesis tries to develop the will as a constructive force, aiming at internal harmony and merging with the universal will. Arica training, an eclectic system devised in Chile but incorporating Eastern teachings, combines diet, sensory awareness, exercises, meditation, and interpersonal analysis; it is reminiscent of G. I. Gurdjieff's Institute for the Harmonious Development of Man, which dates back to the 1920s.

In some therapies, verbalization greatly decreased—or even disappeared—in favor of altered states of consciousness and manipulations of the body. We shall discuss those in a later section.

Multiperson Therapies

Group therapy is identified not by its content but by its format. Group therapies can deal with intra- or interpersonal problems, or use cognitive, abreactive, or behavioral techniques, but the group setting itself can produce special useful effects.

Louis Wender, the father of one of the authors of this book, was one of the originators of psychoanalytic group psychotherapy and convincingly prejudiced him in its favor. As the story was recounted to his son, the idea of group psychotherapy came to Louis Wender as a result of a serendipitous observation born of necessity. In the early 1930s, Wender had been appointed director of a small psychiatric hospital that wished to provide intensive psychiatric care for severe neurotics (probably a mélange of the psychiatric illnesses we have discussed here). Generously staffed with a secretary, a nurse, a gardener, and a cook, Wender found himself in the impossible position of having to give intensive psychiatric care to forty people by himself. Despite psychoanalytic training, he remained a flexible thinker. Regardless of the analytic emphasis on the emotional as opposed to the cognitive components of psychological therapy, Wender decided that one service he could render was to educate his patients in dynamic psychology as a group by focusing on types of problems that he knew the individual patients had. He therefore planned a series of talks on current psychiatric theory about how people developed problems and how they might solve them. In carrying out his plan, he was influenced by discussions with his friend and collaborator Paul Schilder, a highly creative and innovative psychiatrist.

Wender found that several useful effects derived from these early group efforts. To begin with, psychologically relevant education and a demystified understanding of themselves were welcomed by patients—a finding that has been made repeatedly since, most clearly in transactional analysis and in some of the cognitive therapies. His next observation was more surprising: the interaction among the patients was itself extremely powerful. They provided one another with considerable support. Patients in individual psychotherapy often worry about their degree of abnormality. Although many therapists tell patients that their problems are not unique, patients distrust such reassurance, believing that they are part of the treatment. Hearing firsthand the stories of others about similar behavior, feelings, and thoughts is, as one might expect, effective in reducing a patient's feelings of isolation.

Next, Wender found that the types of feelings described by patients in analysis, and experienced by them in the transference toward the analyst, came out in full force in the group. People who had trouble with their siblings fought with their peers; those who had difficulties with older men or women were contentious with older members of the group; and so forth.

Another useful feature was that the group did not permit its members to retain self-serving, inaccurate assessments of themselves for very long. The group provided people with feedback concerning their behavior—whether they wanted it or not. This direct feedback circumvented several practical problems of individual therapy. First, the individual therapist is often entirely ignorant of how patients behave outside the office, since she is dependent on their own reports and the subsamples of behavior exhibited in the office. Second, if the individual therapist tells the patient that people dislike him because he is a self-aggrandizing bastard, or that men are continually propositioning her because she is constantly sending out come-on signals, the therapeutic relationship may be endangered; but once the patient is firmly established as a member of a group, the other members can get away with such frank revelations without, in most instances, threatening the continuation of therapy.

Nor is the group's function limited to criticism. When people change their behavior and act more mature, and less neurotic, or in other ways make themselves more attractive to their fellows, the group also gives positive reinforcement, which supports more adaptive behavior.

What Louis Wender had devised for expediency had ironically turned out often to be more effective than what it was presumably a poor substitute for. Wender felt that he had come across something quite important, but, less garrulous than his son, did not actively proselytize for the new form of therapy. Group therapy did not catch on until the middle and late 1940s, when an inadequate supply of therapists could not meet the psychiatric needs of World War II. Since then, it has grown rapidly and has become an accommodating vehicle for a variety of therapeutic systems.

The important discovery made repeatedly since Wender and Schilder first experimented with group therapy is that it may very well be more effective than the individual psychotherapies for treating neuroses. It is interesting to compare Wender's and Schilder's early formulations of the effective components of group psychotherapy with those listed some thirty years later by a contemporary student of the field, Irvin Yalom. Yalom, like Jerome Frank, sees the curative processes in group therapy as cutting across different therapies. Among these processes are education of the patient, in the form of didactic instruction by the leader and observation of and testimony from other patients; the amplification of hope—that is, the usual expectations that the doctor will be helpful are greatly enhanced by the presence of hopeful others who enthusiastically recount how much therapy has done for them (regardless of the evidence); and the patient's development of an awareness that his or her problems are not unique.

Still another feature of group therapy that distinguishes it from individual therapy is the opportunity to be both doctor and patient, giving as well as receiving help. Aside from recent arguments that altruism may fulfill an inborn biological need (E. O. Wilson, 1975), being an effective helper contributes to one's self-esteem.

The opportunity to confess and the catharsis that follows, intrinsic ingredients of all individual therapies, take on a special tinge in a group—as in evangelical Christianity (both early and contemporary) and Communist societies. It takes courage to confess before one's peers, and absolution from the many exceeds absolution from one, especially when the many are not being paid to extend it.

As Wender and Schilder found, the group also provides a rich medium in which people can reexperience and experiment with their difficulties in human relations. This includes the opportunity to learn how one acts, to learn how one's perceptions may differ from those of others, to learn from others how one's actions are perceived, and to learn, through imitation as well as experimentation, how to interact with people in more satisfying and productive ways.

Different schools use the group in different ways. Although there are few data on the effects of these differences, we will describe how various psychotherapies have used the format in attempting to forward varying therapeutic aims.

The most effective utilization of the group approach, we believe, has been made by the interpersonal psychotherapies. The group setting provides an excellent laboratory in which the patient's human relationships can be observed "in vivo" (in the real world) rather than "in vitro" (in an artificial setting such as individual psychotherapy). In the individual psychotherapist's office, the therapist is limited to the patient's perception of his social reality. The psychiatrist not only expects the patient to have a distorted image of reality but also hopes that by working with the patient he may alleviate or eliminate these distortions and thus learn about the true world in which the patient lives. In particular, he thinks that by observing the patient's distortion of the therapist he can isolate the patient's overall distortions. This calls for a remarkable degree of objectivity in the therapist, and the requirement that the training of therapists must include their own analysis is aimed at producing such objectivity.

All of us, however, neurotic or not, see the world through our own distorting lenses, and it is impossible for any therapist, regardless of his training, to learn about the patient's real world if he confines himself to the patient's reports. If he has the opportunity to see the patient in a group, he can more accurately observe the patient's behavior with other people. Armed with this information, he can more readily determine the actual nature of the patient's behavior and the environmental events and forces that elicit and sustain it. Focusing on the real world in group therapy—and the related couple and family therapies—is a major, probably useful, innovation in the treatment of neurotic and mislearning problems.

Although the most widely applied types of group psychotherapy have been based on interpersonal theories, several specialized techniques have also been employed in the group format, notably gestalt therapy, rational-emotive therapy, and transactional analysis. Gestalt therapy focuses on increasing self-awareness, utilizing all the cues the body gives itself, including physical responses, dreams, and interpersonal behaviors. The group may facilitate the emergence of behavior patterns and thus increase the individual's opportunity to recognize the structure of her personality.

Therapeutically, the major innovations are the utilization of the experiment and the recognition of multiple selves in the patient. This refers to the patient's consciously trying new forms of behavior within the group setting—a form of role-playing. The patient may role-play with other members, who may take the part of a patient, a spouse, and so on, but he may also role-play with a fantasied other or with another whose part he takes. For example, a patient might argue with her mother, who she imagines is in an empty chair, then move to that chair and answer back, playing the role of the mother. Since she is best acquainted with the styles involved, this may be more effective than assigning the role of the mother to another member of the group.

The idea that all persons have component selves—each relatively complete and independent—who cooperate or oppose one another may have therapeutic usefulness. Psychiatry recognizes a rare illness, multiple personality, in which alternating selves claim to represent the person (popularly described in *Sybil* and *The Three Faces of Eve*). What gestalt therapy has recognized is that most people seem to have less well differentiated but still identifiable multiple selves. Concretely, what gestalt therapists do is to ask patients to role-play their conflicting attitudes, values, or wishes. A patient might be asked, for example, to conduct a dialogue between his conscientious, socialized, law-abiding self and his carefree, impulsive, consequences-be-damned self. When patients act this way, each part may have its own posture, gesticulations, tone of voice, and vocabulary, and in addition, the patient may experience the two sets of emotions alternately and vividly. As he alternates between two or more selves, the patient may come to realize or experience whole parts of himself that appear to be complete (a minor form of multiple personality) and shut off from ordinary awareness. This is demonstrable. What remains to be documented is whether such awareness will allow him to provide a rapprochement between conflicting parts of himself. In gestalt therapy, the group plays a comparatively secondary role compared to its function in other group therapies, often merely observing, like a Greek chorus; gestalt therapy thus constitutes an interesting admixture of intrapersonal individual therapy and interpersonal group therapy.

Rational-emotive therapy emphasizes the cognitive weakness behind many of the emotional reactions that bring people to therapy. In group settings, the participants can compare their irrational, self-defeating modes of thinking—such as unrealistic self-denigration or exaggeration of the importance of particular goals—with those of the others, and can garner hope and courage as well as rational comment.

In transactional analysis, the major innovation is the rephrasing of psychoanalytic therapeutic concepts in comprehensible language. In discussing the components of the personality, psychoanalysis uses such terms as the *id* (ostensibly the unconscious portion of the mind, a caldron of primitive desires yearning for expression), the *ego* (the more reasonable, more mature portion of the mind), and the *superego* (the conscience, which helps the ego to master the unruly id). Transactional analysis talks about the same functions as the child, the adult, and the parent in the self, terms which have more immediate meaning to the patient. Furthermore, as in gestalt therapy, the patient is taught to recognize that when he functions in a particular mode—that is, like a parent, adult, or child—not only does he have the attitudes and values peculiar to that mode but his total behavior and consciousness change. In the child state, he not only experiences the wishes of a child but acts and talks like a child. When he is in the state of a critical parent, he not only declaims in speech full of "oughts" and "shoulds" but also adopts the posture, gestures, and feelings of an adult reprimanding a child.

In addition, transactional analysis focuses on repetitive, stereotyped, disadvantageous patterns of action (similar to the irrational ideas focused on by the cognitive therapists), which are referred to as tapes, supposedly ground-in behaviors learned in the family setting. The manipulative aspects of the repetitive behavior patterns are called games. Individual dynamics (the child, adult, and parent), games, and tape-like behaviors can be accurately and quickly observed in the natural environment of the group. The group facilitates the patient's recognition of these patterns and provides a laboratory in which he can experiment with new, more comfortable and effective ways of behaving with others.

Another group technique that should be mentioned is psychodrama, which was developed more than sixty years ago by J. L. Moreno. In this procedure, often used with psychotic inpatients, a patient acts his life role in company with others, who are assigned the parts of important figures in his life, before an audience that comments on his behavior. By taking multiple parts, the patient can learn the effects of his behavior on others, empathize with others' feelings toward himself, and experiment with new forms of behavior. To the extent that the patient can become involved with playing his own role—analogous to what happens in method acting—he may be able to reexperience his feelings intensely, which may both increase his self-awareness and facilitate changes in his behavior. Despite its age, psychodrama has not spread widely and its effectiveness remains unevaluated (although its techniques have been borrowed heavily by gestalt therapy). Moreno was a great innovator and many modern techniques are direct adaptations of his work.

One further adaptation of the group method that has had a major impact in the past two decades is the encounter group. The characteristics that differentiate it from group therapy are its brevity (often only a lengthy day, a weekend, or a series of weekends, or perhaps a week or two in residence), the use of exercises (formalized procedures such as forming circles, touching and hugging, physically breaking through restraints, interpersonal games), and its emphasis on growth rather than pathology. Some of its techniques—such as protracted marathons (sessions many hours in length) and specialized exercises—have been incorporated into group therapy as devices to hasten or intensify emotional reactions. Most encounter groups try to foster frankness and intimacy, as opposed to artificial social conventions.

The success of the encounter-group movement may be a comment on the pathology of our society, just as chlorination of water is a comment on our lack of forethought in keeping sewage out of the reservoirs.* Alienation, isolation, and lack of opportunity for close relations with others are so widespread that we seem to need special places and circumstances in which to establish human contact.

Although encounter groups do not identify themselves as therapy, an exceptionally able study of the effects of different styles of encounter groups on the participants may shed some light on various types of group therapy (Lieberman, Yalom, and Miles, 1973). Because the investigators used random assignment, the range of types of students who were the subjects in the various groups was likely to be similar, and therefore the results carry weight (without random assignment, differing outcomes might simply reflect the selection of different kinds of groups by different kinds of people). As many clinicians had thought, warm, non-intrusive, clarifying approaches were associated in this study with positive responses and not with casualties. Approaches involving hostile confrontation without adequate protection of weaker

---

*Harold Greenwald, former president of the National Psychological Association for Psychoanalysis, has commented: "An encounter group is a therapeutic procedure wherein psychopaths teach obsessionals how to behave like hysterics."

members *were* associated with casualties as well as with positive responses. Passive, cold, uninformative, or overstructured leadership was associated with the subjects' lack of interest in the procedures.

Because encounter groups have the ability, at least in the short run, to hurt, it is possible that in other circumstances they may help. Apparently, most of them are not inactive. What they might do in the long run is unclear. The potential participant should be aware that hostile, intrusive, aggressive forms of leadership can be psychologically damaging, probably by accentuating demoralization and feelings of helplessness. Interventions intended to provide new insights sometimes turn out to be a kind of psychological karate. Before participating, it is wise to find out whether the approach is supportive and paced to the rate of the group members, as opposed to one in which a domineering leader attempts to force his views on others.

In *couple therapy* and *family therapy,* as their names imply, therapists see couples or families together. An important aspect of such therapy, which it shares with group therapy, is the opportunity for the therapist —and the patient—to get a better idea of the patient's behavior in the real world. However, because couple and family therapy differ in the ways they conceptualize the origins and maintenance of psychological dysfunctioning and, therefore, in the methods of dealing with such problems, we will discuss them separately.

Couple therapy emerged out of marital counseling but encompasses premarital couples and increasing numbers of common-law couples. Although the kinds of problems that bring people to individual therapy can affect how two people get along, a couple will have distinctive ways of living together which may have evolved gradually, may be a result of the interaction of these particular personalities, and may have a life of their own. Couple therapists have focused on three distinctive aspects of relationships: (1) communication; (2) expectations; (3) stylized patterns of behavior.

A striking discovery by couple therapists is that, frequently, marital partners have never learned to talk to each other. Of the traits that interfere with clear communication, the first is simply failing to say what is on one's mind. One's motivation can be justified discretion, but in addition many people have never learned to say what they are thinking. This can often be explained on the basis of childhood conditioning, but the explanation is unimportant. What is important is their failure to say what they want and how they feel. Since wishes and emotions often do not go away even if not spoken, these people frequently feel frustrated and angry. They hope that somehow their mates can read their minds, and they justify their dissatisfaction by seeing their spouses as insensitive clods.

Consequently, inducing marriage partners to reveal themselves to each other has been found therapeutically useful. To their surprise, they discover—if they exercise minimal tact—that the results are usually not catastrophic and that often their spouses are likely to gratify their requests.

A second communication skill that can readily be taught is that of checking out or obtaining feedback. This involves inquiring, after one has said something, what one's spouse heard, since the message received may not be the message sent. The psychiatrist conducting individual therapy commonly observes that the upset person often does not receive simple factual communications accurately. Accordingly, we painfully learn the necessity of inquiring of the patient, "What did you hear me say?" or "What do you think I meant?" The accomplished communicator soon learns the virtue of this sort of verification, which avoids confusion and arguments over neutral messages that might be misperceived as hostile.

The third major impediment to communication is mind reading. Two people who have lived together for a long time sometimes unconsciously believe they have developed a kind of extrasensory perception and can read each other's mind. Based on this erroneous tacit assumption, they often act to the discomfort of the other or react inappropriately. The belief in mind reading may be a carry-over from childhood, when we are often surprised that our omniscient parents know so much about our wishes and plans. Carried into adult life, the belief is the source of much grief. The obvious remedy is encouraging members of passive couples to inquire of each other what their wishes and feelings actually are.

These three easy therapeutic techniques often suffice to remedy habitual patterns of miscommunication. Note the behavioral orientation. The focus is not on how the patterns of miscommunication arose but merely on ridding the participants of them.

The area of expectations in couple therapy embodies the idea that most of us behave by generalizing from limited information. We act toward or expect to be responded to on the basis of our past experience with persons of comparable age, sex, orientation, and national origin. If we have grown up with seductive mothers or fathers who demand inordinate psychological payment for every minor concession, we are likely to approach our wives or husbands with similar and probably incorrect expectations and with accompanying misperceptions. The requesting husband may be misperceived as the demanding father. When the unreal expectations and the misperceptions result in incongruous responses, the marriage is headed for trouble. The remedy, as usual, is first diagnosis and then clarification. Partners have to be taught that they may not be seeing reality but rather what has gone on in the past. Using this insight, the couple can be induced to try new patterns of behavior based on what is occurring and not on what occurred when they were younger. These new patterns often produce new successes, new feelings, and more realistic attitudes.

Sex therapists have come to realize that two of the major sources of sexual maladjustment are faulty communication and incorrect expectancy. Since many couples are, understandably enough, culturally inhibited in communicating about their sexual feelings, simple procedures of teaching them to tell each other what they like or dislike in sexual activities can be very helpful. Similarly, understanding that one's sexual expectations and desires may be quite different from those of the partner can also be useful. Although specific sexual information and procedures may also be necessary, improving communication and clarifying expectancies are two of the most effective techniques for dealing with mutual sexual maladjustment.

The couple therapist also focuses on behavioral patterns and values within the marriage—that is, who does what, who sets the rules, and who expects what to be done by whom. Marriages sometimes founder not over major issues such as love but over everyday issues such as who squeezes the toothpaste tube in the middle—although the therapist must of course be alert to the possibility that a minor complaint masks an unspoken major issue. Couples often harbor considerable ill will over whose friends are seen, who does what chores around the house, who spends more time with the children, who decides how money is to be spent, who initiates sexual activity, and who doesn't flush the toilet. Because people are so various, a couple whose wants coincide completely is rare indeed.

The labor-relations-contract approach is often satisfactory in resolving a couple's differing patterns and expectations. The principle employed is that of trade-off. Reminding couples that marriage may be made in heaven but has to be administered on earth may bring them to see that their host of petty grievances can be resolved not by more loving but only by bargaining. In the extreme, behaviorists have taught couples to reinforce each other for changes in behavior —for example, the wife may award the husband tokens for helping with the dishes or child care; these tokens may be exchanged for bedtime privileges that are more to his taste than hers. This highlights as well as caricatures the old-fashioned message concerning the importance of compromise. Compromise can of course be applied not only to concrete concerns and practices but also to interpersonal behaviors. A husband who is excessively authoritarian and infantilizing may be taught that his wife needs autonomy and less babying. This in turn will result in greater rewards for him rather than a sulky mate with a constant headache.

The use of behavioral techniques emphasizes the fact that many couple therapists believe that marital maladjustments are based not on early childhood traumatization and warp but on mutual, unconscious, self-defeating and self-perpetuating behavior. Thus, the therapists direct attention to self-sustaining attitudes and processes in the present rather than to events of the distant past.

Finally, genuine psychiatric illness sometimes affects the roles of marriage partners in a way that can needlessly aggravate the effects of the illness. For instance, the person who is depressed—and therefore separation-anxious and dependent—may induce the spouse to become excessively protective and compliant. Such behavior patterns may become self-perpetuating, so that even when the depression is successfully treated chemically, the distorted relationship continues. For this reason, it may be useful to work with both partners to prevent the development or continuation of maladaptive behaviors learned in the context of psychiatric illness.

An increasing number of biological psychiatrists also find the participation of the spouse advisable because the healthy spouse can often perceive subtle manifestations of the illness that the patient does not recognize. Spouses can also objectively describe behavior of diagnostic value and monitor for effects of biological treatment better than many patients.

Family therapy blossomed in the early 1960s, when belief in the psychological causes of schizophrenia was strong. Some family therapists proposed the startling theory that schizophrenia was not a disease but only a manifestation of pathology within the family. They saw the schizophrenic as a scapegoat—they called him the "identified patient"—and implied that the family neutralized or discharged its pathology by projecting it upon one unfortunate member, who subsequently became ill. Illness of individual members was seen as a symptom of the family sickness. The data on the genetic transmission of some forms of schizophrenia do not support the scapegoat theory.

A less radical claim, and one undoubtedly worth consideration, is that family values and patterns of behavior may initiate and sustain maladjustive behavioral patterns in the members. If one can discover maladaptive learned patterns within families, one may be able to change them and thus change the disturbed behavior of the participants. This has recently been demonstrated in children with various medical illnesses. In diabetes, for example, the emotional state of the patient affects his metabolism, and psychological upset can precipitate acute episodes of the illness. Moreover, management of the illness depends on rigid adherence to a specific diet and faithful administration of insulin. Children from disrupted families may not take their medication, may break their diets, and become embroiled in family upsets. Working with the family to diminish family conflict—especially that related to the child's adherence to the requisite medication and diet regimen—is associated with decrease in acute medical complications.

Similarly, much behavioral deviation in offspring can be viewed as reactions to parental principles of upbringing, yet parents may be totally unaware of what they are doing to their children. The parents may have unconsciously adopted behavioral patterns that reward and reinforce undesirable behavior, and that punish and therefore negatively reinforce desirable behavior. Their children may behave quite predictably with regard to the reward and punishment, but if the parents do not know they are dispensing it, they are unaware that they are initiating or sustaining their children's deviant behavior. For example, a parent may voice dismay over a preadolescent's precocious sexual experimentation but may actually reinforce it by unconscious expressions of pleasure at the evidence of a sexy offspring. Talking to the parents may be inadequate to disclose such patterns, since the parents do not realize what they are doing. Observing the family, either in the doctor's office or in the home, may enable the family therapist to discover the relevant patterns and to change them. Traditional psychoanalytic therapy with individuals prohibited the therapist from seeing other family members, and, in retrospect, it is embarrassing to see how theory overran common sense. All mothers know that it is usually difficult to determine who caused the fight when both participants are present; it is impossible when only one is.

In effect, the approach is based on child guidance, but with an emphasis on the role of reinforcement in molding children's behavior, and an awareness that parents may be unconscious of their behavior patterns. Family therapy with adolescent and adult offspring is based on the same principles.

Family therapy with the nearest relatives of severely ill patients may also help them to accept the patient's limitations, to vent their anxiety and grief, and to lessen their feelings of guilt (see Boszormenyi-Nagy and Framo, 1965; Minuchin, 1974).

Behavior Therapies

The behavior therapies are easier to summarize than the other forms of psychological treatment. One reason is their youth: as specific treatments for fearfulness and anxiety, they are only about twenty years old.

A second reason is the seeming clarity of their theories and practices. The proponents of behavior therapy initially claimed that their model of psychiatric illness and techniques of treatment were directly based on animal experimentation, particularly the branch concerned with learning. This assertion has since been questioned by animal behaviorists. The similarities between animal and human neuroses, and between laboratory cures for animal neuroses and consulting-room cures for humans, are not clear and simple. However, even if the claim that behavior therapies are scientific while other therapies are not turns out to be incorrect, behavior therapists still have performed several scientifically useful functions. First, they have attempted to specify as accurately as possible the problems they treat. Too often, psychiatrists have categorized patients' ills uninformatively—for example, as anxiety neurosis or character disorder—and have vaguely judged the efficacy of the psychotherapy in terms of insights gained rather than behavior or emotional state altered. Second, the behavior therapists have specified and quantified their interventions, indicating what they did, for how long, to what end, and in what fraction of patients. Even when they report on single cases, their data are more credible because sometimes they can alternately stop and start symptoms and behavior in concert with the use or withdrawal of behavior therapy techniques. (Of course, the usefulness of these procedures may not be due to the hypothesized mechanisms.) Whatever the validity of their theories, these specifications have been a boon to all those who would see psychiatry become more of a science.

Desensitization, the type of behavior therapy first used with phobias, is based on the premise that anxiety is a learned fear response which has arisen because of an association between some relatively neutral environmental stimulus (event) and another, painful environmental event. The bitten child fears dogs, the person who has almost drowned fears deep water, and the child tyrannized by the mother fears women. The theory arises from the demonstration that one can generate fears in laboratory animals by pairing a painful event, such as a shock, with a previously neutral event, such as a buzzer. Under these circumstances, the animal apparently develops a fear of buzzing. If one then repeatedly sounds the buzzer without shocking the animal, his fear of the buzzer goes away. That such pairings play an important role in most human anxieties seems quite unlikely, since many humans have developed phobias that seemingly have no basis in traumatic experience.

From the animal model, the behavior therapists predicted that contact with objects that were similar to but less frightening than the phobic stimulus would gradually diminish the fear. In the laboratory rat, a soft buzzer might produce less anxiety than a loud one. By gradually increasing the loudness of the buzzer, without further shocks, one could eliminate the rat's fear of buzzers. Thus, the child who is afraid of dogs would first be allowed to play with a toy puppy, then with a live puppy, then with a friendly bigger dog. Eventually, he might be able to walk past a fenced yard containing an enraged Irish wolfhound.

Since direct contact with frightening stimuli may be hard to arrange for people who are afraid of airplanes, mothers-in-law, or elephants, the desensitizers turned to presenting the frightening stimulus in imagination. The subject would be asked to imagine several objects in progressive degrees of fearfulness. To help decondition the patient, she was first hypnotized, or, if that proved difficult, taught muscular relaxation, techniques which are ostensibly incompatible with fear and which promote sangfroid or indifference to the feared object or situation by reciprocal inhibition. Simply stated, the subject was exposed to previously frightening objects or situations—in reality or in imagination—only when he was in a state of increased calm and imperturbability.

One interesting aspect of desensitization is that it produced results quite different from those predicted by parts of psychoanalytic theory. Psychoanalysts argue that phobias are the product of unconscious fears and conflicts. The person who is afraid of dogs might really be afraid of his father, his rival for his mother; the dogs may be a symbolic representation of this castration anxiety. Accordingly, some psychoanalysts have predicted that removal of a fear by behavioral techniques would not cure the patient, that the fear would manifest itself in other symptoms—such as increased anxiety or inability to handle one's job. This prediction has not been borne out. In most instances, for whatever reasons, desensitization is not followed by the appearance of new fears (Lazarus, 1965).

Desensitization was simple to describe, tedious to employ, and initially very successful. The sessions were often few (say, ten) and the recovery rate was at first reported as very high (around 90 percent). As with any new therapy, time has diminished its luster and potency, and desensitization now takes longer, has a lower recovery rate, and includes an increasing number of backsliding patients. (Klein has recently reviewed all controlled studies of desensitization with phobics. Strikingly, of thirteen studies, only two showed desensitization to be more effective than the other therapy [Klein et al., in press].) The belief that desensitization is an outstanding form of therapy for phobia is, thus, unwarranted.

In addition to phobias, an early target of behavior therapy was generalized timidity and anxiety. On theoretical grounds that were far from clear, some behavior therapists reasoned that non-assertiveness increased general fearfulness, anxiety, and possibly depression. Working on this assumption, they encouraged assertiveness and often gave direct behavioral homework assignments arranged on a scale of gradually increased difficulty and forcefulness. The first assignment might be to say hello to a neighbor, and later ones might be to take spoiled canned goods back to the grocery, or, still later, to express an opinion at a political meeting. Eventually, the patient might get to the point where he could defend his girlfriend, telling a bully not to kick sand in her face. This therapy marked the entry of the behaviorists into the area of more complex interpersonal relationships, which they pursue with increasing interest.

More recently, acting on the theory that many people's social anxieties come from a lack of interpersonal skills, behavior therapists have been offering direct tutelage and practice in human relations. They would argue, for example, that the college student who is afraid to call up a young woman does not have unconscious fears of castration but has never developed a "line." Thus, the behavior therapist will explore with the student several possibly effective "lines," have him practice them in a contrived situation in which a female confederate plays the role of the girl at the other end of the phone, and then have him try them out in the real world. Reputedly, such techniques are effective in overcoming the social anxiety of many timid people. The perception of anxiety as the result of ignorance and lack of practice rather than of obscure unconscious forces is a tremendously important switch in direction in even a part of psychological theory.

It is possible that the theory is wrong, however, even though the practice may be effective. Just as phobias that may not have been produced by experience have been relieved by desensitization, so timidity that may not come from lack of social learning may respond to assertiveness training. We suspect, in fact, that both the phobias and the timidity have biological components, and that behavior therapy, like other kinds of psychotherapy, helps the patients to cope with these mildly to moderately incapacitating conditions.

In the past fifteen or twenty years, the number of problems to which behavioral approaches have been applied and the number of techniques used have expanded greatly. As mentioned earlier, group confrontation of phobic stimuli in a real situation has been especially rapid in eliminating phobic responses, although the proportion of patients eventually helped by other methods is probably the same, given enough time. The various techniques all have in common a comparatively straightforward and direct approach to concrete problems—sometimes to a questionable degree. One of the procedures we referred to in discussing couple therapy—the marriage contract—exemplifies behavior therapy's profound neglect of subtleties. Having determined from each spouse separately what he or she wants in the marriage and is not getting, the behavior therapist sits down with the couple and draws up a formal agreement. The partners are encouraged to make deals, such as: "If you let my parents visit us for dinner once every two weeks, I'll not complain about your playing golf Sunday mornings." The available case reports are insufficient for one to judge how successful this approach is.

A final illustration of the numerous strategies behavior therapists employ is the "therapeutic environment" with "token economy." Token economies have been used with seriously disturbed patients, such as chronic psychotics and severe retardates. Usually, the token economy is established first: the patient is supplied with minimal comforts, adequate to maintain life but supplying little surplus hedonism. The psychotic may be given plain but balanced meals and a mattress on the floor, but is not given permission to watch television or walk around the hospital grounds. Next, for each patient, behavioral goals are established, and the closer the patient's behavior approximates the goals, the more token money she is given. The money can be exchanged for greater privileges, such as a better bed, more tasteful meals, and the opportunity to watch TV.

A psychotic patient, for example, might carry on a loud conversation with hallucinated companions. He might be given one token for every ten minutes he is quiet or talks reasonably. As he begins to inhibit his bizarre activities, the standards set up for him might change. He might now have to abstain for fifteen or twenty minutes before receiving payment. With this technique of reward—which is a close psychological approximation to piecework pay—the patient's behavior can be shaped. The token economy does not relieve the psychosis or improve the intellectual performance of the retarded, but it does train such people into more seemly and more manageable forms of behavior.

The behavior therapies have passed through their period of uninhibited youthful exuberance and remain in the state of perhaps justified hopefulness. Recently, they have been growing more cognitive and also have been devoting more attention to the relationship aspects of the procedures; the use of such therapies in combination with psychodynamic and other approaches is also becoming more common (Lazarus, 1976).

It is our expectation that behavior therapies will prove useful in altering habits, somewhat useful in combination with other techniques in modifying learned behavioral abnormalities, and least useful in dealing with psychiatric illnesses. As in other psychotherapies, these are distinctions rarely made by the behavior therapists. At present, if patients know what they want changed (fear of flying, headaches), behavior therapies may help them to effect these changes relatively quickly and directly. Because of the brevity of treatment, these therapies are comparatively cheap, and if they are ineffectual, the patient finds out sooner rather than later. This contrasts with other therapies in which the patient may painfully and expensively wait years to reach the same conclusion.

Abreactive and Cathartic Therapies

The abreactive or cathartic psychotherapies bear the closest resemblance to Hollywood's dramatic model of psychotherapy—the process of working out the effects of a disagreeable experience, often forgotten, by reliving and reexpressing the emotions. Abreactive therapies, surprisingly, have qualities in common with inspirational therapies, brainwashing, and religious conversion. Different from each other as these processes appear, they may in fact depend on the same psychological mechanisms.

The abreactive therapies played an important role in the development of psychoanalysis. The earliest psychoanalytic investigations, it will be recalled, were carried out on patients with "hysterical neuroses"—instances where paralyses, loss of sensation, or other phenomena that looked like organic illnesses occurred on the basis of psychological disturbance.

Josef Breuer's discovery that some hysterical patients could be made to remember—and to *relive*—painful psychological experiences they had had in the past showed that people could have complete memories of life experiences to which they had no access in their normal conscious state. Furthermore, these memories were in some instances linked to strong emotions and feelings and continued to affect the patient's psychological functioning.

The therapeutic benefits of this remembering and reliving in hypnosis were described by Breuer and Freud in the history of Anna O., one of the most famous patients in psychoanalytic history. Anna's symptom, paralysis of the arm, had emerged at around the time of the serious illness of her father. Anna remembered fully that she had nursed him through his illness, but only under hypnosis did she remember that while nursing him she felt resentment because her nursing responsibilities had prevented her from going to a ball. At the time she had experienced these feelings of resentment, she had suppressed them—pushed them out of her conscious mind—because she had felt that she must rid herself of such unfilial feelings. Under hypnosis, she spontaneously relived the experiences she had had at that time and remembered that when she had felt the resentment, her arm had been draped uncomfortably over a chair, so that she had had pins-and-needles sensations. When she was able to relive the experience, the odd sensations in the arm disappeared.

Freud applied the same techniques to other hysterical symptoms, with fairly good results. Hysteria, he declared, was a disease of reminiscence—or more accurately, of its absence. Hypnosis enabled people to reexperience, to relive suppressed feelings, and by the process of abreaction or catharsis to end them. Fascinated by this remarkable cure, Freud began to employ it in his treatment of patients with a variety of neuroses, but immediately ran up against the practical barrier that not everyone can be hypnotized. Experimenting with other techniques that would facilitate the patient's recollection of suppressed or repressed memories, he came on the techniques of free association and dream interpretation.

As psychoanalysis broadened its scope, fewer patients came to psychoanalysts with hysterical complaints (the decrease in hysterical patients has never been adequately explained). Analysts found that free association did not have dramatic cathartic effects in people with other forms of psychological difficulty, and psychoanalysis began to draw away from catharsis as a therapeutic technique.

Abreactive and cathartic techniques underwent a period of decline in psychiatry until World War II. At that time, psychiatrists observed a phenomenon similar to what had been called shell shock in World War I. Soldiers with shell shock had reacted to either a prolonged stay at the front or a near-miss—such as a nearby bomb explosion that killed some of the sufferer's friends—with such symptoms as paralysis, inability to talk, trembling, and fearfulness. Some neuropsychiatrists believed that loud or violent explosions produced actual changes in the nervous system.

The psychiatrists of World War II found, however, that the nature of the psychological experience rather than any physical change produced the war neurosis. The near-miss experience—in which, for example, the soldier was the only survivor from a burning tank or a jeep blown up by a mine—lay behind traumatic neuroses and the development of psychological problems. In many instances, as in the hysterics of Freud's era, the victim could not remember his traumatic experience, and abreactive or cathartic therapy, in the form of hypnosis or the barbiturate sodium amytal, could facilitate his remembering and reexperiencing the critical event. This catharsis was often followed by the disappearance of the symptoms, especially if accompanied by a medical discharge. In other words, traumatized soldiers in World War II behaved like 1890 hysterics: abreaction or catharsis was followed by recovery.

Even more interesting was the discovery that if the traumatic war neurotic reexperienced *any* intense emotion, his symptoms might be relieved. For example, he might have developed mutism following his escape from a burning tank, but that mutism might be relieved if he reexperienced the anger or fear he had felt at other times on the battlefield. Intense excitement, the release of intense emotion, tended to relieve psychological symptoms even if the experienced emotions were unrelated to the traumatic event. Another important property of these abreactive experiences was that they worked better for acute problems than for chronic ones.

The possible relation of these cures of traumatic neuroses to treatment of the far more common nontraumatic neuroses has been looked at closely by William Sargant, an English psychiatrist. During World War II, having noticed the therapeutic effect of intense emotional experience in the treatment of traumatic neuroses, Sargant became interested in the general role of such emotion in the generation and changing of psychopathology, beliefs, and behavior. He went on to examine Pavlovian conditioning, Communist brainwashing, and the religious practices of various Christian sects, and found that intense paroxysms of emotion and drastic change in people seemed to go together.

Pavlovian conditioning, as is well known, refers to the experiments in the area of conditioned reflexes by the spiritual and scientific ancestor of modern behaviorists, Ivan Pavlov. To review Pavlov's familiar work briefly, he observed that if the presentation of food to a dog was repeatedly preceded by a conditional stimulus, such as the sound of a buzzer, the animal would respond to that stimulus as he would to the food and would begin to salivate in response to the sound of the buzzer. The animal had developed a conditioned reflex. Pavlov elaborated his initial studies by hunting for the kinds of factors that made the reflex more or less permanent, or that could eliminate it.

Sargant believed that the techniques for changing conditioned reflexes in dogs might be useful in changing the psychology of humans; accordingly, he studied the techniques that Pavlov found most effective in changing conditioned reflexes in dogs and compared them with the practices used to try to change the attitudes, values, and beliefs of human beings.

Pavlov had found that when his dogs were stressed by hunger, by physical exhaustion, by increased intervals between the stimulus and the reward, or by being forced to make fine distinctions between reward and nonreward conditions, breakdowns would occur in their conditioned reflexes. With increasing stress, there were four degrees of breakdown. In the first stage, the animal lost the ability to discriminate. If he had learned that a buzzer signified food and a bell did not, under conditions of stress he would lose the ability to discriminate between bell and buzzer and would salivate equally to both. The human equivalent might be a battle-fatigued soldier who is as upset by the buzzing of a mosquito as he was by the sound of a shell exploding nearby. In the second stage of breakdown due to stress, the reaction to stimuli is actually reversed. The dog now salivates at the bell and does not salivate at the sound of the buzzer. The human being is overjoyed with a minor blessing and indifferent to a major one.

The final two phases are the ones Sargant feels are most relevant to human behavior. In the ultra-paradoxical phase of brain activity, many positive conditioned reflexes suddenly become negative, and previous negative conditioned responses (learned avoidances) suddenly switch to positive. The dog will begin to hate its master. In humans, a dramatic alteration in personal, political, and religious values often ensues: men abandon previous attachments, give up modes of life, and become attached to ideals, faiths, and persons they previously disliked. A person formerly indifferent to God, for example, may be converted to a fundamentalist religion, or a former member of the Communist Party may now feel that she was misled and become a right-wing Republican.

Finally, the dog—and presumably the man—may enter the hypnoidal state, which is similar to the state seen in humans who are very good hypnotic subjects. In this stage,

> the brain stops computing critically the impression received. New impressions, new commands, new ideas become suddenly impera-

> tive, in their need of acceptance and ring absolutely true; and, moreover, are often completely immune to all the normal processes whereby the brain examines critically most of the new impressions received, compares them with all its stored impressions and experiences, and decides on the basis of past knowledge and present balanced judgments, whether the new ideas are likely to be true or false. New ideas can then be accepted and believed in which are totally at variance with the individual's other past and present experiences and beliefs. [Sargant, n.d., p. 11]

In other words, sufficient stress applied in a particular way can neutralize the individual's rational judgmental ability and may cause him intensely to espouse ideas, beliefs, values, and feelings that were previously foreign or offensive to him; perhaps an artificial temporary derangement of the "Ah-ha" mechanism, referred to in our discussion of delusions.

There is, of course, a wide gap between the psychology of salivation in dogs and the psychology of salvation in people. There are no canine parallels for intellectual challenge, group support, or promised redemption. Sargant may be wrong. However, an examination of the conditions under which brainwashing and conversion occur offers useful data.

Sargant's hypothesis is clear-cut: experiences that engender sufficiently strong feelings can result in a change of ideas, even though the feelings bear no logical resemblance to those ideas. The same techniques can be used to make a man a true believer or an atheist, a Communist, an anarchist, or a fascist. Almost any idea can be implanted. One application of this principle is in brainwashing. The techniques of brainwashing illustrate the kinds of stresses that seem to favor profound behavioral changes. First, the individual is subjected to physiological stress: he may be deprived of sleep and food, and allowed to use the bathroom only on an irregular schedule. He is denied autonomy, with his behavior completely controlled by his interrogators. He is denied individuality by being deprived of his name, status, and identifying possessions. He is kept in isolation, which denies him support from the group to which he belongs and keeps him from strengthening his beliefs by checking with others. He is kept confused by his interrogators, who alternately challenge, agree, threaten, and comfort. Lastly, he cannot escape from the situation, so that the experience is one of complete physiological and psychological exhaustion. Relief, salvation, the reception into a state of grace are promised and given only when he changes his beliefs in the prescribed manner.

Sargant observes that many of these techniques were applied by John Wesley and his associates in the powerful evangelical movement of Methodism. In prolonged meetings, individuals were repeatedly threatened with damnation if they did not believe and promised eternal bliss if they did. The behavior and conversion of the most easily persuaded catalyzed that of the more recalcitrant.

Under stress and pressures, the beliefs of many of us do change. We are all familiar with examples, from Patty Hearst to Charles Colson. However, some dogs—and some men—are prone to backsliding after conversion. If new habits or modes of thought are to be maintained after intense emotion has generated such changes, repeated reinforcement must occur. The bourgeois student who adopts the beliefs of his Communist girlfriend may relapse to his previous state unless he is given continuous booster shots of party doctrine. Similarly, religious converts frequently backslide following a dramatic conversion. One investigator states that only about half of religious conversions are maintained at the end of one year, and only 15 percent permanently (Frank, 1974, p. 82). Wesley systematically monitored conversions, regularly conducting small group meetings to preclude a loss of belief. The Chinese Communists constantly held political group meetings to maintain the faith of the populace, many of whom still remembered some of the advantages of the previous system.

If Sargant is right, the success of religious evangelicals and political brainwashers is a reflection of the construction of the canine and human minds. The psychotherapeutic relevance is that analogous techniques may be useful in altering disturbed behavior.

Before we examine the related therapies, one further aspect of Pavlov's work, discussed by Sargant, is worth mentioning. Pavlov found that some dogs were easy to recondition, while others were more difficult. If the stresses are great enough, however, even the most resistant dogs can be broken down. Dogs that are difficult to break down are likely to maintain the changes produced under stress, while weaker, less resistant dogs change easily and may equally easily lose their new habits. There are some data suggesting that people behave similarly. Hysterics appear to change easily but do not maintain the change for long. Compulsives bend with difficulty but persist in their changes. One might expect that compulsives, if won over to any belief, would make more persistent and ardent true believers.

Primal-scream therapy and *est* are examples of procedures that make use of abreaction mechanisms. The former, devised by Arthur Janov, is based on the implausible assumption that most psychological dysfunction is a result of stymied screams of protest and frustration that should have occurred in infancy. The theory is that a suitable opportunity to protest in later life will drain the psychic pus and restore the sufferer to health. In practice, the individual is sequestered for several days, so as to be removed from contact with important people in his life, and then enters therapy. The therapist then makes considerable effort to work the patient into a fevered state of emotionality. In this state, the idea that suffering derives from hitherto strangled screams can be implanted with effect. After reaching a pitch of emotional excitement, the participant is enjoined to yell his head off. Ostensibly, this produces relief. And not surprisingly, in view of our discussions of the likelihood of backsliding with the abreactive methods, follow-up visits are deemed therapeutic. There are no objective data on the effectiveness of primal-scream therapy.

In Werner Erhard's *est,* which does not describe itself as a therapy but implies that it can bring about helpful change, the mechanisms used are deprivational. Participants are kept in a large room for many hours (as in a traditional revival meeting), are forbidden to take their drugs of dependency, including cigarettes, alcohol, and coffee, are allowed to go to the bathroom only after long intervals, are kept for long stretches without food, and can interact with one another only upon instructions from the "trainers" who lead the meetings. Does this recall the Victorian grammar school? Sleep is curtailed, meetings take place in marathon fashion, and the trainers systematically harangue the participants into a state of childlike humiliation. A variety of exercises is employed, some confessional—but what is most important is the overall approach. Out of this experience of complete dependence, some people emerge reporting that they see their lives differently—particularly in the areas of self-responsibility, acceptance of the inevitable, and heightened self-esteem. Follow-up visits are strongly encouraged, as is that the participants become proselytizers. Social psychologists have shown that we are more likely to maintain beliefs we have been forced to defend, so perhaps the best way to ensure constancy is make a converter out of the converted.

The numerous secular, mystical, and divine movements that have proliferated during the past decade supply abundant additional examples of related techniques in action. The Reverend Sun Myung Moon, Hare Krishna, Synanon, and Dianetics, to name only a few, all depend on practices that bear a close resemblance to those discussed.

But an interesting problem remains. Why do some people get better when their beliefs are changed? In some instances, the answer is obvious. If the convert is firmly convinced that she will now go to heaven rather than hell, of course she feels better. But why should it be therapeutic to scream with abandon? As with all psychotherapies, to some extent believing that one can cure oneself if only one follows directions is comforting. The belief that one is helpless is demoralizing. The belief that one is in control is un-demoralizing. Animal experimentation bears this out. Animals taught to control painful experience—e.g., taught how to avoid a shock—behave normally. Animals who are taught that a shock is unavoidable may later not be able to learn how to avoid the shock and may exhibit disturbed (neurotic) behavior. If abreaction itself is irrelevant to the healing and only a way of convincing the sufferer that he is doing something, then the comfort produced by abreaction should be short-lived. We will return to this issue at the end of the section.

A major therapeutic component of the inspiring subgroup of abreactive therapies probably depends on the fact that we have evolved as social animals. The effectiveness may stem not only from the expression of feeling but also from the simultaneous entrance into and participation in a group of true believers. Participating in and belonging to groups obviously meets a deep need in many people, and as we know, modern society has decreased the availability of large family or tribal groups. Working together toward a common goal produces warm feelings toward others and a sense of union with the group. Feelings of membership with our religious group, our ethnic group, our college, our team, our political party, our country are accompanied by feelings of warmth, security, superiority, and pride. One can see the therapeutic impact of converting anyone to a belief system that makes her a member of a group, particularly if she has no other strong ties.

Pleasure in group participation is so prevalent and so strong that seemingly it must have biological as well as social antecedents. One explanation might be that man is raised in a family group and seeks group participation in later life as a substitute for his early environment. Or the phenomenon might stem from an innate social regulatory mechanism developed through evolution. If membership in the primate group increased the probability of survival of the individual, the paleolithic Rotarians and their descendants would have had the best chance of survival.

Still another possibility is that the group—the tribe, the herd, the crowd—somehow serves to disinhibit individuals and intensify their emotional experience. Much has been written attesting that the crowd has less conscience than its individual members and that it promotes emotional contagion. Intense, disinhibited feeling combined with a sense of participation produces euphoria in many people, and euphoria itself is reinforcing. As in susceptibility to conditioning, however, people vary in the satisfaction they obtain from merging with a group.

Though the question of who benefits from group participation and who does not is obviously very important, especially clinically, it has not been evaluated.

One final comment about the permanency of participatory feelings: both the effects of conversion and the good feelings that stem from immersion in the group are often relatively transient. The therapy convert—like his religious fellow or the member of the weekly bowling league—must be periodically recharged by renewed participation in the group. As one would anticipate, the convert to a particular brand of therapy devotes considerable energy to identifying himself with his psychotherapeutic sect. Many who seemingly have benefited from psychotherapy identify strongly with the kind they have experienced. Furthermore, they are eager to convince others that theirs is the best. This need for convincing others characterizes not only the abreactive therapies but other forms as well. One may infer that in many instances the need to believe is correlated with the need to associate with, participate with, and draw strength from other converts. It may well be a characteristic of all successful psychotherapies.

State-Altering Therapies

During the 1960s and 1970s, an extraordinary interest developed in altered states of consciousness and mechanisms for producing them. Countless techniques and practices have been suggested for achieving relief or enlightenment, many enjoying only a temporary prominence. We will describe a few of the major ones.

The interest in altered states of consciousness flowered at about the time of the introduction of the psychedelic drugs, such as LSD. Experimentation with these drugs convinced both users and serious scientists that mystical experience could be produced by chemical means rather than by years of arduous spiritual training. Accompanying the interest in drug-induced altered states of consciousness was a rediscovery of Eastern mysticism. Perhaps spurred by an increasing belief that psychedelic drugs damaged the brain or the chromosomes, some members of the younger generation then eagerly took the lead in practicing the spiritual exercises of various non-Western religions.

Perhaps the best-known of these exercises has been transcendental meditation, but it is related to a variety of others—old and new, scientific and quasi-scientific, mundane and mystical—with approximately the same goals of reduced tension and peace of mind; sometimes the goal is expressed philosophically or theologically as becoming at one with the universe.

Hypnotism. When hypnotism originated as mesmerism in the eighteenth century, it was at first erroneously believed to result from a mystical force termed "animal magnetism." During the suceeding two hundred years, its popularity and respectability have alternately waxed and waned. Its career has been compared to that of the streetwalker of romantic novels who is rescued from her sordid circumstances to lead an honorable existence but who inevitably backslides.

Hypnosis has never been satisfactorily explained. It is not related to the power of a hypnotist over a subject, since all of its effects can be generated through autohypnosis. What is known is that it is not sleep—and may not represent any special state of consciousness at all. One investigator, Theodore Barber, has found that all of the usual effects of hypnosis can be induced simply by asking the subject to pretend, to imagine, to try as hard as she can, to produce the desired result. Induction of hypnosis with suggestions of sleep, of heaviness, of entering a trance, may not be necessary.

This observation does not explain the remarkable phenomena that occur in perhaps 10 to 25 percent of people who are hypnotized, such as anesthesia to pain sufficient to perform major surgery, visual and auditory hallucinations, the apparent ability to control portions of the autonomic nervous system, and the voluntary control of some emotional responses and sensations. Some students of hypnotism have proposed that even such changes may be the results of motivation and role-playing—that is, unconscious simulation due to a desire to please the hypnotist.

As we know from its role in the development of psychoanalysis, hypnosis has often been used as a specific aid to forms of psychotherapy. In addition to its use in the recovery of repressed material, it has been utilized to produce images or visual fantasies "constructed" to be of therapeutic value. A patient blocked by a problem, for example, might be induced to visualize himself in the future looking back at the problem as if he had successfully solved it. The fantasy might produce not only optimistic feelings but also a way of solving the problem. Or a patient might be asked to relive under hypnosis a painful period in her life and then to relive it with modifications in which the outcome was successful. Both techniques—which presumably can be applied only to that part of the population susceptible to deeper forms of hypnosis—have been repeatedly described anecdotally as dramatically helpful.

The following case history illustrates the successful therapeutic use of hypnotism. This case, a kind of scenario reminiscent of psychiatric movies of the 1940s, is both dramatic and atypical. Although unusual, it is an example of the occasionally startling potency of psychological techniques.

Gail Q.

Gail was referred at the age of twenty-eight by her family physician, who could find no physiological basis for her chronic abdominal pain. It had begun suddenly during Gail's junior year in college, but she could not link it to any events in her life. Because standard and detailed exploratory techniques provided no clues, the therapist (Paul Wender) decided to hypnotize Gail to see if he could recover memories related to the appearance of the pain.

Gail was an excellent hypnotic subject. After agreement on a set of finger signals, she was placed under hypnosis, asked to relive the period under investigation and instructed to signal the physician when she had completed reexperiencing the time period. Gail was completely silent for about five minutes and then began to show signs of emotional arousal. Her face became red, her respiration rate increased, and the arteries in her neck began to pulsate vigorously, indicating that her heart rate had gone up. After fifteen or twenty minutes, she signaled that she had lived through the episode. She was then requested to relive the experience again, but this time from an outside position—as if the period of her life was being played on a stage or movie screen. Another twenty minutes went by, with the same physiological reactions. Then Gail was asked if she could perceive any psychological experiences associated with the pain. When she signaled that she *had* found such a relationship, she was instructed to relive that period differently, directing herself, on the basis of her insight, to alter the events related to the development of the pain. Another twenty minutes passed, but this time with no sign of increased physiological activity. An hour had now gone by, during which Gail had not uttered one word. Still under hypnosis, she was told that she would awaken at a prescribed time, that she could remember these experiences if she chose to do so, and that she had the option of telling or not telling the psychiatrist about her experiences.

When Gail awoke, she was without pain for the first time in six years. She did remember what had happened and willingly described her experiences. Gail was the adopted daughter of a professor of mathematics (father) and a lawyer (mother) who had three natural children. Her siblings were brighter than she was and had been very successful academically. Although motivated to succeed in line with her parents' expectations, Gail felt herself no match for her siblings. She felt that she had been loved by the parents as if she had been their natural child and was more disappointed in her performance than they were. Because she drove herself academically, she was able to enter what she considered a lackluster college, where she strove mightily to obtain decent grades. In her third year she found herself in over her head. During the spring examination period she found it necessary to work laboriously, sleeping only two to four hours a night and spending most of her time studying. In this context, her pain developed.

She had not remembered the experience prior to the induction of hypnosis, nor had she noticed the obvious relationship between the experience and the pain. When she observed herself in hypnosis, she made the obvious connection. In her third reliving under hypnosis, she had told herself that she must come to terms with the fact that she was not as smart as her siblings, that her parents loved her, and that her failure to perform as well as her brother and sisters would not result in the loss of their love. In imagination, she had relived this period, studying less hard for her examinations.

A case like this is as puzzling as it is dramatic. Most adolescents whose parents expect too much from them do not develop abdominal pain when they do not live up to parental expectations. Moreover, most students who become tense and uptight during academically stressful periods do not develop persistent anxiety, depression, or pains. The development of Gail's pain may be physiologically understandable: when very anxious, some people secrete excessive hydrochloric acid in their stomachs and may develop gastric or intestinal irritation or ulceration. However, Gail's X rays at the age of twenty-eight disclosed no abdominal abnormalities despite the persistent pain. In addition, most people who develop symptoms during periods of stress remember both the symptoms and the stress. The reasons why Gail repressed her experience, why she continued to have symptoms, and why the symptoms responded to this novel form of treatment remain totally unclear. Such rapid and effective treatment for specific problems is rare, and prospective patients cannot usually expect results of this kind.

Successful treatment by hypnosis is like finding one black swan. It proves that not all swans are white. But it tells us nothing about how many black swans there are.

Persons who have a learned maladaptation and who are good hypnotic subjects may derive considerable benefit from relatively brief hypnotherapy. However, hypnotists do not report their failures as often as they do their successes; the question of who can benefit, and under what circumstances, as usual remains unanswered.

Hypnotism has also been used to directly "suggest away" bodily symptoms believed to have been psychologically caused, and to produce states of relaxation following recovery from hypnotic trance. Since these induced changes seem to be relatively short-lived, prolonged beneficial effects are not possible unless the hypnotist produces them several times a day or the subject is taught to self-induce hypnosis. The usefulness of autohypnosis—self-hypnosis—to induce relaxation and peace of mind is mentioned in several scientific texts and many lay publications; some physiological changes that may be related to those states, such as decreased respiration and heart rate, have been summarized by researcher Herbert Benson.

One factor suggesting that autohypnotic techniques might not be generally helpful is the limited proportion of people in whom deep hypnotic phenomena can be induced. Lighter hypnotic phenomena, however, such as eye closure and hand levitation, can be induced in a very large fraction of the population—perhaps 80 percent. Conceivably, this level of depth might produce useful autohypnotic calm and peacefulness. The fraction of people in whom it might produce some degree of enduring peace of mind is unknown.

Meditative techniques. The least involved and ornate of the spiritual disciplines that have become popular recently, incorporating neither contortional nor martial skills, has been transcendental meditation. This technique—the repetition to oneself of a one-syllable mantra supposedly assigned on an individual basis—has been widely popularized and apparently widely practiced. Its proponents claim that it reduces anxiety, is good for the body as well as the mind, and is relatively quickly learned; it also is not regulated by the Bureau of Narcotics and Dangerous Drugs. To some, it seems an invaluable contribution of East to West. In fact, as Herbert Benson has pointed out, relaxation techniques of this kind have been a part of both Eastern and Western religions for most of recorded history, appearing not only in yoga and Buddhism but in repetitive prayers and prolonged contemplation by Catholics, Moslems, and orthodox Jews. It seems to be an instance of old wine in new goatskins.

Benson's investigations indicate that the essential elements of effective regular meditation—which he calls the Relaxation Response—are: (1) a quiet environment, (2) a mental device or fixation object used repetitively, (3) a passive attitude, (4) a comfortable position. The choice of fixation object varies, including, most commonly, a word or phrase continually repeated, silently or aloud; the sensation of air passing in and out of the nostrils; the sensation of air passing through the bronchial tree; repetitive body motion (dancing and rhythmic prayer); a flame or a material object; portions of the skin surface.

Some teachers of meditation describe an orderly sequence of expectable subjective phenomena. What fraction of practitioners experience these phenomena, however, and whether they experience them in order, is unknown. Some manuals assert that, after practice, one will experience vivid visual imagery, apparently without induced expectation in the subject. Covert suggestion remains a possibility.

Skill in mastering meditative technique is said to require a great deal of time, even years. Brain-wave studies of Zen monks seem to indicate that over a period of ten to twenty years meditative practices produce unique skills in talented subjects. During periods of relaxation, the introduction of a novel stimulus—e.g., a particular tone—ordinarily changes the brain waves. If the stimulus is repeated several times, its novelty wears off, and the brain waves eventually fail to change. In the tests of the monks, however, they continue to respond to a repeated stimulus as if it were a new stimulus. This corresponds to the claims of mystics that the perfected mystical mind has the ability to react, like that of a young child, to every common stimulus as if it were new.

Whether there are differences in the subjective states achieved by varying techniques of meditation is uncertain. We would guess that the meditative object is less important than the amount of practice. However, the expectations by the subject of what he will experience must play a major role in the different reports. A Christian mystic is likely to phrase his experience in terms of Saviour rather than *satori.* Yet the subjective phenomena themselves seem very similar, and certain aspects of mystical experiences appear to be independent of the culture in which they occur. Moreover, these aspects resemble the phenomena triggered by psychedelic drugs and some psychoses. All this suggests that these experiences depend upon specific, common, physiological mechanisms such as the postulated "Ah-ha!" mechanism.

In addition, Herbert Benson's medical research has indicated that almost any generalized version of meditation—secular or religious—does have measurable physiological effects such as decreased respiration and heart rate, and some decrease in blood pressure in people with hypertension.

Autogenic training. A filial relative of hypnosis, autogenic training was evolved in Germany and is widely known on the Continent. It was devised by Johannes Schultz, a German neuropsychiatrist, who had found hypnosis useful in treating a wide variety of psychological discomforts but too time-consuming. Observing that hypnotic phenomena were at times accompanied by such bodily changes as muscular relaxation, a sensation of heaviness and warmth in the limbs, and slowed respiration and heartbeat, Schultz devised a highly systematized technique in which someone successively gives himself suggestions for each of these changes. A patient would focus on warmth, gradually moving from one to all of his limbs; next on heaviness; and so forth. The program was to be performed several times a day for several months. Autogenic training has been widely employed for psychosomatic and psychological difficulties, and German scientific reports state that it has been quite successful in alleviating symptoms in a variety of circumstances. Since the studies did not use control groups, however, we cannot determine the technique's effectiveness with any confidence. It sounds interesting and tedious, and presumably is relatively harmless.

One unexpected aspect of autogenic training is that, with continuing practice, some persons experience vivid, dreamlike episodes similar to those experienced by practitioners of meditative techniques. Teachers of autogenic training and of some meditative techniques regard these experiences as potentially valuable, allowing the individual to reach a submerged portion of himself. Similar phenomena occur in hypnosis and in drug-induced states. Recall of some kinds of psychological material is deemed cathartic, but whether such aspects of autogenic training have any permanent effects remains to be demonstrated.

Body mechanics. Body mechanics—or body therapies—such as the techniques of the Reichians, bioenergeticists (see Lowen), and Rolfers, are based on the idea that psychological and body functioning interrelate in two ways: not only does the mind affect the body but the body also affects the mind. Manipulation of the body and breathing (exercise, dance, massage, pummeling) can sometimes produce intense, vivid, cathartic emotional experiences. Whether this is of any long-term value is unclear. Some people insist that body therapies have helped them after more traditional therapies had failed.

Although no experimental evidence is available, these therapies should not be highhandedly dismissed. There are at least three reasons for believing that they might be useful. First, they often alter the patient's breathing patterns, which corresponds to traditional meditative processes that do have measurable physiological relaxing effects. Second, as the James–Lange Hypothesis proposed (independent ideas from William James and Danish physiologist C. Lange) at the end of the last century, there is some possibility that, at least in part, emotional states may result from physiological reactions as well as produce them. In its pure and largely discredited form, the theory maintained that a distressing situation led automatically and mechanically to a bodily change, such as crying, and that the feeling of sadness was due to our experiencing this physiological change. Common language reflects some belief in the theory, as when we talk of being uptight, tight-assed, or loose. These words are used in a double sense to convey both a physical and an emotional state. We cannot dismiss the possibility that a change in bodily reactions to events may produce different feelings. Put your chin out, pull your stomach in, march forward vigorously, and watch your depression and feelings of low self-esteem vanish.

Alterations in posture and movement, moreover, have been traditionally used in durable mystical-training practices. The most obvious is yoga, but there is also tai chi, the dancing Sufi dervish, and the Zen alternate meditation. In the latter, the individual is enjoined to become fully aware, during daily life, of himself and his surroundings. The awareness of body (as well as environment) is ostensibly good and useful. Since these practices may possibly have persisted on the basis of their utility, we infer that bodily posture and movement may affect the emotional state of the participants.

Muscular relaxation. As noted, relaxation of the voluntary (skeletal) musculature is a concomitant of hypnosis and an aim of autogenic training. The particular technique called progressive muscular relaxation was developed forty years ago as a direct method of anxiety reduction, and according to the clinical reports (there are no large controlled studies), has been applied to a variety of specific and nonspecific complaints. It has been used by behavior therapists as a substitute for hypnosis in desensitization, has been employed by psychiatrists, and has been introduced into obstetrics for pain control (it is the basis of the Grantly Dick-Read method of natural childbirth).

The goal of muscular relaxation is to enable the individual to make his skeletal muscles as limp and flaccid as possible. Toward this end, the person is taught to contract them individually and to relax them subsequently until he gets a feel for the sensation accompanying relaxation. As in autogenic training, therapists expect that it will take several months to master the technique. Like autogenic training and unlike hypnosis, muscular relaxation requires very little professional time. One can apparently master it on the basis of intensive practice, with infrequent coaching sessions directed at commonly occurring problems. Studies of desensitization with or without relaxation have shown no added benefits from relaxation training, thus casting doubt on its utility.

Biofeedback. Methods for inducing state alteration by modern technology are classed under the general heading of "biofeedback." These techniques have claimed to offer instant enlightenment through electronics (an update of "better living through chemistry").

The various technical devices inform an individual about bodily states of which he is not normally aware—e.g., brain waves, heart rate, skin conductivity, and blood pressure. Such physiological variables, which are controlled by the so-called autonomic nervous system, fluctuate considerably from moment to moment and can be readily measured.

It had long been believed that the autonomic nervous system was not subject to voluntary control by self-instruction, despite the apparent ability of certain Eastern fakirs to control heart rate. Such claims were largely ignored, considered false, or explained as the consequences of voluntary alteration of respiration.

One of the major tenets of the two-process animal-learning theory has been that some bodily functions—e.g., the movement of the skeletal musculature—are under voluntary control and subject to learning via reward, punishment, and instruction, but that others react only automatically to external stimuli (cold, heat, fear) and are not subject to voluntary control. Pavlov had discovered that the experimenter could bring some involuntary bodily functions under *his* control, but seemingly it was impossible to teach the dog—or human being—to control his own salivation, or analogous bodily functions, through reward or punishment.

Much of the interest in biofeedback techniques has resulted from dramatic experiments that seemed to contradict the two-process theory, but repeated attempts to replicate these experiments have not been successful. The experiments involved paralyzing rats with curare, keeping them alive with artificial respiration, and using electrodes attached to the pleasure centers of the brain to give them rewarding stimulation for random changes in heart rate. Supposedly, the rats were trained to raise or lower their heart rates—and later to control other functions, such as constriction and dilation of blood vessels in the ear—in response to particular signals. In the absence of replication, however, learning theorists now doubt the validity of the experiments.

At approximately the same time, investigators were exploring the effects of informing an individual of the state of her own brain waves. The living brain generates very small amounts of electrical voltage (roughly 10 to 150 millionths of a volt), which can be recorded by the electroencephalograph (EEG). Several major wave forms have been found to correlate roughly with states of arousal. For example, in deep sleep the voltages are very large (perhaps 150 millionths of a volt) and occur at a frequency of approximately four per second. In some persons, the so-called alpha frequency (eight to thirteen cycles per second) is associated with a state of lessened arousal or attention. Similarly, in states of wakefulness and arousal, the brain generates about 10 millionths of a volt at frequencies of about fifteen to thirty cycles per second (beta).

By connecting an EEG to simple electronic equipment, one can provide a visual or auditory signal whenever the subject's brain is generating a particular wave frequency. Untrained subjects told to "keep the light or sound on," but not told that the experimenters were trying to increase their alpha frequency, could learn with practice to increase the fraction of time during which their brains were generating alpha waves. Not everyone could acquire this skill, and not all those who did could increase the percent of alpha substantially. Some of those who increased their alpha time reported subjective changes, including a sense of pleasant relaxation and well-being.

However, alpha waves may merely be associated with unfocused visual attention. If you tell people to close their eyes, approximately 90 percent will develop alpha waves. If you then place towels in front of their faces and have them open their eyes, the alpha waves immediately go away. After a while, however, they come back even with the eyes open. If you tell the subject to focus on the texture of the towel, the alpha waves disappear. Apparently, also, everyone's alpha waves increase in a pitch-dark room. People who are generating more alpha waves may have learned how to defocus their visual attention. Similarly, the early reports that the alpha state is accompanied by decreased anxiety and feelings of well-being have not been substantiated.

A study of experienced Zen practitioners *suggests*, if true, that EEG biofeedback might have long-term effects. Students who had practiced Zen for ten to twenty years and were judged successful by their teachers continued to maintain alpha frequencies with their eyes open, generated these waves from the front as well as the back of the head (unlike the usual situation), and manifested voltages that greatly exceeded the normal range.

This might all be secondary to a hypertrophied ability to remain visually defocused with the eyes open. Much Zen training consists of sitting before a wall, which could well stimulate prolonged defocusing. Further, this does not indicate that EEG biofeedback is equivalent to Zen meditation. Nonetheless, the observation suggests that years of practice can produce striking changes in brain-wave patterns and that such changes may be associated with other changes in psychological reactivity. Or they may not.

The physiological variables with which biofeedback can be used are as numerous as those that can be measured. Another popular variable is muscular tension. Even when a muscle is at rest—as when one is lying down—sensitive instruments demonstrate that the muscle fibers continue to contract at a low rate. Many persons who believe themselves to be relaxed have above-normal levels of resting muscular activity. Autogenic training and muscular relaxation attempt to reduce this activity to a minimum, assuming that reducing muscular tension reduces anxiety. By the use of powerful muscle-tension amplifiers, one can demonstrate to the subject his continued muscular activity while resting. He can then be taught to diminish this activity to a subnormal level, which might conceivably be a useful general antidote to anxiety. The technique has also been used, with varying degrees of success, for other conditions, such as tension headaches produced by spasm of neck and scalp muscles. Its usefulness in combating states of general anxiety has not been documented. Confirmation requires experiments similar in length to the long periods required for autogenic training and muscular relaxation.

Experiments are currently attempting to use these techniques to alter abnormal EEGs in epileptics, to lower blood pressure in hypertensives, and to eliminate cardiac irregularities. The degree and duration of such effects are unknown.

Biofeedback methods must be used over longer periods of time before we can come to any conclusions about their usefulness in medical disorders and psychiatry. It is important to remember that advocates of each new method in psychotherapy start out by promising a quick cure but after a while begin to claim that months and years of such treatment are needed for maximum effectiveness. One possibility is that patients who are not helped drop by the wayside—often early in therapy—leaving therapists with only a group of true believers who may or may not have been helped by the techniques. Such an experience could convince therapists that long-term treatment is necessary and that if those who left had only persevered, they too would have been helped. Plainly, this criticism applies as well to all the other psychotherapies we have discussed.

The basis of the appeal of biofeedback seems to be that it has promised instant mystical expertise via modern technology, a sort of Zen science. What takes the Zen master twenty years to accomplish is promised through American know-how to be available within a few weeks. Enthusiasm for such modern techniques should be tempered by the same caution necessary in approaching all forms of psychiatric treatment. Our desire for wisdom and serenity continues to exceed our abilities to produce them.

CHAPTER 9

What Path for the Sufferer?

The position we have advanced in this book not only is of importance to the psychiatric theoretician but is of the utmost practical importance to the person with psychological distress who is seeking relief.

Our major point is that the sufferer from biogenic psychological illness can expect maximum benefit from chemical treatment. There is no good evidence that psychotherapy alone is of even slight benefit to the severely schizophrenic patient, the biologically depressed patient, or the bipolar (manic-depressive) patient. There is clear evidence that medication, with psychological therapy as an adjunct, is the optimal treatment for the agoraphobic patient, or the patient with spontaneous panic attacks. And there is increasing evidence that medication is the treatment of choice for the hysteroid dysphoric and the adult hyperactive.

The fact that medication is of documented effectiveness in these disorders does not imply that *additional* psychological treatment is of no value. Even when properly treated, the patient suffering from a biogenic illness is also likely to have as complications of the illness personal limitations and realistic unhappiness that will *not* respond simply to medication. In many instances, he will require a combination of medication, psychological therapy, training in new social habits, and possibly a change in style of life. The sufferer whose unhappiness largely has a realistic base—the partner in a bad marriage, the person in a job for which he has no taste, the housewife atrophying in the suburbs—may need a change in life setting, but may be unable to recognize the problem or muster the energies necessary for such a change. Psychological therapy *may* provide the necessary boost, but so may a variety of other psychologically potent forces such as religious groups, social organizations, consciousness-raising groups, and encounter groups. In addition, overcoming various learned maladaptive behaviors often requires psychological therapies. What kinds of limitations and mislearning respond to what kinds of psychological therapies is of critical importance but is a question that cannot yet be answered.

The position we have advanced is different from that accepted by most lay persons and many practitioners. Until recently, the psychiatric atmosphere has been highly pro-psychotherapy and relatively anti-drug. Until the 1960s, as indicated in earlier chapters, American psychiatry was dominated by psychoanalytic thinking. Young physicians were eager to go into training programs that provided a firm grounding in psychoanalytic therapeutic techniques. Half the chairmen of departments of psychiatry were psychoanalysts. The exclusively organic school converted few disciples: its explanatory system was weak and its therapeutic resources relatively limited.

The flavor of the times is captured in a classic study, conducted more than twenty years ago, which investigated the relationship between social class, psychiatric illness, and treatment (Hollingshead and Redlich, 1958). Upper-class patients received more intensive psychotherapeutic treatment than lower-class patients, who usually had either minimal psychotherapy or drug treatment. This was cited as evidence that once again the lowly were being shortchanged. The affluent got first-class treatment; the poor and blue-collar groups got second-class treatment. The phenomenon was explained not only by the ability of the upper classes to pay the healthy sums that long-term psychotherapy requires but by the prejudices of the psychotherapists, who preferred verbal, psychologically minded, ethnically similar patients who shared their mores and values. The implication was that intensive psychotherapy was the treatment of choice for most psychiatric patients and that the decision to deny it to the lower classes was reached not for medical but for socioeconomic reasons. It is ironic, then, that many of those who were given medication for three months may have had more appropriate treatment than their upper-class counterparts who underwent depth analysis for five years.

The common view of the time was advanced by one of the most prominent psychiatric statesmen, Karl Menninger, who, in a book written with two colleagues, *The Vital Balance* (1963), stated that there were no separate psychiatric illnesses. Menninger argued that there were only degrees of psychological disorganization and threats to disintegration of mental functioning. The disorganization might be produced externally—e.g., by grief—or internally—e.g., by conflicts between warring components of the mind. The disorganization and the attempts to master it produced the psychiatric symptoms. Greater illness, Menninger continued, was simply a manifestation of greater dyscontrol; lesser illness, a manifestation of lesser dyscontrol. Basically, he maintained, there was only a quantitative difference between the mental dyscontrol associated with irritability or mild anxiety and that which produced schizophrenia. He described schizophrenia as an example of "extreme states of disorganization, regression, and reality repudiation which . . . represent a penultimate effort to avoid something worse, viz., [maximal] dysorganization—malignant anxiety and depression eventuating in death, often by suicide" (Menninger, p. 250). All forms of dyscontrol were supposedly responsive to the same universal remedy: psychotherapy. For Menninger there was one disease and one treatment.*

One of the historical contributants to the popularity of the exclusive psychogenic approach was the spread of psychoanalytic therapy from psychoanalysts to the nonmedical professions. Among the reasons were the long training required in psychoanalysis proper, the few patients psychoanalysts could see (an analyst who confines himself to his profession may treat only a few hundred people in the course of a lifetime), and the high fees charged by psychoanalysts (which attracted other professions and also tempted patients willing to try a related version at a lower cost); above all, it was a kind of therapy that did not seem to require medical knowledge and was vague enough to lend itself to a variety of professional offshoots. Psychologists and social workers—and eventually pastors and nurses—became second-class psychoanalysts who were excluded from the inner sanctum but were able to attract large clienteles of patients seeking psychotherapy. Because the background of many of these practitioners has been in nonmedical theories of personality and in theories of learning, virtually all gave little attention to biological variability and the role it played in individual psychological problems.

At the same time, our culture developed an antimedication bias, since medication was misunderstood as coercive restraint, both among professionals and among lay persons. The antimedication position is maintained by some psychiatrists as well as by many nonphysician

---

*And for Thomas Szasz—of *The Myth of Mental Illness*—there are *no* diseases and one treatment.

psychotherapists. In medicine, the most opposition and/or indifference comes from the psychoanalytic schools. Many psychoanalysts are socially and intellectually removed from the field of medicine as a whole, and despite the fact that many are scholars within their own area, they resist the implications of what has been happening in psychobiology and psychopharmacology.

Attempts to deal with all mental illnesses psychoanalytically were reasonable sixty years ago, when no treatments were very promising and analysis was a new and unexplored technique that held out possibilities. Psychoanalysis did indeed provide the opportunity for detailed, unique, in-depth, longitudinal observation of the behavior of ill people, thus stimulating the development of interesting hypotheses. But it never tested these hypotheses through the formal mechanisms of scientific research—controlled experimental studies. As newer groups have come along with other intriguing hypotheses, analysts have been left in the dubious position of having nothing to defend their ideas with except their tradition. Of course, one of the intellectually charming things about psychoanalysis is that originally it was *anti*-tradition. Ironically, psychoanalysis is now the establishment.

It is common today for psychoanalysts and psychoanalytic psychotherapists to judge the suitability of patients for psychoanalytic treatment not in terms of the patient's symptom picture and, therefore, possible underlying disease but in terms of adequate intelligence, psychological-mindedness, good ego strength (i.e., not being grossly ill), willingness to enter psychodynamic treatment, and adequate insurance coverage. Since many depressive disorders, separation anxieties, bipolar affective illnesses, and misdiagnosed borderline states occur in people of good intelligence, psychological-mindedness, fair ego strength, willingness to undergo psychodynamic treatment, and good insurance coverage, the psychoanalyst who does not use the full panoply of drugs, or the nonphysician therapist who does not consider referring patients to physicians for drug administration, may not be giving his patients the best possible treatment.

Psychoanalysis and related treatments have also been described as research techniques, methods for exploring personality, but as stimulating as that kind of experience may be, most patients do not seek therapy just for the sake of the analytic exploration itself.

As the research evidence regarding the effectiveness of drug therapy has become more compelling, psychologists, social workers, and pastoral counselors have found themselves in an uncomfortable position, since until recently their training and their professional societies have not emphasized advances in neurochemistry and psychopharmacology. Those psychologists, social workers, and pastoral counselors who have recognized the possible role of biological components in a great range of mental illnesses—and many of these therapists have resisted such recognition—have had to come to terms with the training gaps and legal status that prevent them from dispensing biological treatments. Inevitably, rationalization, motivated perception, and the pocketbook are likely to play a part in the ardent defense of the nonbiological position by some therapists who are not physicians. An unfortunate aspect of this is that many psychologists and social workers are not adequately trained to distinguish patients with biological disorders, although a few special training programs are beginning to try to remedy this deficiency.

Psychiatrists with a psychogenic outlook are often similarly insensitive. We and our colleagues have compiled a large, informal list of patients who have received unsuccessful, interminable psychotherapy conducted by psychiatrists, psychologists, and social workers, and who responded promptly and dramatically to appropriate treatment with medication.

The most unfortunate aspect of the current situation is that there is sufficient psychotherapeutic work available for all therapists. As we have said repeatedly, patients with biological disorders who have been successfully treated medically frequently need psychological treatment, and the large segment of the patient population that is unhappy for nonbiological, psychological reasons can be treated optimally only through psychological techniques. Cooperation, not competition, would be in the patient's and the therapist's best interests. To quote Alfred Whitehead: "A clash of doctrines is not a disaster—it is an opportunity."

The lay person's opposition to medical treatment of psychiatric disorders comes from several directions. First, the middle and upper classes are suffering from cultural lag. Nurtured on psychoanalysis and sustained by the promises of gestalt therapy, transactional analysis, primal scream, and other therapies, most educated people still believe that psychotherapy is the treatment of choice and that treatment with medication is an inferior modality.

A second source of resistance can be best understood philosophically. Historians of thought (including Freud, in 1917) have pointed out that modern man has been dealt three major blows to his vanity. The first came from Copernicus, who posited that the earth went around the sun and not the sun around the earth. Our planet was not the hub of the universe by God's designation. The second blow came from Darwin, who held that we were descended from ape-like creatures and not from Adam and Eve. (Or, in Mark Twain's words, that we were a little lower than the angels and a little higher than the French.) The third blow came from Freud, who argued against our feelings of autonomy and free will. We were not fully in control of our behavior but were, to varying degrees, controlled by our unconscious minds. Unlike Copernicus and Darwin, Freud offered us a sop. If we underwent psychoanalysis, we might become aware of the unconscious determinants of our behavior and thus learn to control them to some extent.

The biological theory of mental illness offers a fourth blow. It implies that sometimes one cannot by oneself control moods and behavior psychologically. This is contrary to many theological and philosophical positions—and also to a few psychotherapeutic ones, such as those of Szasz and Glasser—which hold that we are completely responsible for our feelings and acts. We have presented clear evidence that in many circumstances one *can't* control oneself. One must sometimes abdicate control—or recognize that one has already involuntarily abdicated control; and people who want to believe in free will or an exclusive psychological determinism find this very hard to accept.

Third, the lay person tends to regard medications as concealing or suppressing the symptoms of a disorder rather than as attacking the impairment. One typically depressed patient, for example, who only after considerable resistance accepted antidepressant medication, recovered dramatically and then returned to the psychiatrist, saying, "Now, let's get into psychotherapy, *really* get to the bottom of this problem, and solve it once and for all." To the therapist, the patient's statement was ironic; there is no systematic evidence that psychotherapy does get to the root of the problems of the biological depressives. Psychological treatment may help the patient understand the need to continue the medication, relieve her anxieties, give the person a perspective on psychological problems that may be complicating his life, and permit the maximizing of those gains.

Like the patient cited, many lay persons base their attitude toward psychiatric drugs on their experience with alcohol and barbiturates, which do indeed conceal problems. They relieve emotional stress in a nonspecific way, and their effect on the ill person is similar to their effect on the normal person. In both instances, they produce some degree of befuddlement and stupidity. As a result, the individual is not concerned about things that would ordinarily bother him, and his anticipatory anxiety is decreased. The so-called minor tranquilizers such as Librium and Valium are considerably less intoxicating but share some of the same actions in that they are also nonspecific inhibitors of worrying and anticipatory anxiety, and their effects on normal and ill people are quite similar.

The mechanism of action of the antidepressants and antipsychotics seems to be more complicated than that of the minor tranquilizers. Lithium, for example, normalizes both mania and some forms of depression. Further, it acts as a prophylactic against both mania and depression in patients who have bipolar affective illnesses. The use of lithium seems to help in the adjustment of complicated control circuits in the brain. It attacks malfunction at a more basic level. But it does not cure. When lithium is stopped, its actions are stopped, although relapse does not occur immediately.

We think, therefore, that the antipsychotics, the antidepressants, and lithium are not masking the symptoms of an illness. They are relieving the symptoms by normalizing some deep malfunctioning closely related to the underlying causes. They are not second-class therapies. They are the best we have now. They contrast to the sedative-hypnotic drugs such as barbiturates, Miltown, Librium, and Valium, which *are* masking symptoms and are *not* acting on what we believe are brain functions related to basic underlying causes (although they have clear symptomatic value).

To reiterate, the major psychiatric drugs produce benefits only in persons suffering from specific psychiatric diseases; they do *not* relieve common, garden-variety anxieties that are psychologically produced. They do not produce good feelings in the healthy. Unlike the minor tranquilizers, in more than twenty-five years on the market, they have not been abused. (Some persons may indeed take antipsychotic drugs without a doctor's prescription; they are usually psychotics successfully medicating themselves without the blessing of a physician.) Although some of the newer minor tranquilizers are much less abusable than the barbiturates, they can be used as intoxicants, as reflected in a Greenwich Village graffito: "Give me Librium or give me Meth."

Another difference between the major drugs and the usual sedatives and barbiturates is that patients do not become tolerant to the former. When barbiturates are given over a period of time, the dosage must be escalated in order for the same benefits to occur. If they are then abruptly terminated, the patient may suffer withdrawal symptoms, a sign that the body has become physiologically dependent on the drug. If the barbiturate was prescribed for anxiety, the anxiety may now be worse than before treatment.

Recent studies of the chronic administration of benzodiazepines, such as Librium and Valium, indicate that many patients experience all the benefit they are going to get after the dosage has been adjusted within the first six weeks. They can then be maintained for prolonged periods on such drugs without becoming tolerant to them or requiring an escalation of dosage. The horror stories about patients who have become addicted to Valium refer almost exclusively to patients who were already chronic alcoholics or who had spontaneous panic attacks.

With the major psychiatric drugs, if the illness has disappeared, the medication may be withdrawn *without* an immediate recurrence of the illness—that is, schizophrenic or depressive symptoms will not abruptly become worse than before treatment. Schizophrenic symptoms generally do not reappear for at least another six weeks, although the patient may develop other symptoms if the main drugs are abruptly terminated, such as headache, nausea, or malaise. Many patients are chronically afflicted with schizophrenia or a mood disorder and must take medication on a permanent or semipermanent basis. For such unfortunate persons, medication is a must if symptoms are to be relieved, and in this sense an individual may be dependent on medication for his well-being. But his dependency is not addictive: it is similar to that of the diabetic on insulin, the patient with pernicious anemia on vitamin B_{12}, or the epileptic on anti-epilepsy medication.

Finally, a major source of public concern is that drugs are overused. The minor psychiatric medications may be overused, but even this is not clear. Minor tranquilizers are prescribed by many general physicians—often in desperation—when confronted with numerous patients who are anxious, depressed, with or without detectable physical illness. The minor tranquilizers often provide relief, and this, combined with the fact that many psychological problems are reactive to transient life circumstances and therefore short-lived, gives both the patient and the physician a measure of satisfaction. Perhaps their use could be diminished if effective psychological treatment for psychological difficulties were more certain, but this is also guesswork. Several studies indicate that the general population uses minor tranquilizers episodically for situations of marked stress and that most people are prone to *under*use rather than *over*use them.

In a national survey in 1970–71, for example, 15 percent of the adults sampled reported using a minor tranquilizer or daytime sedative during the past year (2 percent had used antidepressants, and similar small percentages had used other drugs, for a total of 22 percent). Fewer than 40 percent of all psychotherapeutic drug users had used medications regularly for at least two months. In the same sample, 27 percent of those surveyed reported high psychic distress (largely anxiety and depression) and 33 percent had been high on an index of life crises during the same year. About 32 percent of those with high psychic distress and 22 percent of those with a high level of life crises had used psychotherapeutic drugs (largely, minor tranquilizers). Of those with low psychic distress and a low level of life crises, about 11 percent had used psychotherapeutic drugs. Altogether the figures indicate that drug use is highest among those with symptoms appropriate to such use, and that only a minority of those who might benefit from psychotherapeutic drugs—particularly minor tranquilizers—use them (Mellinger et al., 1974).*

The major psychiatric medications are also very probably *under*used. Our knowledge of the frequency of depression and the amount of antidepressant medication prescribed suggests that a large number (perhaps two-thirds) of depressed persons either are not receiving treatment or are receiving inadequate treatment. Studies of symptomatic volunteers illustrate the extent of untreated sufferers. Symptomatic volunteers are people who are symptomatic but have not on their own initiative presented themselves for psychiatric care. Researchers find them by advertising for people who have untreated psychological complaints, sometimes receiving responses from hundreds of people with symptoms comparable to those of patients under psychiatric treatment (Covi et al., 1979). In such studies, depression and anxiety self-rating scales are published in a newspaper advertisement and subjects scoring above a cutoff point indicative of depression or anxiety are invited to participate (see Brauzer and Goldstein, 1973). The researchers have found that the typical volunteer has been suffering from such symptoms for about two years, has seen a general practitioner and received minor tranquilizers, has failed to benefit from these drugs, and has decided to live with the symptoms. The volunteers obtain significant relief of symptoms from the medications administered in the course of the studies. There are many such untreated but treatable walking wounded.

In summary, treatment with medication is not necessarily second-class treatment. Treatment with major medication is in fact the treatment of choice, the best treatment, for some psychiatric illnesses. Response to major psychiatric medications is evidence, ipso facto, that a patient suffers from major psychiatric illness; we say this because the medications are ineffective with normals, persons suffering from realistic unhappiness, or persons with learned maladaptations. Patients with psychiatric illnesses who have been successfully treated with med-

*In response to a Food and Drug Administration request, drug companies recently added to their instructions to physicians regarding minor tranquilizers a statement to the effect that the stress of everyday life usually does not require such treatment. This decision was not made on the basis of any new information.

ication may need additional help to overcome learned maladaptations and realistic unhappiness.

Medication is usually considered an adjunct to psychological treatment, but the reverse is probably nearer the truth. Psychological treatment may be a useful adjunct to medication. Further, in major illnesses where psychological treatment as well as medication is desirable, the medication may also play an essential role in moving the patient to a point where psychotherapy can begin—that is, in reducing thought distortion, emotional malfunctioning, or inappropriate behavior sufficiently so that the patient can benefit from talking and thinking about the difficulties.

An essential aspect of optimal therapy is correct diagnosis. The knotty problem for the ill person is discovering what kind of problem(s) he or she has. In general, the prospective patient is more likely to obtain a correct diagnosis from a physician—a psychiatrist—than from a psychologist or social worker. We use the phrase "more likely" because many psychiatrists have not been sufficiently trained in either systematic diagnosis or biological psychiatry and regard biological treatment as applicable only to the most seriously disturbed patients. The majority of psychologists and social workers do not have an adequate background in biological psychiatry. Therefore, many patients who turn for help to such independent practitioners may well be incorrectly diagnosed and treated. A clinic with an admissions procedure involving diagnosis by psychiatrists, and a staff that includes psychologists and social workers, is often in a good position to offer correct alternative treatments.

Because of the variability of diagnoses and treatments, the patient should attempt the difficult task of questioning the prospective physician about his theoretical stance. Some physicians may regard this as presumptuous and will conclude that the patient either is manifesting severe resistance to acknowledging the psychological basis of his problems or is displaying an interest in matters in which he has no competence. In that case, the patient can diagnose the physician as authoritarian, dogmatic, and insecure and should look elsewhere.

The prospective patient should have a full discussion with the physician, exploring the psychiatrist's theoretical background, therapeutic plan, and the way in which the therapy would be carried out and evaluated. We think it is important to inquire about the psychiatrist's policy regarding the use of medication. An increasing number of psychiatrists will find this acceptable. Some now choose to make a contract with patients—that is, they specify the duties of both participants, the frequency of the meetings, and the point at which progress will be evaluated in order to determine whether treatment should continue.

Like most physicians, we do not think that it is generally a good idea for patients to diagnose themselves. The prospective patient can, however, make some diagnostic observations on himself and report them to the psychiatrist. First, he can compare his signs and symptoms to those in the biological psychiatric syndromes described in this book: the schizophrenias; the disorders of mood—unipolar depression and bipolar manic-depressive illness; separation anxiety; hysteroid dysphoria; panic attacks; adult or childhood hyperactivity. A second important marker is the presence of any such psychiatric illnesses in brothers, sisters, or parents. The patient should remember, for example, that he may be miserable because he was raised by a depressed mother but it is equally tenable that he is miserable because she supplied him with depressive genes. In general, if an ordinary competent life is suddenly interrupted by psychiatric symptoms, a biological cause must be suspected.

The response to treatment provides some partial data with regard to the correctness of the diagnosis. Rapid amelioration of a long-standing condition after drug administration would seem to confirm both the diagnosis that led to this prescription and the utility of the medication. There is a certain amount of trial and error in drug prescription, however, and it is not unusual for patients to respond to the second or third medication prescribed rather than to the first. Further, failure to respond to all known biological treatments does not mean that the problems are necessarily nonbiological in origin. It may simply mean that a useful biological treatment has yet to be devised. If a patient has repeatedly failed to respond to biological treatments, however, it is certainly incumbent on the doctor to review the entire situation for the possibility of misdiagnosis and mistreatment.

Analogously, failure to respond to psychotherapy does not necessarily mean that one's problems are not psychological, since these failures may stem from differences in people's ability to change their entrenched ways, or possibly a mismatch between patient and therapist or therapy.

To make matters all the more confusing, it is conceivable that the patient who is apparently responding to medication is actually demonstrating a nonspecific placebo effect. However, such effects are often relatively transient. Similarly, a beneficial response to psychotherapy may occur in conditions that are basically organic in origin, but this, too, is usually transient.

It is our clinical impression that individuals in whom psychotherapy will prove useful show marked changes in six months to a year. If changes do not occur by then, or if the patient feels that his psychiatrist or other therapist does not understand or is not helping the problem, it is eminently reasonable and proper to discuss this with the therapist and request a consultation. The statement that a treatment program should be reevaluated every six months may seem radical, but our experience has been that many patients who do not show distinct progress within this period of time may have major biological components to their difficulties.

An important practical question is whether drug treatment or psychotherapy should be tried first. This is the sort of issue that has been discussed in game theory and involves what is called the payoff matrix. One evaluates the advantages and disadvantages of the four possible options: (1) The patient has a biological illness and is given only drug treatment. (2) The patient has a biological illness and is given only psychotherapy. (3) The patient does not have a biological illness and is given only drug treatment. (4) The patient does not have a biological illness and is given only psychotherapy.

What are the relative costs in time, money, and personal hazards? Drug treatment is specific, not time-consuming, and cheap, and can be evaluated in four to six weeks. If the patient falls into category 1, he will have optimal treatment. If he falls into category 3, he will receive inappropriate treatment, but this will be determined cheaply and fairly rapidly. If he is in category 2, he may waste considerable time and money. If he is in category 4, he will have appropriate treatment.

One additional major question concerns category 3—not having a biological illness but receiving drug treatment. Treatment with the major psychiatric drugs is not entirely safe but is safer than treatment with many commonly used agents. All drugs produce side effects—occasionally fatal ones. With the major psychiatric drugs, the risks when used in therapeutic amounts and with recommended precautions (see Appendix) are low, probably much lower than the risk of anesthesia in routine surgery such as for a hernia. These risks must be compared with those of category 2, having a biological illness that is treated by psychological, not pharmacological, means. The risks in untreated or inappropriately treated biological illnesses are substantial. In addition to the symptoms themselves, they include personal difficulties such as divorce, job or academic failure, and, in extreme cases, suicide. Such risks are in general far greater than those incurred in ingesting a foreign chemical substance.

Many psychiatrists do not use the therapeutic strategy of an initial rapid trial of medication but reserve drug treatment for psychotherapy failures. We find it difficult to understand why, for indicated illnesses, one should embark on a lengthy, expensive course of treatment without first testing the possible effectiveness and greater efficiency of an inexpensive reparative medication.

It is a mild consolation that the situation is slowly changing. The exclusively psychogenic view is beginning to wane. But many psychiatric training programs—indeed, those that many young physicians consider most desirable—continue to emphasize the psychoanalytic understanding of the personality and psychoanalytic techniques of treatment. Because it is no longer possible to ignore the dramatic effects of medication, drug therapy is taught during the first year of training, when the resident must contend with the seriously ill, hospitalized psychiatric patients. However, the importance of drug therapy is associated only with psychotics, who many psychiatrists expect will play only a small part in their later practice. Advanced training in the second and third years tends to emphasize psychotherapy, with its intricate and demanding requirements, and to neglect the continued necessary attention to drug therapy for a wide range of patients.

Nonetheless, some programs are beginning to utilize the biopsychiatric approach. For some young psychiatrists trained in such programs, our discussion of genetics, neurochemistry, and pharmacology contains nothing new. In the older generation, too, we are not unique in being unable fully to accept—perhaps, we've been told, because of negativism, oedipal problems, or learning disabilities—the psychoanalytic doctrines we were taught. But there are not many of us around yet.

The fall-off in the attraction of psychoanalysis for the medically trained has resulted in a decrease in high-quality applications for training to psychoanalytic institutes. The prestigious American Psychoanalytic Association, which in the past has admitted only M.D.s for clinical training, is now considering allowing psychologists to enter as full-fledged candidates—a sign of the times.

The paucity of adequate training in both the biological and the psychological aspects of psychiatric illnesses makes finding well-rounded therapists difficult—not only for the patient but for us. It is a recurrent personal experience of ours that when asked to refer a patient for treatment in a distant city, we must ponder long and hard in order to locate appropriate psychiatrists. We have no difficulty locating a physician for a patient with clear-cut biological problems or a reputable psychotherapist for someone with clear-cut personal limitations or maladaptations. Unfortunately, often the patient's problem is an indeterminate mixture requiring careful biological and psychological evaluation, and finding a physician for such a patient is extraordinarily difficult.

The foregoing may sound arrogant. We hope it does not. Often, the best we can do is to refer the patient to two persons—a physician skilled in the use of medication and a psychotherapist skilled in the use of psychological treatment. In such instances, the referral must also consider the attitudes of the physician and psychotherapist; an insular contempt or disdain in either would weigh against effective collaboration.

Despite our emphasis on medication, we hope that our discussion of the threefold nature of unhappiness and of the uses of psychotherapy has made it clear to the prospective patient that medications are far from being a panacea for all the ills of mankind. An understanding of the differences among mental illness, maladaptation, and realistic unhappiness is essential. This book has been designed to help the sufferer decide how to search for the appropriate solution (or palliative) for his or her problems: normalizing medication; psychotherapy; or a change in life patterns.

Appendix

The Use of Medication in the Treatment of Psychiatric Illness

In the discussion of the major psychiatric illnesses, particularly the mood disorders and the schizophrenias, we have mentioned the drugs most useful in their treatment: the antidepressants (the MAO inhibitors and the tricyclic antidepressants), lithium, the major tranquilizers, and the minor tranquilizers. Drugs are marketed by pharmaceutical companies with a *"physician* packet insert" explaining the structure, mechanism of action, therapeutic effects, and side effects of the drug. It has been proposed that, in the future, medication be dispensed to patients with a *"patient* packet insert" with information useful in maximizing the therapeutic benefit of the drug. Since this information is not currently available, we would like to provide here the "patient packet inserts" that we distribute in our private practices. Drug doses must always be individualized, and since amounts vary for the different drugs, we cannot tell the patient/reader how much of which drug he will probably be taking. This information will have to be supplied by the patient's physician. What we have done is to provide specific information that we hope will enable the prospective psychopharmacological drug consumer to derive maximum benefit from the drug prescribed for him.

All patients receiving psychological or psychiatric care should have a complete medical evaluation to rule out possible organic causes for their difficulties. Patients taking prescribed medication should have not only this initial medical evaluation but also medical reevaluations, as recommended by their physician on the basis of current indications.

Tricyclics and MAO (Monoamine Oxidase) Inhibitors

These two groups of medications are the agents most commonly used in the treatment of some forms of depression in adults; as mentioned in the text, they are used in other psychiatric problems as well. Both have been used for approximately twenty years. Unlike stimulants (such as the amphetamines), the tricyclic antidepressants and MAO inhibitors have no mood-elevating effect on those who are not suffering from psychiatric problems. They are non-habit-forming.

One of the important characteristics of these drugs, of which the average patient is often not fully aware, is that they do *not* have an immediate effect. Even in patients for whom they prove highly beneficial, the effects rarely begin before one or two weeks and often reach their maximum level only when the medicines are taken for four or five weeks. Since the dosage is increased at intervals of approximately one week, it may be three or four weeks before the optimal dose level is determined. It is usual, therefore, not to be able to estimate the maximal effects of the medications until about six weeks after they are begun, although some benefits can be seen in four weeks. The standard procedure is to begin at a low dose, which is usually given once daily at bedtime; the MAO inhibitors are sometimes given in the morning if they produce wakefulness rather than sedation. The amount is gradually increased, often every week, until beneficial effects are produced or side effects become annoying.

These drugs are almost entirely safe when given under medical supervision, but precautions must be observed. Both groups of medication frequently produce a *lowering* of blood pressure; in fact, some of the MAO inhibitors have been used in the treatment of high blood pressure. The lowering of blood pressure is not very great in people with normal blood pressure, but patients taking the drug should be aware of it. The most common effect is a slight drop in blood pressure when the patient stands up suddenly, which produces a feeling of light-headedness. When first getting up in the morning, therefore, or when standing after having knelt down, a person on these medications should arise relatively slowly. The effect is not observed in all patients.

In the MAO inhibitors, one major precaution must be observed. They will cause sudden high blood pressure in *some* people *if* taken together with certain other medications or foods. These substances are ordinarily metabolized by the body, but in the presence of the MAO inhibitors they cannot be metabolized at as rapid a rate and their accumulation tends to raise blood pressure. The patient taking a MAO inhibitor should inform any physician that she consults that she is having such treatment and should not treat herself with over-the-counter drugs without first checking with the doctor. Most over-the-counter drugs are safe, but some remedies, such as cold, hay-fever, sinus, and reducing preparations, may cause an elevation of blood pressure in combination with MAO inhibitors. Some foods contain very high amounts of chemicals that can produce high blood pressure in a small fraction of the people taking MAO inhibitors. Although the risk is very small, the patient having such medications should not eat these foods. The foods to exclude are:

beer	pickled herring and other pickled products
broad bean pods	
canned figs	raisins
cheese, aged [cream cheese, cottage cheese, etc., are all right]	red wines and sherries
	salted fish
	sauerkraut
chicken livers	snails
chocolate	soy sauce
coffee	yeast products
licorice	

This list of banned foods may very well be excessive. The only hard clinical data linking foods and hypertension has indicted aged cheeses, such as cheddar and Stilton, and red wine. Experimental work with animals has not made clear the possible danger posed by other foods.

Parenthetically, the mechanism by which aged cheeses produce elevated blood pressure is known. The cheeses contain a large amount of tyramine, a substance produced by the fermentation of protein. Tyramine can raise blood pressure but ordinarily does not do so because enzymes in the body break it down into a harmless compound. These protective enzymes are rendered inactive by the MAO inhibitors —in fact, the inactivation may be what makes the inhibitors therapeutically useful. Eating aged cheeses while using these medications may introduce a blood-pressure-raising substance that the body cannot break down.

There is no doubt that these drugs can be dangerous. Before it was known about foods containing tyramine, a few deaths were reported in persons taking MAO inhibitors. Some were probably due to a sudden rise in blood pressure in people with congenitally weak blood vessels in the brain. When these episodes were carefully scrutinized, however, there seemed to be some basis for believing that most had involved suicide attempts by persons using MAO inhibitors along with other drugs (see Klein and Davis, 1969). Risks of this kind can be minimized, but they do exist and must be weighed against the advantages provided by the medicine.

In addition, these drugs, like all powerful medical agents, sometimes produce less critical side effects. They are undesirable and sometimes annoying but usually harmless—such as dryness of the mouth and a tendency to constipation. All these effects tend to decrease in severity after their first appearance and sometimes disappear when patients have taken the drug for some time. Many of the side effects, such as constipation, are treatable by conventional methods.

Occasionally, someone develops an allergy to these drugs, such as a skin rash. Such allergies are fortunately rare, but obviously the patient should report any unusual symptoms to the treating physician.

In a minority of patients taking antidepressants, there is a distinct decrease in sexual drive and capacity. However, this is always alleviated upon the eventual termination of the medication.

As indicated in the chapter on depression, information on possible long-term effects is inadequate. Patients should consult their physicians for a complete discussion of current knowledge.

Lithium

Lithium has been increasingly used in psychiatry in the past ten to fifteen years. Lithium salts were first used in the treatment of patients who were manic, overly excited, or high, but have been found useful in several other psychiatric conditions, such as some depressions and forms of shifting labile mood.

Lithium, like the other major drugs, has very little or no positive effect on persons without psychiatric problems. For this reason, the drug is completely non-habit-forming.

A very small number of people develop some underactivity of the thyroid gland when they take lithium over a long period. This is not a serious condition, and if lithium is proving useful, the thyroid underactivity can be remedied with a small amount of thyroid hormone. As a strict precautionary measure, anyone taking lithium should have periodic thyroid tests. These may be done at the same time that blood is drawn for the determination of lithium levels. Otherwise, lithium can usually be given for long periods without producing any ill effects.

Lithium has been administered to some patients for periods of over five years, in most instances without any serious side effects.

Some recent reports have mentioned damage to the concentrating ability of the kidneys, resulting from chronic lithium treatment. These reports have caused some alarm, but there is no evidence that the kidneys' primary ability to excrete waste products is impaired by lithium.

Of extreme importance in lithium treatment is that the dose for each patient must be regulated on an individual basis. When lithium is administered, the intention is to produce a particular concentration in the blood. It is this concentration that is important, and not the amount of medication that the patient is given daily. If the concentration in the blood is too low, lithium will not produce beneficial effects, and if the concentration is too high, the patient may suffer from side effects. To regulate the dose, therefore, the procedure is to begin the patient at a very low dose, administer it for a few days, take a blood sample to determine the blood level, and then increase the dose as needed. This means that initially the patient must have a blood test each time the dose is increased. As the patient's response to lithium becomes regulated and as his blood level becomes stable, tests may be conducted at less frequent intervals. Practically, this usually means that initially the patient will undergo blood tests every three or four days, then once every week, once every two weeks, once every month, and then perhaps once every three months, or even less often. All lithium is marketed in tablets whose weight is 300 milligrams. Four to six days after lithium treatment is begun, blood will be taken in the morning before the first dose is administered. Thereafter, the physician will contact the patient and inform him of the dose increases that may be necessary.

The procedure in taking the pills and having blood drawn is important. If the patient takes two lithium pills per day, he or she should take one in the morning and one at night. If the dose is increased to three a day, they should be taken morning, noon, and night. As the dose is increased, the medicine should be as equally distributed as possible. (Four tablets per day: 2-1-1. Five tablets per day: 2-2-1, etc.) It is also extremely important that the blood for determining lithium levels be drawn at a specific time. *Blood for lithium levels should be drawn twelve hours following the last dose and before the patient has taken the first dose of lithium in the morning.* If she takes a dose before the blood is drawn, the laboratory values will be confused and the blood values will incorrectly read as higher than they really are.

The concentration of lithium in the blood that the physician is attempting to achieve is roughly 0.8 to 1.4 "milli-equivalents per liter." What the patient should be aware of are the numbers involved—namely, that the desirable levels are usually between 0.8 and 1.4. The exact levels most useful for different patients are still open to some debate, but these are the figures most commonly used. As the patient becomes experienced in lithium treatment, arrangements can be made for him to contact the laboratory directly, have his blood levels reported directly to him, and in turn to contact the doctor. The blood tests are a minor annoyance, but the procedure resembles that used for diabetes.

Once lithium blood levels are stable, they tend to remain so except in unusual circumstances. If a patient becomes ill and develops either diarrhea or vomiting, her metabolism of lithium may be affected and she should contact the treating physician. Similarly, large variations in the intake of table salt may affect the levels of lithium in the blood. If people eat a great deal of table salt, they drive their blood lithium down, and if they lose a great deal of salt—as they may, for example, if they are very active in the summer or are dieting—their lithium values may rise. For people who engage in vigorous physical labor or athletics, it may be necessary to check lithium levels somewhat more often in the summer when sweating is heavy.

Lithium is entirely safe within the dose range used for treatment, but excessive doses may produce sickness and large overdoses may occasionally prove fatal. Although it is unlikely that the patient whose blood levels are checked will build up lithium in his body and become sick, it is wise for him to be aware of some of the symptoms of overdosage. During the initial treatment, some patients develop a need to urinate more frequently, and a mild thirst. Occasionally, there is also mild nausea, loose stools, and a slight tremor of the hands. These symptoms tend to disappear with time. If a big excess of lithium is taken, the patient may develop severe diarrhea, vomiting, appetite loss, drowsiness, sluggishness, muscular twitching, marked tremor, slurred speech, or incoordination. These symptoms do not appear in patients whose doses are carefully regulated and indeed may be produced by such illnesses as the flu or intestinal diseases, but the patient should inform the physician if any of them do develop. If the physician cannot be reached, lithium should be discontinued until a medical evaluation is made.

Finally, as we've mentioned, recent research indicates that lithium may affect kidney functioning. Patients taking lithium should also have occasional tests of kidney function.

The possible side effects are no reason to shy away from treatment with lithium but are an indication of the need for caution. The same cautions hold true for the use of antibiotics in the treatment of infectious diseases, insulin in the treatment of diabetes, and anticonvulsant medicines in the treatment of epilepsy. When used within the correct dosage ranges, these agents are very safe, though large overdoses may produce illness.

Major Tranquilizers

The major tranquilizers are those that have proven effective in the treatment of the most serious of psychiatric disorders—the schizophrenias. They were introduced for severe psychiatric illness approximately twenty years ago, but since then have been found to be effective in some forms of depression and other psychiatric conditions. As is true of most of the effective psychiatric drugs, the major tranquilizers are non-habit-forming or addicting. They have been readily available for twenty years and have never been abused.

There are literally dozens of major tranquilizers, many of them very similar chemically. They are also very similar in effect, with slight differences that may make one or another preferable for an individual patient. Among those most frequently used, and this list is very far from complete, are (brand names in parentheses): chlorpromazine (Thorazine); thioridazine (Mellaril); trifluoperazine (Stelazine); perphenazine (Trilafon); thiothixene (Havane); haloperidol (Haldol). Sometimes physicians will employ still others of this group of compounds if for some reason those most commonly used seem undesirable for a particular patient.

Patients with apparently similar problems vary considerably in the amount of a given major tranquilizer that is necessary to improve their symptoms. Neither the severity of the symptoms nor the size of the individual is a good predictor of how much medicine will ultimately be needed. A very large person with very severe symptoms may sometimes require only a small amount of medication, whereas a small person with mild symptoms may require a very large dosage. It is necessary, then, to begin most patients at a low dosage, realizing that this may be too little to produce benefit, and gradually to increase the amount. Once the desirable dose has been determined, some patients may derive immediate benefit, while others may note continuing improvement over a longer period.

In general, these medications have two effects. At first they often produce a feeling of sleepiness, but after several days or weeks the groggy effect tends to disappear. Not all the major tranquilizers have this effect. The grogginess is not what is being sought, but in order to derive benefit from the tranquilizer, one must sometimes put up with sleepiness for a while.

The doses of different major tranquilizers vary considerably. Thorazine, for example, is usually given in amounts ranging from about 30 to 800 mg. per day. Haldol, which is more potent per milligram, may be given in doses ranging from 0.5 to 20 mg. per day. The difference in actual amount is of no practical importance and is merely a reflection of the different chemical structures of the medications.

In order to simplify the administration of medication, tablets of different sizes are generally used. The physician usually begins with a smaller dose tablet, which permits greater flexibility, and if the dose must be increased, she will substitute larger tablets so that the patient need not take a fistful of pills a day.

The effects of the major tranquilizers last long enough so they can be given in only one dose per day. Medication is usually given at bedtime, approximately one or two hours before the patient retires. The sleep-inducing effect of the medication appears approximately an hour after it is taken and wears off within several hours. If the medication is taken before bedtime, it will assure a good night's sleep and in most instances will not leave the patient groggy the following morning.

Occasionally, the major tranquilizers produce allergic reactions. If allergies develop, they usually do so within the first few weeks or months that the medicine is taken. As with the antidepressants, one of the more common symptoms of an allergic reaction is a skin rash. Another allergic symptom is the development of a severe sore throat, which in rare instances can indicate an allergic reaction that decreases white blood cells and thus decreases resistance to infections. Although sore throats are frequent symptoms in flu-like illnesses and colds, any patient receiving *any* drug who develops a severe sore throat should inform his physician.

An annoying but not dangerous side effect of some major tranquilizers is greater susceptibility in some people to irritation by the sun. A few people will develop an itchy rash. The correct preventive treatment is to wear long-sleeved clothing and avoid exposure to the sun.

A very annoying side effect which develops in many people who require large doses of major tranquilizers and a few very sensitive persons taking small doses consists of symptoms that include some degree of muscular stiffness, shaking, trembling, and restlessness. These are not dangerous but can be extremely bothersome. They can be prevented by giving anti-Parkinsonian drugs with the major tranquilizer; these drugs have no psychiatric effect in themselves but will prevent or relieve the muscular symptoms. Fortunately, in the case of most patients who develop muscular symptoms and who need anti-Parkinsonian medication, such medication can usually be discontinued after a time without the reappearance of the annoying symptoms.

Other patients, however, may have to continue to take anti-Parkinsonian drugs at all times to counteract a disorder called akinesia. Akinesia is characterized by feelings of diminished energy, lack of spontaneity, and apathy, and may be mistaken for an effect of the illness rather than a side effect of medication. It should be emphasized that this group of symptoms rarely develops in patients receiving low doses of major tranquilizers, and when the symptoms do develop, they are no cause for alarm.

Other allergic symptoms can develop, but they occur less frequently. To be absolutely safe, the patient should always notify the treating physician of any unusual manifestations.

If large doses of major tranquilizers are administered continuously for many years, some patients develop a neurological disorder called tardive dyskinesia, usually involving uncontrollable movements of the facial muscles. Because of the possibility of this long-term effect, psychiatrists must monitor chronic drug administration carefully and watch for beginning symptoms. There is evidence that discontinuation of the medications upon the appearance of initial symptoms may reverse the developing tardive dyskinesia. Unfortunately, however, many of these patients require chronic medication to control their psychosis. Under these circumstances, the patients and their doctors are in a dilemma. Patients and family members should discuss comparative benefits and risks with their physician if long-term antipsychotic treatment appears indicated.

Minor Tranquilizers

Among the most widely used and most widely known of the psychiatric drugs are a chemically mixed group referred to as the minor tranquilizers. The most effective are the benzodiazepines. The most commonly used are Librium, Valium, Serax, and Tranxene. Unlike the major tranquilizers and the antidepressants, the minor tranquilizers in general affect in the same way all those who take them, both the symptomatic and the asymptomatic. The minor tranquilizers are effective in diminishing anxiety in most nonschizophrenic and depressed adults. They sedate and render excessively placid those who are not anxious.

Although it is unusual, continued use in increasingly high dosages may produce dependence in some persons—that is, abrupt discontinuation of the medicine will produce withdrawal symptoms such as insomnia, tremor, and agitation. The risk of this is far less than with drugs such as the opiates and barbiturates. If patients find that they are continually increasing their dose of a minor tranquilizer, it is possible that they have an addictive pattern, and this should be thoroughly reviewed with their physician.

The benzodiazepines are metabolized by the body at different rates, which means that some of the drugs need be taken only once or twice a day, or once every other day, while others must be taken several times a day. The physician prescribing the medication will acquaint the patient with the dosage schedule. Because some of the drugs accumulate in the body, they may take several days to have a maximal therapeutic effect.

The minor tranquilizers are in general quite free of either annoying or dangerous side effects. The most common side effects are drowsiness and unsteadiness of gait when the medication is taken initially in too large a dose. All these drugs potentiate the effect of alcohol—that is, they tend to amplify its effect. Those who drink while on minor tranquilizers should do so with caution.

Because of the drowsiness effect, it is also wise, when the drug is first taken, to avoid tasks such as driving a car and operating dangerous machinery. After a few days, the individual frequently becomes tolerant to this side effect of the medication while continuing to derive benefit from the effects on anxiety. At that time, he may resume his usual activities.

As with all other medications, physical changes or symptoms that indicate an allergy or other abnormal reaction—such as a skin rash or a sore throat—should be reported to the physician.

References

Adler, A. Selections (1907–37). In H. L. Ansbacher and R. R. Ansbacher, eds., *The Individual Psychology of Alfred Adler.* New York: Basic Books, 1956.
American Psychiatric Association. *Diagnostic and Statistical Manual of Mental Disorders,* 1st ed., 3d ed. Washington, D.C.: American Psychiatric Association, 1952, 1980.
Bachrach, A. J., and Pattishall, E. G., Jr. "An Experiment in Universal and Personal Validation." *Psychiatry* 23 (1960): 267–70.
Barber, T. X. *Hypnosis: A Scientific Approach.* New York: Van Nostrand, 1969.
Beck, A. T., Rush, A. J., Shaw, B. F., and Emery, G. *Cognitive Therapy of Depression.* New York: Guilford Press, 1979.
Benson, H. *The Relaxation Response.* New York: William Morrow, 1975.
Berne, E. *Games People Play.* New York: Grove Press, 1964.
Blachly, P. H. "Effects of Decriminalization of Marijuana in Oregon." In *Chronic Cannabis Use,* edited by R. L. Dornbush, A. M. Freedman, and M. Fink, *Annals of the New York Academy of Science* 282 (1976): 405–15.
Bleuler, E. *Dementia Praecox or the Group of Schizophrenias.* Translated by J. Zinkin. New York: International Universities Press, 1950.
Block, J. *Lives Through Time.* Berkeley, Cal.: Bancroft Books, 1971.
Boszormenyi-Nagy, I., and Framo, J. L., eds. *Intensive Family Therapy.* New York: Harper & Row, 1965.
Brady, J. P., and Brodie, H. K. H., eds. *Controversy in Psychiatry.* Ch. 18, "Genetic Counseling for Psychiatric Patients," contributions by R. R. Crowe; S. S. Kety, S. Matthysse, and K. K. Kidd; and R. R. Fieve and M. Young. Philadelphia: Saunders, 1978.
Brady, J. P., and Lind, D. L. "Experimental Analysis of Hysterical Blindness: Operant Conditioning Techniques." *Archives of General Psychiatry* 4 (1961): 331–39.
Brauzer, B., and Goldstein, B. J. "Symptomatic Volunteers: Another Patient Dimension for Clinical Trials." *Journal of Clinical Pharmacology* 13 (1973): 89–98.
Breuer, J. See Freud, Vol. 2.

Burnham, D. L., Gladstone, A. I., and Gibson, R. W. *Schizophrenia and the Need-Fear Dilemma.* New York: International Universities Press, 1969.

Burr, W. A., Falek, A., Strauss, L. T., and Brown, S. B. "Fertility in Psychiatric Outpatients." *Hospital and Community Psychiatry* 30 (1979): 527–31.

Burton, R. *The Anatomy of Melancholy* (1621), edited by F. Dell and P. Jordan-Smith. New York: Tudor Press, 1955.

Cade, J. F. J. "Lithium Salts in the Treatment of Psychotic Excitement." *Medical Journal of Australia* 2 (1949): 349–52.

Cadoret, R. J. "Evidence for Genetic Inheritance of Primary Affective Disorder in Adoptees." *American Journal of Psychiatry* 135 (1978): 463–66.

Cantwell, D. P. "Genetic Studies of Hyperactive Children: Psychiatric Illness in Biological and Adopting Parents." In R. R. Fieve, D. Rosenthal, and H. Brill, eds., *Genetic Research in Psychiatry.* Baltimore: Johns Hopkins University Press, 1975.

Corson, S. A., Corson, E. O., Arnold, L. E., and Knopp, W. "Animal Models of Violence and Hyperkinesis." In G. Serban and A. Kling, eds., *Animal Models in Human Psychobiology.* New York: Plenum Press, 1976.

Covi, L., Lipman, R. S., McNair, D. M., and Czerlinsky, T. "Symptomatic Volunteers in Multicenter Drug Trials." *Progress in Neuropsychopharmacology* 3 (1979): 521–33.

Dworkin, R. H., Burke, B. W., Maher, B. A., and Gottesman, I. I. "A Longitudinal Study of the Genetics of Personality." *Journal of Personality and Social Psychology* 34 (1976): 510–18.

Eisenberg, L. "School Phobia: A Study in the Communication of Anxiety." *American Journal of Psychiatry* 114 (1958): 712–18.

Ellenberger, H. F. *The Discovery of the Unconscious: The History and Evolution of Dynamic Psychiatry.* New York: Basic Books, 1970.

Ellis, A., and Harper, R. A. *A New Guide to Rational Living.* Englewood Cliffs, N.J.: Prentice-Hall, 1975.

Erikson, E. H. *Childhood and Society.* New York: Norton, 1950.

Eysenck, H. J. *Fact and Fiction in Psychology.* New York: Penguin, 1965.

———. *Eysenck on Extraversion.* New York: Halsted Press, 1973.

Eysenck, H. J., and Eysenck, S. B. G. *Manual of the Eysenck Personality Inventory.* London: University of London Press, 1964.

Fink, M. *Convulsive Therapy: Theory and Practice.* New York: Raven Press, 1979.

Fink, M., Kahn, R. L., and Green, M. A. "Experimental Studies of the Electroshock Process." *Diseases of the Nervous System* 19 (1958): 113–18.

Fisher, S., and Greenberg, R. P. *The Scientific Credibility of Freud's Theories and Therapy.* New York: Basic Books, 1977.

Frank, J. D. *Persuasion and Healing,* rev. ed. Baltimore: Johns Hopkins University Press, 1973. New York: Schocken Books, 1974.

Freud, A. *Normality and Pathology in Childhood.* New York: International Universities Press, 1965.

Freud, S. *Standard Edition of the Complete Psychological Works.* 24 vols. London: Hogarth Press, 1953–74.

"Fraülein Anna O," by J. Breuer, Vol. 2.
"Psycho-Analytic Notes on an Autobiographical Account of a Case of Paranoia (Dementia Paranoides)" (1911), Vol. 12.
"On Narcissism: An Introduction" (1914), Vol. 14.
"A Difficulty in the Path of Psycho-Analysis" (1917), Vol. 17.
"From the History of an Infantile Neurosis" [the "Wolf Man"] (1918), Vol. 17.
"The Psychogenesis of a Case of Homosexuality in a Woman" (1920), Vol. 18.
New Introductory Lectures on Psycho-Analysis (1933), Vol. 22.
"Analysis Terminable and Interminable" (1937), Vol. 23.
Friedan, B. *The Feminine Mystique.* New York: Dell, 1977.
Fromm, E. *The Art of Loving.* New York: Harper & Row, 1956.
Fromm-Reichmann, F. *Principles of Intensive Psychotherapy.* Chicago: University of Chicago Press, 1950.
Gendlin, E. *Focusing.* New York: Everest House, 1978.
Gittelman-Klein, R., and Klein, D. F. "Controlled Imipramine Treatment of School Phobia." *Archives of General Psychiatry* 25 (1971): 204–14.
Glasser, W. *Reality Therapy: A New Approach to Psychiatry.* New York: Harper & Row, 1965.
Goodwin, D. W., Schulsinger, F., Møller, N., Hermansen, L., Winokur, G., and Guze, S. B. "Drinking Problems in Adopted and Nonadopted Sons of Alcoholics." *Archives of General Psychiatry* 31 (1974): 164–69.
Gottesman, I. I. "Genetic Variance in Adaptive Personality Traits." *Journal of Child Psychology and Psychiatry* 7 (1966): 199–208.
Gray, J. A. "The Psychophysiological Nature of Introversion-Extraversion: A Modification of Eysenck's Theory." In V. D. Nebylitsyn and J. A. Gray, eds., *Biological Bases of Individual Behavior.* New York: Academic Press, 1972.
Gross, M. L. *The Psychological Society.* New York: Simon and Schuster (Touchstone Edition), 1979.
Grosz, H. J., and Zimmerman, J. "Experimental Analysis of Hysterical Blindness: A Follow-Up Report and New Experimental Data." *Archives of General Psychiatry* 13 (1965): 255–60.
Harlow, H. F. "The Nature of Love." *American Psychologist* 13 (1958): 673–85.
Herink, R., ed. *The Psychotherapy Handbook: The A to Z Guide to More Than 250 Different Therapies in Use Today.* New York: New American Library (Meridian), 1980.
Heston, L. L. "Psychiatric Disorders in Foster Home Reared Children of Schizophrenic Mothers." *British Journal of Psychiatry* 112 (1966): 819–25.
Hollingshead, A. B., and Redlich, F. C. *Social Class and Mental Illness.* New York: Wiley, 1958.
Holmes, O. W. *The Young Practitioner: Medical Essays 1842–1882.* Boston: Houghton Mifflin, 1889.
Horney, K. *Neurosis and Human Growth.* New York: Norton, 1950.
James, W. "What Is Emotion?" *Mind* 19 (1884): 188–205.

———. *The Principles of Psychology* (1890). New York: Dover Publications, 1950.
———. *The Varieties of Religious Experience* (1902). New York: New American Library, 1958.
———. *The Will to Believe.* Cambridge, Mass.: Harvard University Press, 1979.
Janov, A. *The Primal Scream—Primal Therapy: The Cure for Neurosis.* New York: Putnam's, 1970.
Jaspers, K. *The Nature of Psychotherapy: A Critical Appraisal.* Translated by J. Hoenig and M. W. Hamilton. Chicago: University of Chicago Press, 1964.
Jung, C. G. *The Portable Jung,* edited by S. Campbell. New York: Viking Press, 1971.
Kagan, J, *The Growth of the Child: Reflections on Human Development.* New York: Norton, 1978.
Kallmann, F. J. *The Genetics of Schizophrenia.* New York: J. J. Augustin, 1938.
Kanter, J., and Lin, A. "Facilitating a Therapeutic Milieu in the Families of Schizophrenics." *Psychiatry* 43 (1980): 106–19.
Kernberg, O. F. *Borderline Conditions and Pathological Narcissism.* New York: Jason Aronson, 1975.
Kessler, S. "Psychiatric Genetics." In *American Handbook of Psychiatry,* 2d ed., Vol. 6, *New Psychiatric Frontiers,* edited by D. A. Hamburg and H. Keith H. Brodie. New York: Basic Books, 1975.
Kety, S. S., and Kinney, D. K. "Biological Risk Factors in Schizophrenia." Unpublished.
Kety, S. S., Rosenthal, D., Wender, P. H., and Schulsinger, F. "Mental Illness in the Biological and Adoptive Families of Adopted Schizophrenics." *American Journal of Psychiatry* 128 (1971): 302–06.
Kierkegaard, S. *A Kierkegaard Anthology,* edited by R. Bretall. New York: Random House, 1946.
Klein, D. F. *Psychiatric Case Studies: Treatment, Drugs and Outcome.* Baltimore: Williams & Wilkins, 1972.
———. "Endogenomorphic Depression: A Conceptual and Terminological Revision." *Archives of General Psychiatry* 31 (1974): 447–54.
———. "A Proposed Definition of Mental Illness." In R. L. Spitzer and D. F. Klein, eds., *Critical Issues in Psychiatric Diagnosis.* New York: Raven Press, 1978.
———. "Psychosocial Treatment for Schizophrenia, or Psychosocial Help for People with Schizophrenia?" *Schizophrenia Bulletin* 6 (1980): 122–30.
———. "Anxiety Reconceptualized." In D. F. Klein and J. Rabkin, eds., *Anxiety: New Research and Changing Concepts.* Proceedings, 70th annual meeting, American Psychopathological Association (March 1980). New York: Raven Press, 1981.
Klein, D. F., and Davis, J. M. *Diagnosis and Drug Treatment of Psychiatric Disorders.* Baltimore: Williams & Wilkins, 1969.
Klein, D. F., Gittelman, R., Quitkin, F., and Rifkin, A. *Diagnosis and Drug Treatment of Psychiatric Disorders: Adults and Children,* 2d ed. Baltimore: Williams & Wilkins, 1980.

Klein, D. F., Zitrin, C., Woerner, M., and Ross, D. "Psychotherapy of Phobia: Behavior Therapy vs. Supportive Therapy," in press.

Kohut, H. *The Analysis of the Self: A Systematic Approach to the Psychoanalytic Treatment of Narcissistic Personality Disorders.* New York: International Universities Press, 1971.

Kraepelin, E. *Clinical Psychiatry: A Text-book for Students and Physicians.* Translated and adapted from the German edition by A. R. Deifendorf. New York: Macmillan, 1921.

Kretschmer, E. *Physique and Character* (1925), 2d ed. London: Routledge and Kegan Paul, 1936.

Lacan, J. *Ecrits: A Selection.* Translated by A. Sheridan. New York: Norton, 1977.

Laing, R. D., and Esterson, A. *Sanity, Madness, and the Family: I. Families of Schizophrenics.* New York: Basic Books, 1965.

Lange, C. "The Emotions" (1885). In K. Dunlap, ed., *The Emotions.* Baltimore: Williams & Wilkins, 1922.

La Rochefoucauld, F. *The Maxims of La Rochefoucauld.* Translated by L. Kronenberger. New York: Vintage Books, 1959.

Lazarus, A. A. "Behavior Therapy, Incomplete Treatment, and Symptom Substitution." *Journal of Nervous and Mental Disease* 140 (1965): 80–86.

———. *Multimodal Behavior Therapy.* New York: Springer, 1976.

Levinson, D. J., et al. *The Seasons of a Man's Life.* New York: Alfred A. Knopf, 1978.

Lewin, K. *Resolving Social Conflicts: Selected Papers in Group Dynamics.* New York: Harper, 1948.

Lieberman, M. A., Yalom, I. D., and Miles, M. B. *Encounter Groups: First Facts.* New York: Basic Books, 1973.

Lowen, A. *The Betrayal of the Body.* New York: Macmillan, 1967.

Marks, I. M. "Behavioral Treatments of Phobic and Obsessive-Compulsive Disorders: A Critical Appraisal." In M. Hersen, R. M. Eisler, and P. M. Miller, eds., *Progress in Behavior Modification,* Vol. 1. New York: Academic Press, 1975.

Marks, I., Bird, J., and Lindley, P. "Behavioral Nurse Therapist, 1978—Developments and Implications." *Behavioral Psychotherapy* 6 (1978): 25–35.

Masters, W. H., and Johnson, V. E. *Human Sexual Inadequacy.* Boston: Little, Brown, 1970.

May, P. R. A. *Treatment of Schizophrenia.* New York: Random House, 1968.

Mellinger, G. D., Balter, M. B., Parry, H. J., Manheimer, D. I., and Cisin, I. H. "An Overview of Psychotherapeutic Drug Use in the United States." In E. Josephson and E. E. Carroll, eds., *Drug Use: Epidemiological and Sociological Approaches.* New York: Hemisphere Publishing, 1974.

Mendlewicz, J., and Rainer, J. D. "Adoption Study Supporting Genetic Transmission in Manic-Depressive Illness." *Nature* 268 (1977): 327–29.

Menninger, K., with Mayman, M., and Pruyser, P. *The Vital Balance: The Life Process in Mental Health and Illness.* New York: Viking, 1963.

Mijuskovic, B. *Loneliness in Philosophy, Psychology, and Literature.* Atlantic Highlands, N.J.: Humanities Press, 1979.

Minuchin, S. *Families and Family Therapy.* Cambridge, Mass.: Harvard University Press, 1974.

Morel, B. A. *Traité des dégénérescences physiques, intellectuelles et morales de l'espèce humaine* (1857). New York: Arno Press, 1976.

Moreno, J. L. *Psychodrama.* New York: Beacon Press, 1946.

Morris, J. B., and Beck, A. T. "The Efficacy of Antidepressant Drugs." *Archives of General Psychiatry* 30 (1974): 667–74.

Murphy, H. B. M. "The Advent of Guilt Feelings as a Common Depressive Symptom: A Historical Comparison on Two Continents." *Psychiatry* 41 (1978): 229–42.

Novak, W. *High Culture: Marijuana in the Lives of Americans.* New York: Alfred A. Knopf, 1980.

Parloff, M. B., Wolfe, B., Hadley, S., and Waskow, I. E. *Assessment of Psychosocial Treatment of Mental Disorders: Current Status and Prospects.* Washington, D.C.: Institute of Medicine, National Academy of Sciences, 1978. Revised version in press, McGraw-Hill.

Paul, G. L., and Lentz, R. J. *Psychosocial Treatment of Chronic Mental Patients: Milieu versus Social-Learning Programs.* Cambridge, Mass.: Harvard University Press, 1977.

Perls, F., Hefferline, R. F., and Goodman, P. *Gestalt Therapy: Excitement and Growth in the Human Personality.* New York: Delta, 1965.

Peter, L., and Hull, R. *The Peter Principle.* New York: Bantam, 1970.

Prusoff, B. A., Weissman, M. M., Klerman, G. L., and Rounsaville, B. J. "Research Diagnostic Criteria Subtypes of Depression." *Archives of General Psychiatry* 37 (1980): 795–801.

Rank, O. *Will Therapy.* New York: Norton, 1978.

Reich, W. *Character Analysis.* New York: Farrar, Straus and Giroux, 1972.

———. *The Discovery of the Orgone: The Function of Orgasm.* New York: Farrar, Straus and Giroux, 1966.

Reite, M. L. Quoted in *Medical World News,* Jan. 21, 1980, pp. 52–53.

Rifkin, A., Quitkin, F., Carrillo, C., Blumberg, A. G., and Klein, D. F. "Lithium Carbonate in Emotionally Unstable Character Disorder." *Archives of General Psychiatry* 27 (1972): 519–23.

Rogers, C. *Client-Centered Therapy: Its Current Practice, Implications, and Theory.* Boston: Houghton Mifflin, 1951.

Rogers, C. R., Gendlin, E. T., Kiesler, D. J., and Truax, C. B., eds. *The Therapeutic Relationship and Its Impact: A Study of Psychotherapy with Schizophrenics.* Madison: University of Wisconsin Press, 1967.

Rolf, I. "Structural Integration." *Journal of the Institute for the Comparative Study of History, Philosophy, and the Sciences* 1 (1963), no. 1.

Rosenthal, D., Wender, P. H., Kety, S. S., Welner, J., and Schulsinger, F. "The Adopted-Away Offspring of Schizophrenics." *American Journal of Psychiatry* 128 (1971): 307–11.

Rush, A. J., Beck, A. T., Kovacs, M., et al. "Comparative Efficacy of Cognitive Therapy and Pharmacotherapy in the Treatment of Depressed Outpatients." *Cognitive Therapy and Research* 1 (1977): 7–37.

Rutter, M. *Maternal Deprivation Reassessed.* New York: Penguin Books, 1972.

Sargant, W. *Battle for the Mind.* New York: Harper, 1957. Reprinted, Perennial Library, Harper & Row paperbacks, n.d.

Scarr, S., and Weinberg, R. A. "The Influence of 'Family Background' on Intellectual Attainment." *American Sociological Review* 43 (1978): 674–92.

Schilder, P. "Results and Problems of Group Psychotherapy in Severe Neurosis." *Mental Hygiene* 23 (1939): 87–98.

Schofield, W. *Psychotherapy: The Purchase of Friendship.* Englewood Cliffs, N.J.: Prentice-Hall, 1964.

Schuckit, M. A., Goodwin, D., and Winokur, G. "A Study of Alcoholism in Half Siblings." *American Journal of Psychiatry* 128 (1972): 1132–36.

Schulsinger, F. "Psychopathy: Heredity and Environment." *International Journal of Mental Health* 1 (1972): 190–206.

Schultz, J. H., and Luthe, W. *Autogenic Training: A Psychophysiologic Approach in Psychotherapy.* New York: Grune & Stratton, 1959.

Seligman, M. E. P., and Hager, J. L. *Biological Boundaries of Learning.* New York: Appleton-Century-Crofts, 1972.

Shaywitz, B. A., Cohen, D. J., and Bowers, M. B., Jr. "CSF Monoamine Metabolites in Children with Minimal Brain Dysfunction: Evidence for Alteration of Brain Dopamine." *Journal of Pediatrics* 20 (1979): 67–71.

Smith, M. L., Glass, G. V., Miller, T. I. *The Benefits of Psychotherapy.* Baltimore: Johns Hopkins University Press, 1981.

Snyder, S. H. *The Troubled Mind.* New York: McGraw-Hill, 1976.

Southard, E. E., and Garrett, M. C. *The Kingdom of Evils* (1922). New York: Arno Press, 1973.

Spitzer, R. L., Endicott, J., and Gibbon, M. "Crossing the Border into Borderline Personality and Borderline Schizophrenia." *Archives of General Psychiatry* 36 (1979): 17–24.

Strupp, H. H., and Hadley, S. W. "Specific vs. Non-specific Factors in Psychotherapy." *Archives of General Psychiatry* 36 (1979): 1125–36.

Stunkard, A., and Mendelson, M. "Obesity and the Body Image: I. Characteristics of Disturbances in the Body Image of Some Obese Persons." *American Journal of Psychiatry* 123 (1967): 1296–1300.

Stunkard, A., and Burt, V. "Obesity and the Body Image: II. Age at Onset of Disturbances in the Body Image." *American Journal of Psychiatry* 123 (1967): 1443–47.

Sullivan, H. S. *The Interpersonal Theory of Psychiatry.* New York: Norton, 1953.

Suomi, S. J., and Harlow, H. F. "Social Rehabilitation of Isolate-Reared Monkeys." *Developmental Psychology* 6 (1972): 487–96.

Szasz, T. S. *The Myth of Mental Illness: Foundations of a Theory of Personal Conduct.* New York: Hoeber-Harper, 1961.

Targum, S. D., Dibble, E. D., Davenport, Y. B., and Gershon, E. S. "The

Family Attitudes Questionnaire: Patients and Spouses View Bipolar Illness." *Archives of General Psychiatry*, in press.

Thomas, A., and Chess, S. *Temperament and Development.* New York: Brunner/Mazel, 1977.

Toffler, A. *Future Shock.* New York: Random House, 1970.

Vandenberg, S. G. "Hereditary Factors in Normal Personality Traits (as Measured by Inventories)." In J. Wortis, ed., *Recent Advances in Biological Psychiatry*, Vol. 9. New York: Plenum Press, 1967.

Webb, J. *The Harmonious Circle: The Lives and Work of G. I. Gurdjieff, P. D. Ouspensky, and Their Followers.* New York: Putnam's, 1980.

Weissman, M. M., and Myers, J. K. "Affective Disorders in a U.S. Urban Community: The Use of Research Diagnostic Criteria in an Epidemiological Survey." *Archives of General Psychiatry* 35 (1978): 1304–11.

Weissman, M. M., and Paykel, E. S. *The Depressed Woman.* Chicago: University of Chicago Press, 1974.

Wender, L. "The Dynamics of Group Psychotherapy and Its Application." *Journal of Nervous and Mental Disease* 84 (1936): 54–60.

Wender, P. H. "On Necessary and Sufficient Conditions in Psychiatric Explanation." *Archives of General Psychiatry* 16 (1967): 41–47.

———. "Vicious and Virtuous Circles: The Role of Deviation Amplifying Feedback in the Origin and Perpetuation of Behavior." *Psychiatry* 31 (1968): 309–24.

———. *Minimal Brain Dysfunction in Children.* New York: Wiley, 1971.

Wender, P. H., Rosenthal, D., and Kety, S. S. "A Psychiatric Assessment of the Adoptive Parents of Schizophrenics." In D. Rosenthal and S. S. Kety, eds., *The Transmission of Schizophrenia.* Oxford: Pergamon Press, 1968.

Wender, P. H., Rosenthal, D., Kety, S. S., Schulsinger, F., and Welner, J. "Crossfostering: A Research Strategy for Clarifying the Role of Genetic and Experiential Factors in the Etiology of Schizophrenia." *Archives of General Psychiatry* 30 (1974): 121–28.

Wender, P. H., and Wender, E. H. *The Hyperactive Child and the Learning Disabled Child.* New York: Crown, 1978.

Wheelis, A. *The Quest for Identity.* New York: Norton, 1958.

White, R. W. "The Experience of Efficacy in Schizophrenia." *Psychiatry* 28 (1965): 199–211.

Whitehead, A. N. *Science and the Modern World* (Lowell Lectures, 1925). New York: Macmillan, 1929.

Willis, T. *The London Practice of Physick* (facsimile of 1692 ed.). Boston: Milford House, 1973.

Wilson, E. O. *Sociobiology: The New Synthesis.* Cambridge, Mass.: Harvard University Press, 1975.

Wilson, G. "Introversion/Extraversion." In T. Blass, ed., *Personality Variables in Social Behavior.* New York: Wiley, 1977.

Wittgenstein, L. *Philosophical Investigations.* Translated by G. E. M. Anscombe. Oxford: Blackwell, 1953.

Wood, D. R., Reimherr, F. W., Wender, P. H., and Johnson, G. E. "Diagnosis and Treatment of Minimal Brain Dysfunction in Adults: A Preliminary Report." *Archives of General Psychiatry* 33 (1976): 1453–60.

Yalom, I. D. *The Theory and Practice of Group Psychotherapy*, 2d ed. New York: Basic Books, 1975.

Zeiss, A. M., Lewinsohn, P. M., and Muñoz, R. F. "Nonspecific Improvement Effects in Depression Using Interpersonal Skills Training, Pleasant Activity Schedules, or Cognitive Training." *Journal of Consulting and Clinical Psychology* 47 (1979): 427–39.

Zitrin, C. M., Klein, D. F., and Woerner, M. G. "Treatment of Agoraphobia with Group Exposure in Vivo and Imipramine." *Archives of General Psychiatry* 37 (1980): 63–72.

Index

abreactive and cathartic therapies, 284, 294, 310–12, 315–18
abulia, 116
acheiropody, 165
adaptability, 70–1, 233
Adler, Alfred, 31, 228, 247, 263, 287, 292
adolescents, 75–7, 80–1, 93, 98, 104, 117, 232, 244, 251; and schizophrenia, 106, 109–10, 121–2; IQ of, 238; and sex, 246–7; *see also* children
adoption, research on, 132, 183, 186–90, 195, 240, 251–2; schizophrenia and, 172–6, 186; and bipolar illness, 179–80
adrenaline, 146, 200
affective disorders, 40, 44, 86, 119, 153–4, 176, 189; vs schizophrenia, 127, 130; *see also* depression *and* melancholia
affective vulnerability, *see* schizophrenia, borderline
agammaglobulinema, 226–7
aggression, 203, 209
agoraphobia (ics), 93–7, 204–5, 208, 252; and psychotherapy, 262; *see also* anxiety, separation
akinesia, 351
alcohol, 85, 96–7, 147, 158–9, 352; effect of, 19, 66, 82–3, 217–18, 223, 334
Alcoholics Anonymous, 272, 280
alcoholism (ics), 66, 71, 82–4, 148, 159, 172, 186, 189–90, 252, 293, 336; as personality disorder, 76, 186,
210, 216–18; and hyperactivity, 78–80; treatment of, 82, 162; biological and social components of, 84, 186–7, 189–90, 195–6, 251–2, 256
Alzheimer's disease, 22
American Psychiatric Association, 58, 67, 89n, 133
American Psychoanalytic Association, and candidates, 341
amphetamines, 66, 225; and hyperactivity, 77, 106, 146, 162, 214–15, 220; effects and uses of, 82, 146, 162, 199–203, 218–19, 255–6, 344; research on, 146, 162; psychosis, 160–2, 219
"Analysis Terminable and Interminable," 30–1, 250
Anatomy of Melancholy, The, 63
anemia, 164–5; sickle-cell, 164–5, 192–3
anhedonia, 59–60, 115–16, 128–30, 178
Anna O., 290, 311
anorexia nervosa, 64
antisocial personality, 74–80, 89, 102, 183, 186, 188, 190, 216–17, 240; treatment of, 76, 217, 251; biological and psychological components of, 187–90, 210, 231, 251–2; *see also* personality disorders
anxiety, 7, 10–12, 19, 25, 28, 40, 49–50, 64, 67, 78–9, 87, 101–2, 104–5, 107–8, 132, 146, 230, 240, 244, 254, 292, 306–8, 322, 337; treatment of, 50, 205–6, 208; drugs and alcohol

363

and, 82, 96, 147–8, 334–5; and psychotherapy, 261–2, 269; anticipatory, 82, 95–7, 99, 145, 269, 334–5; generalized, 94–6, 98, 251; separation, 53, 65, 93, 202, 204–9, 212, 227, 240–1, 252; *see also* panic
appetite, *see* food
Arica training, 294
armadillos, 171–2
arthritis, 20–1
association, impairment of, 113–14
asthma, treatment of, 146
atropine, and psychosis, 158
autism, 115
autogenic training, 323–5, 328
autointoxicants, 158–9, 161
avoidance conditioning, 95–8
avoidant personality disorder, 92–3
Axelrod, Julius, 143

Bachofen, Johann, 25
Bachrach, Arthur, 69
Barber, Theodore, 319
barbiturates, 96–7, 143, 158, 217–18, 334–5; *see also names of*
Beck, Aaron, 293
behavior therapies, 10–12, 97, 99–100, 102, 126, 205, 260–2, 279, 284, 291, 294, 304, 306–10
Benson, Herbert, 322–3
benzodiazepines, 149, 335, 351–2
Berne, Eric, 31, 289, 293
biofeedback, 325–8
biogenic amines, 199–203, 209–10, 215, 218, 220
biological components, 13, 15–16, 16n, 17, 20, 23–5, 30–6, 39, 41–3, 48, 51–3, 57–9, 63–4, 74–5, 84, 88, 118, 126–7, 160, 163, 186–7, 189–90, 195–6, 203–4, 209–11, 214, 217, 219, 226–31, 243–4, 250–2, 256, 260, 268, 270, 272–89, 333–40; *see also* genetics *and* psychological disorders
biological vulnerability, 138, 250–1
biopsychiatric approach, 20, 24, 36–7, 253, 283, 341
blackmail, 73, 93

Bleuler, E., 113–14, 176
blood pressure, *see* hypertension
blood sugar, 4, 21
body therapies, 260, 324–5
brain, 16, 22–3, 118, 145, 151, 197–8, 215, 220, 222; damage to, 19, 117–18, 177–8, 186, 188, 190, 225; chemistry of, 147, 160–1; stimulation of, 198–202; of dogs, 215; alpha waves of, 326–7; syphilis of, *see* paresis
brainwashing, 310, 312–15
breast cancer, 165–6, 275
Breuer, Josef, 26, 290, 310–11
Briquet's Syndrome, 187
Burnham, D. L., and colleagues, 129
Burton, Robert, 63

caffeine, effects of, 98
Cantwell, Dennis, 190
carbon dioxide, and anxiety, 146
Castaneda, Carlos, 158
catatonia, 116–17
celiac disease, 177
certainty, 222–4
Charcot, Jean, 25–7
cheese, aged, MAO inhibitors and hypertension, 345
chemicals, *see* drugs *and names of*
Chess, Stella, 238
children, 72–6, 93, 102, 104, 177, 217, 220, 240–1, 244, 305; and sexuality, 29, 35, 246–7, 284–5; and depression and personality disorders, 52–3, 180–4, 188–90; and schizophrenia, 105–6, 109, 121, 216; intellectual development of, 238–9; and hyperactivity, *see* hyperactivity; *see also* adolescents *and* school phobia
chlorpromazine, 137, 147–50
cocaine, effects of, 82, 201–2, 218
cognitive therapies, 155–6, 261, 279, 293–5, 299
Colson, Charles, 315
coma, insulin and, 144
compensatory devices, 228
compulsive personality disorder, 27–8, 99–100, 315
computer, 36–7

Confucius, 265
conscience, *see* guilt
consciousness, 202, 318
conversion reactions, 91, 128
convulsive therapy, *see* electroconvulsive therapy
Copernicus, 333-4
Corson, Samuel, 214-15
couple therapy, 297, 301-4
criminality, 190-1, 251-2
culture, 24, 45, 111, 183-4, 189, 221-2, 233, 248-9, 291-2

Darwin, Charles, 333-4
Delay, Jean, 147
delusions, 108-13, 128; and medication, 108-10, 136, 150, 219; and psychedelic drugs, 157-8; and schizophrenia, 112, 118, 121, 132, 160; explanation of, 221-6
dementia praecox, 23-4, 105-6, 166; *see also* schizophrenia
demonic possession, 101
demoralization, 42, 138, 186, 253-7, 267, 270, 292, 301; treatment of, 66, 199, 255-7, 261; psychotherapy, 256-7, 269, 271, 281
Deniker, Pierre, 147
dependency, 93, 209, 227, 244, 247
depression, 41-4, 66, 78, 93, 102, 104-5, 132, 160, 178, 183-6, 199-202, 205-6, 209, 220, 227, 232, 240, 244, 250, 254-5, 292-3, 337; causes of, 19, 25, 39-40, 42-3, 132, 226; treatment of, 25, 41, 43, 46, 58-60, 65-6, 80, 135-6, 144, 150-3, 155-6, 202, 206, 208, 215, 217, 256, 261, 270, 279, 293, 335, 337, 344, *see also* psychotherapy, *and* drugs, antidepressant; biological and psychological, 25, 42-3, 51-3, 58, 63, 151, 178, 180-4, 202-3, 208-9, 254-6, 267, 270; vital or physiological, 41, 43-59, 85, 178-80, 182, 185, 202-4, 207-8, 215-17, 226, 254-5, 260-1, 281; nonvital or neurotic, 42, 44, 58-63, 80, 178, 180, 182-5, 199; life experiences and, 43, 59, 182-5; unipolar (endogenous), 44-5, 59, 65, 153, 179, 182, 279; bipolar, 44, 58, 153, 335; definition of, 46; psychotherapy and, 46, 59-65, 93, 151, 154, 185-6, 260-1, 270, 281; case histories of, 46-52, 60-5; masked, 63-6; diagnosis of, 64, 66; and schizophrenia, 116, 119-20; borderline, 179; hysteroid dysphoria and, 210, 212; and pleasure, *see* pleasure
depressive character, 42, 58-60, 180, 251
desensitization, 10, 12, 16, 306-8, 325
despair, 207-8, 267; *see also* unhappiness
Dexedrine, 77, 160, 213
diabetes, 21, 143, 172, 192, 305
diagnoses, 338-9
Diagnostic and Statistical Manual, 67, 89n
Dianetics, 316
Dick-Read, Grantly, method, 325
dissatisfaction, *see* unhappiness
dogs, 214-15, 312-15, 326
dopamine, 160-1, 215-16, 219-20
dream interpretation, Freud and, 27
drug therapy, teaching of, 341
drugs, 12, 70, 72, 76, 81-2, 96-7, 103, 116, 136, 145, 156-7, 198, 203, 225, 283; and mental illnesses, 13, 17, 227, 251-2, 261-2, 268; abuse of, 66, 71, 76-80, 82-4, 161, 210, 217-19, 256; and schizophrenia, 121, 127-8, 134-8, 143-4, 146-7, 150; experiments with, studies and testing of, 128, 154-6, 159, 274, 277; new, 142; risks vs benefits of, 153-7, 161-2; mimicking of mental illness by, 157-9; and beliefs and convictions, 222-4; effects of various kinds of, 334-6; "patient packet inserts" for, 343
drugs, antidepressant, 41, 53, 60, 80, 99, 120, 150-1, 201, 204-6, 208, 251-2, 255-6, 334-5, 343; and panic, 12, 13, 97, 217; and depression, 47-8, 51-3, 59, 61, 64-5, 80, 151, 153, 208-10, 215, 217, 227, 261, 270, 337; effects of, 48-9, 55,

199–202, 206, 346, 350; and hysteroid dysphoria, 86, 212–13; and schizophrenia, 124, 136; discovery of, 150; deaths from, 153–4; value and studies of, 156–7
drugs, anti-Parkinson, 124, 350–1
drugs, antipsychotic, 55, 60, 94, 146–50, 152, 219, 335; experimentation with, 149–50; and schizophrenia, 104, 107–10, 112, 120, 124–5, 134–8, 144, 153, 159, 172, 194, 220, 225; long-term effects of, 137, 351; value of, 156; *see also* tranquilizers, major
drugs, maintenance, 51, 88, 136
drugs, monoamine oxidase (MAO) inhibitors, 86, 88, 151–2, 199, 200, 212–13, 343; uses, dosage, and effects of, 344–6
drugs, psychedelic, 111, 117, 119, 157–9, 161–2, 219–20, 318, 323
drugs, psychiatric vs standard, 156–7; uses and effects of, 335–7, 340
drugs, sedative, 96–7, 143, 335
drugs, stimulant, 80, 107, 146, 213, 216, 218; and hyperactivity, 60, 76–7, 79–80, 214, 216, 251; effects of, 199, 202, 344; and demoralization, 199, 255–7
drugs, tricyclic, 58, 86–7, 150, 201, 212, 215, 343; uses, dosage, and effects of, 344
Dworkin, Robert, and twins, 244
dyslexia, 106, 130

efficacy, 235, 253, 279
Eisenberg, Leon, 205
electroconvulsive therapy (ECT), 58–9, 61, 64–5, 87, 135, 144–5, 138, 151
electroencephalogram (EEG), 5, 151, 188, 326–8
Ellis, Albert, 290, 293
Ellis, Havelock, 26
emotionally unstable character disorder, 80–2, 135–6, 153, 251
encounter groups, 260, 294, 300, 300n, 301

Endicott, Jean, survey of, 133
environment, 232, 237, 244–5, 248, 257; and heredity, *see* heredity
epilepsy, 5, 94, 102, 144, 222
Erhard, Werner, 224, 316
Erikson, Erik, 32
est, 224, 315–16
ether, 158, 222
euphoria, 39, 40, 43, 57–8, 80, 317; drugs and, 200–3
evolution, and heredity, 192
exhibitionism, 56–7, 89
Exorcist, The, 101
explosive personality disorder, 102
extraversion/introversion, 241–3
Eysenck, Hans, 241–3

families, 178–9, 184, 186–90, 233–4, 238, 246–7, 253; and schizophrenia, 126–7, 132, 166–70, 173–6, 178–9, 226, 251; therapy, 297, 301, 304–5
father, relationships with, *see* parents
fear, 11–12, 19, 230, 306–7
Fechner, Gustav, 25
Feminine Mystique, The, 234
Fink, Max, 151
flooding, 12
"focusing," 293
folie à deux, 168
food (appetite), 43, 59, 199–200, 218, 254, 345
Food and Drug Administration, 337n
Frank, Jerome, 266, 272, 281, 296
free association, 27, 29, 35
Freemasons, psychotics and, 24
Freud, Anna, 205
Freud, Sigmund, 6, 239–40, 333; thoughts and beliefs of, 16, 16n, 27–32, 34–7, 141, 226, 236, 250–1, 263; and mental illness, 20, 25–7, 250–1; works of, 27, 30. 32, 289; and infantile sexuality, 29, 35, 246–7, 284–5; and hysterics, 30, 35, 91, 116, 311–12; differences with, and criticisms of, 31–4, 289; and psychoanalysis, 31–2, 35–6, 334; and homosexuality,

35, 181–2, 239; and separation anxiety, 206; and transference, 286–7; and Anna O., 290, 311; and "Wolf Man," 289
Friedan, Betty, 234
Fromm, Erich, 32, 289, 292
Fromm-Reichmann, Frieda, 168
Future Shock, 233

Galen, 240
Games People Play, 31, 293
Gendlin, Eugene, 293
genetics, 13, 163–7, 170–6, 178, 180, 186–90, 192–6, 203, 226; and schizophrenia, 126–7, 132, 166–70, 172–6, 178, 186, 219, 304; and mental illness, 163, 250–2; environment and, *see* heredity and environment; *see also* biological components and phenocopies
gestalt therapy, 260, 268, 279, 288–90, 293, 298–300, 333
Gilbert, W. S., 219
Gittelman-Klein, Rachel, 205
Glasser, William, 293, 334
Goodwin, Donald, 189
Gottesman, Irving, and twins, 243
Gray, J. A., 243
Greenwald, Harold, 300n
Gross, Martin, 229–31
group therapy, 90, 97, 99, 107, 124, 128, 260, 288, 293–301, 309
groups, satisfaction from, 317–18
Growth of the Child, The, 249–50
growth-promoting therapy, 273–4
guilt, 45, 72–5, 82, 99, 107, 151, 183–4, 205, 230, 253–4
Gulliver's Travels, 110
Gurdjieff, G. I., institute of, 294

Hadley, S. W., 281
Haldol, 349–50
hallucinations, 108–9, 111–12, 120–1, 123, 125, 128, 132, 169, 289; and medication, 108–9, 120, 136, 150, 219; and schizophrenia, 111, 118, 121, 136, 159, 220; and psychedelic drugs, 111, 157–60, 219–20; auditory, 111, 159–60, 219–20; visual, 220
Hare Krishna, 316
Harlow, Harry, 183
hashish, 222
Hearst, Patty, 315
heredity, 23, 105, 250–2; and environment, 163–5, 170, 172–7, 186, 188–91; *see also* genetics
heroin, 82, 84, 148, 159, 218
Heston, Leonard, 173
histrionic personality disorder, 89–90
Holmes, Oliver Wendell, 264–5
homosexuality, 35, 181–2, 239
Horney, Karen, 289
Huntington's chorea, 164
hyperactivity, 74, 76–80, 98, 116, 187, 189–90, 210, 214–16, 250, 261; and medication, 60, 76–7, 79–80, 106, 136, 146, 162, 214–15, 220, 268; and children, 60, 76–8, 81, 106, 146, 178, 186–7, 190, 214, 216, 220, 240, 251; case histories of, 78–80; and psychotherapy, 80, 268
hypertension, 160, 192, 200, 323, 344–6
hyperventilation syndrome, 4
hypnosis, 25–7, 91, 311–13, 319–25; and psychotherapy, 319; case history of, 319–21
hypochondria, 130–1
hypoglycemia, *see* blood sugar
hysteria (ics), 25–8, 30, 35, 67, 90–1, 116, 130, 289, 311–12, 315
hysteroid dysphoria, 59, 60, 84–90, 178, 199, 210–14, 226; treatment of, 60, 86–8, 136, 211–13, 251, 268; characteristics of, 75, 84–6, 210–13; case histories of, 86–8; rejection and, 210–13; and psychotherapy, 211, 261, 268

illness, 13, 20–1, 41; mental: 20, 23–4, 40, 138–9, 160, 163, 166, 191, 195, 197, 199, 229, 250–2, 270, 292; theories about, 19–36; definition of,

19, 250; "exclusively organic" and "exclusively psychogenic," 19–20, 24–5, 36; causes, nature, and treatment of, 13–17, 29, 141–3, 145–6, 166, 252–3; psychological contributions to, 226–7; biological component of, 230, 250, 252, 333–4; and psychotherapy, 253, 268, 273; and psychoanalysis, 289, 332; *see also* schizophrenia *and other kinds of*
imipramine, 150
impotence, 56–7
inferiority complex, 31, 228, 247, 287
inspirational therapies, 310
insulin, 143–4
interpersonal and related therapies, 260, 278–9, 284, 287, 289–94; and group therapy, 297–8; *see also* couple therapy *and* family therapy
intrapersonal therapies, 284, 290, 294, 298
introversion, *see* extraversion
invalidism, 138, 292
iproniazid, 151, 200, 202
isolation, sensory, 169

James-Lange Hypothesis, 324
James, William, 184, 222–3, 259
Janov, Arthur, 315
Jaspers, Karl, 105
Johnson, Virginia, 246, 262
Joyce, James, 129
Jung, Carl, 31, 129, 241, 263, 287

Kagan, Jerome, 249–50
Kallmann, Franz, 167–8
Kernberg, Otto, 89n
Kesey, Ken, 145
Kessler, S., 174
Kety, Seymour, 173, 176–7
Kierkegaard, Søren, 231n
Kinney, Dennis, 176
Klein, D. F., 80, 94, 127, 147–9, 204–5, 212, 279, 308
Kohut, Heinz, 89n
Kraepelin, Emil, and mental illness, 20, 22–4, 35–6, 43–4, 176; and dementia praecox, 23–4, 109–10, 113, 166

Krafft-Ebing, Richard von, 26
Kretschmer, Ernst, 167
Kuhn, Roland, 150

Laborit, H. M., 147
Lacan, Jacques, 287
Laing, R. D., 33–4
La Rochefoucauld, François de, 240
Levinson, Daniel, 232
Lewin, Kurt, 33
Librium, 97, 149, 334–5, 351
limitations, inborn, 237
lithium, 55, 57–8, 81, 102, 203, 251, 343, 347–8; uses, dosage and effects of, 152–3, 335, 346–9
Locke, John, 32
London Practice of Physick, The, 119
LSD, 158–60, 220, 318; effect of, 161–2, 222, 224–5

madness, 105, 117, 119, 166, 168; *see also* dementia praecox, illness, mental, *and* schizophrenia
malaria, and genetics, 193
malingering, 91
mania, 41, 44, 54–5, 57–8, 119, 152–3, 201, 203, 227, 240, 335; case histories of, 54–8; *see also* manic-depressives
manic-depressives, 179, 194–5, 199, 229–30, 252; *see also* mood
marijuana, 66, 83–4, 87–8, 119, 222
marriage, 262, 309; *see also* couple therapy
Maslow, Abraham, 290, 293
Masters, William, 246, 262
masturbation, 112, 115, 122, 183
May, Philip, 144
medication, effectiveness of, 329–30, 332–9, 341–2; positions against, 331–4, 336; and medical evaluation, 344; *see also* drugs
medicine, 264–7; *see also* physicians
Mednick, Sarnoff, 173n
Meduna, Ladislas von, 144, 146
megavitamin therapy, 137–8

melancholia, 43, 45, 63, 119; *see also* affective disorders
Mellaril, 216
Menninger, Karl, 330–1
mescaline, and norepinephrene (noradrenaline), 158
Mesmer, Franz, 25
"meth," 160
methadone, 84
methamphetamine, 77
methylphenidate, 77
Metrazol, 144
Mijuskovic, Ben, 231n
Miltown, 149, 335
mislearning (maladaptation), 231, 238–9, 245–50, 252, 254, 256, 267, 290, 292, 321; psychotherapy and, 268–70; and group therapy, 297; and family therapy, 304–5
mongolism, 23
monkeys, 183, 206–7
mood, disorders of, 15, 18, 23–4, 39–66, 111, 138, 145, 153, 176, 178–86, 199–210, 268, 336, 343; *see also specific kinds of;* lability of, 78, 80, 212; changes in, and schizophrenia, 119
Moon, Sun Myung, 316
Morel, Bénédict, 105, 108
Moreno, J. L., 299–300
morphine, 82, 143, 148, 162, 218
mother, relationship with, *see* parents
multiple-person therapies, *see* group therapy
Myth of Mental Illness, The, 331

narcissism, and psychotherapy, 89
National Institute of Mental Health, 194, 260, 262
National Training Laboratories, 33
need-fear dilemma, 129
neuroleptics, *see* drugs, antipsychotic
neuroses, 6, 12, 15–16, 27, 67, 130, 229–31, 286; and schizophrenia, 127, 130, 133; group therapy and, 296–7; traumatic and nontraumatic, 311–12
neurotransmitter, 198, 200–1, 219, 249
niacin, and schizophrenia, 138

nitrous oxide, 222–3
norepinephrine (noradrenaline), 158, 160–1, 215

observation and discovery, 142
obsessions, 130
obsessive-compulsive disorder, 27–8, 101–2, 262, 289
Oedipus complex, 29, 34
Office of Strategic Services (OSS), tests used by, 68
One Flew Over the Cuckoo's Nest, 145
opiates, 143, 219
opium, 82, 147, 218
organic causation and treatment, 139, 143, 146

panic, 3–13, 64, 87, 94–9, 208, 216–17, 251, 268, 336; *see also* anxiety
paranoia, 103, 118, 157, 168, 219, 222
parents, relationship with, 8–10, 28, 56, 61, 122, 124–5, 204–7, 239, 247–8, 253, 285, 290–1, 302, 305
paresis, 22, 143
Parkinson's disease, 215
Parloff, Morris, 260
Parnate, 152
Pattishall, Evan, 69
Pauling, Linus, 177
Pavlov, Ivan, 214–15, 312–15, 326
Paykel, Eugene, 209
pellagra, 22
penicillin, 143
Perls, Frederick, 289, 293
personality, 31, 184–5, 234, 237–47, 252, 298; biological factors and, 228, 242–4; constitutional (inborn) differences in, 230, 237–41, 244–5; extraversion/introversion dimension of, 241–3; *see also* mislearning
personality disorders, 23, 39, 67–103, 116, 132, 138, 184, 186–8, 199, 210–19; definition of, 67–8; *see also individual types of*
Peter Principle, 100
peyote, 222
phenocopies, 39, 164–5, 175–8, 187–8, 190, 203, 213, 228, 270

phenothiazines, 146–7, 149, 161
phenylketonuria (PKU), 23
pheochromocytoma, 4
phobia, 10–12, 97–9, 130, 231, 262, 279, 289, 306–9
phocomelia, 165
physicians, and treatment and cure, 271–7; questioning of, by patient, 338–9
placebo, 65, 79–80, 155–7, 270, 275–80, 339
pleasure, 100, 104, 132, 199–201, 208, 218, 254; pursuit and experience of, 41–2, 52, 59–60, 82, 85, 116, 121, 199–202, 208
polymorphic balance, 193
prevention, types of, 271–2
primal scream therapy, 260, 268, 278–9, 315–16, 333
problems, human, varieties of, 15, 17
psilocybin, 147
psychiatry (ists), 77, 91–2, 102, 137, 141–3, 157, 166–7, 197, 230, 257; resistance to, 4, 6, 7, 10; beliefs about and biases of, 14–15; and mental illness, 22–36, 43; and four "A's," 113–16; and schizophrenia, 126, 133–4; and unhappiness, 234–6; and goals, 271–3; and research and experiments, 274–8; as evaluator, 282–3; training of, 341; *see also* physicians *and* psychoanalysis
psychoanalysis, 6–12, 87, 96–7, 260, 284–93, 299, 307, 310–11, 319, 332; various views of, 31–6; non-physicians and, 32, 331; domination of, 330, 333, 341; decreased attraction of, 341; *see also* psychiatry
psychodrama, 299–300
psychodynamics, 139, 141–2, 205, 210, 217
psychological (psychiatric) disorders, 13, 15, 17–20, 22–36, 43, 53–4, 58, 60, 63–4, 74, 76, 104–5, 113, 127, 151, 153–4, 204, 210, 226–8, 230–1, 250–2, 270, 308; *see also* biological components
Psychological Society, The, 229

psychotherapy, 6, 12–13, 17–18, 26, 33, 84, 87–8, 128, 260–2, 269, 288, 341; number, names, and kinds of, 33, 259–60, 279, 281, 283–4, 288–90, 318; effectiveness and uses of, 157, 260–8, 270, 279–81; patients suited for, 261; inappropriate, 271–2; and specific goals, 271–4; and treatment, 271–9; professional qualifications for, 281–3; categorizing of, 283–4; theories about, 329–30, 333–4; as adjunct to medication, 329, 333–4, 338; response to, 339–40; uses of, 342; *see also* psychoanalysis, *and under names of various illnesses*
punishment, 73–4, 79

Quest for Identity, A, 16

Rank, Otto, 287
rational emotive therapy, 268, 290, 293, 298–9
Rauwolfia serpentina, *see* reserpine
reality therapy, 293
Reich, Wilhelm, 324
Reite, Martin L., 183
rejection, 74–5, 85, 88, 104, 210–13, 227
relaxation, 10–13, 322, 325, 328
religion, 26, 116, 183, 189, 246, 255, 312, 318, 322; conversion and, 224–5, 259, 310, 313–16; and psychoanalysis, 287–8
reserpine, 146–7, 159–61, 200
retardation, 22–3, 174
rheumatic fever, 117–18
Ritalin, 77
Rogers, Carl, 33, 263–4, 290, 293
Rolfing, 268, 324
Rorschach test, 68–9
Rosenthal, David, 173

sadness, *see* unhappiness
Sakel, Manfred, 143–4
Sargant, William, 312–15
Schilder, Paul, 295–7
schizoid-eccentric, 127, 132, 134

schizoid personality disorder, 103-4, 127, 132, 167-8, 171, 251
schizophrenia, 5, 15, 18, 23, 39, 43-4, 60, 81, 86, 92, 94, 105-39, 144, 172, 175-8, 186, 189, 191-4, 199, 216, 219-26, 232, 252, 290, 304; case histories of, 105-15, 117; attributes of, 107, 110-18; psychotherapy and, 121, 135, 144, 168, 260-1, 268, 281; treatment and drugs for, 121, 137-8, 143-4, 146-7, 153, 159, 193-4, 220, 268, 336, 343, 349, *see also* psychotherapy and medication, 134-8, 143-4, 146-7, 150-1, 153, 157-9, 161, 336, 343, 349; and psychedelic drugs, 157-9, 220; psychological transmission of, 168-70, 175; twins and, 170-2; adoption and, 172-6, 251; and hysteroid dysphoria, 210-11; biological component in, 229-30, 250; families and, *see* families; and genetics, *see* genetics; *see also types of, immediately following, and* delusions, hallucinations, illness, mental, madness, phenocopies, *and under items throughout*
schizophrenia, acute, 118-21, 133, 225; case histories of, 119-20; and medication, 134-5, 137-8; and adoption studies, 176; and biological vulnerability, 250
schizophrenia, borderline (ambulatory, pseudoneurotic), 126-34, 167, 178-9, 193, 251; affectively vulnerable, 127, 130, 134-6, 176, 179; diagnosis of, 132-3; schizotypal group, 127, 132, 134, 136, 251; case histories of, 127-32; attributes of, 129-30, 132-4; and medication, 135-6; and adoption, 176
schizophrenia, chronic (process), 103-4, 109-10, 118, 121-6, 132-3; and medication, 121, 124, 135-8, 151, 268; case histories, 121-26 and psychotherapy, 124; long-term care of, 126, 135; attributes of, 129; and adoption, 172; and psychological forces, 178; fertility of, 194

schizophrenia, paranoid, 103, 107, 118, 122-3; and amphetamines, 160-1
school phobia, 6, 8-9, 53, 65, 107, 204-5, 207-8
Schuckit, Marc, 189
Schulsinger, Fini, 173, 188
Schultz, Johannes, 323
self-esteem, 202-4, 228, 235, 247, 270; and demoralization, 253-4; psychotherapy and, 269-70
self-evaluation, 40-1, 75
Seligman, Martin, 255
Serax, 351
serotonin, 158, 160, 200, 215
sex, 26, 29, 35, 43, 47, 85, 90, 199, 200, 218, 246-7, 254, 262, 284-5, 293, 303; feelings and anxieties about, 6-10, 28; and schizophrenia, 120, 122-6, 128-31; children and, *see* children
shame, 72-4, 254
Shaywitz, Bennett, 215
shock therapy, *see* electroconvulsive therapy
signs, 20-1, 25, 30, 58
sleeping, 44, 47, 49, 51-2, 54-5, 59, 106-8, 199, 200
slums, and drugs, 82-4
Smith, M. L., 281
Snyder, Solomon, 230-1
socializing, methods of, 73
sociopath, 76, 78
sociotherapy, drug-free programs of, 84
sodium amytal, 312
somatic therapy, 58, 61-2
Southard, Ernest, 15
"speed," *see* drugs, stimulant, *and* amphetamines
Spitzer, Robert, 133, 167
state-altering therapies, 284, 318, 325; *see also individual kinds of*
streptomycin, 274
stress, developmental, 232-3
Strupp, H. H., 281
Stunkard, Albert, 204
suicide, 79, 90, 93, 186; and depres-

sion, 43, 45–7, 49–50, 58, 60, 151, 153–4, 186; and hysteroid dysphoria, 85, 87–8; and schizophrenia, 122, 135, 186; and psychotherapy, 154
Sullivan, Harry Stack, 168, 211, 247–8, 289–90
Sybil, 298
Sydenham, Thomas, 20–1, 23
symptoms, 20–1, 24, 26–9, 42, 111–12; physiological and psychological causes of, 25–6, 28; and hysteria, 25, 27–8, 30; groups of, 35; of depression, 45, 58, 60, 63–4; and schizophrenia, 107, 110–18
Synanon, 84, 272, 316
syndromes, 20–1, 23–4, 67, 82, 93
Szasz, Thomas, 33–4, 230, 331n, 334

talking therapies, 290, 293
tardive dyskinesia, 137, 351
technology, and malaise, 233; empirical, 262; modern, 293–4, 325, 328
thalidomide, effects of, 165
Thematic Apperception Test, 68–9
therapy, *see individual kinds of*
Thomas, Alexander, 238
Thorazine, 5, 349–50
Three Faces of Eve, The, 298
timidity, 308
tobacco, effects of, 83, 159
Toffler, Alvin, 233
Tofranil, *see* imipramine
tranquilizers, 5, 6, 12; minor, 50, 56, 65, 97–8, 149, 334–7, 337n, 343, 351–2; major, 87, 146–50, 343, 349–51, *see also* drugs, antipsychotic; discovery of, 274; uses, dosage, effects, and names of, 349–52; *see also under names of*
transactional analysis, 260, 268, 289, 293, 295, 298–9, 333
transcendental meditation, 318, 322–4
transference, 284, 286–7, 295
Tranxene, 351
treatment, 271–9, 338–41
Troubled Mind, The, 230

tuberculosis, iproniazid and, 151
twins, 170–2, 178–9, 242–4
tyramine, 345

unconscious, Freud and, 16, 17n, 27–9, 334
unhappiness, 233, 235–6, 244–7, 249, 252; causes and sources of, 42, 231–7, 231n, 252–3, 267–70; realistic, 82, 231, 237, 250, 252, 263, 269–70, 273, 290; threefold nature of, 231, 250, 342; personal, 231–2; situational, 232
U.S. Senate and psychotherapy, 280–1
Unnamed Quartet, 186–8, 195, 199, 216
"ups," *see* drugs, stimulant *and* amphetamines

Valium, 4, 7, 97, 149, 334–6, 351
Vandenberg, S. G., 243
Varieties of Religious Experience, The, 259
virginity, guilt and, 184
Vital Balance, The, 330
voyeurism, 56–7

Wagner-Jauregg, Julius von, 143
Watson, John, 32
Weissman, Myrna, 209
Welner, Joseph, 173
Wender, Louis, 294–7
Wender, P. H., 78, 80, 172–3, 186, 215, 320
Wesley, John, 315
Wheelis, Allen, 16
White, Robert W., 235, 253
Wilde, Oscar, 70
Willis, Thomas, 119, 166
Wilson, Glenn, 241
Wittgenstein, Ludwig, 276
world view, 248–9

Yalom, Irvin, 296

Zeiss, Antonette, 279
Zen, 325, 327–8